Foreword

We are e*Essentia*created at Los A pediatri where th

Our hope in the creation of this book is to give clinicians and injured children an essential handbook, useful in every practice setting. This book does not replace a comprehensive textbook, but we hope you find it a helpful guide in your clinical practice.

Acknowledgements

We want to thank all of our faculty editors from the Department of Emergency Medicine at Los Angeles County Harbor-UCLA Medical Center for their commitment to resident education and for providing their expertise, guidance, and time to ensure that this project would become a reality.

FACULTY EDITORS

Raymen Rammy Assaf, MD, MPH, MIA
David B. Burbulys, MD
Lilly Bellman, MD
Tabitha Cheng, MD
Ilene Claudius, MD
Aubrey Yurie Ferguson, MD
Sheetal Khiyani, MD
Adedamola Ogunniyi, MD
Ryan Pedigo, MD

Katie Rebillot, DO
Mohsen Saidinejad, MD
Supriya Sharma, MD
Manpreet Singh, MD, MBE
David Tanen, MD
Nicole Titze, MD
Shirley Tung, MD
William White, MD, MA

We also want to thank all of our residents, clinical fellows, and medical students who worked very hard to ensure we would have a high yield, quality product that has the potential to improve the care of children nationwide.

In the true spirit of emergency medicine, this has been a collaborative effort, and we could not be more grateful.

Glossary of Abbreviations

AAP	American Academy of Pediatrics
ABCs	airway, breathing, circulation
AMS	altered mental status
ANC	absolute neutrophil count
AVM	arterio-venous malformation
BMP	basic metabolic panel
BNP	brain natriuretic peptide
BP	blood pressure
BPM	beats per minute
BRBPR	bright red blood per rectum
BRUE	brief resolved unexplained event
BSA	body surface area
BMV	bag-mask-valve ventilation
Ca	calcium
CBC	complete blood count
CDC	Centers for Disease Control
CHD	congenital heart disease
CHF	congestive heart failure
CMP	complete metabolic panel
CN	cranial nerve
CNS	central nervous system
COVID	SARS-coronavirus-2 (COVID-19)
CPAP	continuous positive airway pressure
CPR	cardiopulmonary resuscitation
CRP	C-reactive protein
CSF	cerebrospinal fluid
CT	computed tomography scan
CV	cardiovascular
CVAT	costovertebral angle tenderness
CXR	chest x-ray (radiograph)
Ddx	differential diagnosis
DIC	disseminated intravascular coagulation
DM	diabetes mellitus
EBV	Epstein-Barr virus
EKG	electrocardiogram
ECMO	extracorporeal membrane oxygenation
ED	emergency department
FAST	focused assessment with sonography for trauma
GAS	group A streptococcus
GBS	group B streptococcus
GCS	glasgow coma scale
GER	gastroesophageal reflux
GI	gastrointestinal
GLC	glucose
GNR	gram negative rods
GU	genitourinary
H+P	history and physical examination
HA	headache
Hct	hematocrit
HEENT	head eyes ears nose throat
HFO2	high-flow oxygen therapy
Hgb	hemoglobin
Hib	H. influenzae type b
HOCM	hypertrophic obstructive cardiomyopathy
HR	heart rate
HSV	herpes simplex virus
IBD	inflammatory bowel disease

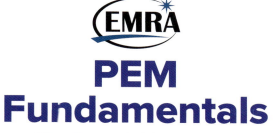

PEM Fundamentals
The Essential Handbook for Pediatric Emergencies

Editor-in-Chief
Cindy D. Chang, MD

Associate Editors
Patricia Padlipsky, MD, MS | **Kelly D. Young, MD, MS**

Los Angeles County
Harbor-UCLA Medical Center
Department of Emergency Medicine

2021 EMRA Board of Directors

President
RJ Sontag, MD

President-Elect
Angela Cai, MD, MBA

Immediate Past President
Hannah R. Hughes, MD, MBA

Secretary/Editor, *EM Resident*
Priyanka Lauber, DO

Speaker of the Council
Tracy Marko, MD, PhD, MS

Vice Speaker of the Council
Ashley Tarchione, MD

Resident Representative to ACEP
Nicholas P. Cozzi, MD, MBA

Director of Education
Deena Khamees, MD

Director of Health Policy
Maggie Moran, MD

Director of Leadership Development
Capt. Yev Maksimenko, MD, MA, DiMM, FAWM, FP-C

Director of Technology
Nicholas Salerno, MD

ACGME RC-EM Liaison
Breanne Jaqua, DO, MPH

EMRA Representative to the AMA
Sophia Spadafore, MD

Medical Student Council Chair
Chiamara Anokwute

REVIEWERS
Deena Khamees, MD | University of Michigan
Nat Mann, MD | Prisma Health
Brian Levine, MD | ChristianaCare
Jamie M. Rosini, PharmD, MS, BCCP, BCPS, DABAT | ChristianaCare

ILLUSTRATIONS
Matthew Holt, BodyRender

EMRA STAFF CONTRIBUTOR
Managing Editor Valerie Hunt

Copyright 2021 | ISBN 978-1-929854-62-2
4950 W. Royal Lane | Irving, TX 75063
972.550.0920 | emra.org

All rights reserved. This book is protected by copyright. No part of this book may be reproduced in any form or by any means without written permission from the copyright owner.

DISCLAIMER
This handbook is intended as a general guide to therapy only. While the editors have taken reasonable measures to ensure the accuracy of the information presented herein, the user is encouraged to consult other resources when necessary to confirm appropriate treatment, side effects, interactions, and contraindications. The publisher, authors, editors, and sponsoring organizations specifically disclaim any liability for omissions or errors found in this handbook, for appropriate use, or for treatment errors. Further, although this handbook is as comprehensive as possible, the vast differences in emergency practice settings may necessitate treatment approaches other than those presented here. Refer to your institution's protocols.

References available at emra.org/guides

ICP	intracranial pressure	PGE1	prostaglandin E1
ICU	intensive care unit	Plts	platelets
ID	infectious disease	PMD	primary medical doctor
IO	intraosseous	PMH	past medical history
IV	intravenous	PO	per os
IVF	intravenous fluids	PO4	phosphorus
KUB	kidney, ureters, bladder (abdominal radiograph)	POC	point of care
		PPV	positive pressure ventilation
LFTs	liver function tests	PRN	as needed
LMA	laryngeal mask airway	ROM	range of motion
LMP	last menstrual period	RR	respiratory rate
LOC	loss of consciousness	RSI	rapid sequence intubation
LP	lumbar puncture	RSV	respiratory syncytial virus
LR	lactated ringer's	RUQ	right upper quadrant
Mg	magnesium	SBI	serious bacterial illness
MRI	magnetic resonance imaging	SJS/TEN	Stevens-Johnson syndrome/ toxic epidermal necrolysis
MRSA	methicillin resistant staph aureus	SVR	systemic vascular resistance
		SVT	supraventricular tachycardia
MVA	motor vehicle accident	Sx	symptoms
N/V/D	nausea/vomiting/diarrhea	TB	tuberculosis
NAT	non-accidental trauma	TBI	traumatic brain injury
NAAT	nucleic acid amplification test	TM	tympanic membrane
		TORCH	toxoplasma, rubella, cytomegalovirus, herpes
NEC	necrotizing enterocolitis		
NG/T	nasogastric / tube	TxS	type and screen
NPO	nil per os (nothing by mouth)	UA	urinalysis
NO	nitric oxide	URI	upper respiratory infection
NS	normal saline	US	ultrasound
OGT	orogastric tube	UTI	urinary tract infection
OR	operating room	Utox	urine toxicology screen
OTC	over the counter	UVC	umbilical venous line
PCP	primary care physician	VBG	venous blood gas
PDA	patent ductus arteriosus	VFib	ventricular fibrillation
PECARN	pediatric emergency care applied research network	VTach	ventricular tachycardia
		VP	ventriculoperitoneal
		XR	x-ray (radiograph)

Contents & Contributors

QUICK REFERENCE TABLES
All chapters by Cindy D. Chang, MD, Kelly D. Young, MD, MS, and Patricia Padlipsky, MD, MS

1. Normal Vital Signs by Age...1
2. Weight by Age..1
3. Pediatric GCS %..2
4. Equipment Sizing...2
5. Common Pediatric Medication Dosages..4
6. Ventilator Settings...11
7. Immunizations..13
8. Developmental Milestones..14
9. Teeth Chart..16
10. Return to School...17
11. Tips & Tricks for Examining Children..18

RESUSCITATION
Section editor Patricia Padlipsky, MD, MS

1. PALS: Dysrhythmias (John J. Campo, MD)...21
2. Neonatal Resuscitation (John J. Campo, MD)....................................25
3. PALS: Shock (Alexander S. Grohmann, MD)......................................27
4. Airway Management (Alexander S. Grohmann, MD)..........................31
5. Vascular Access (Zachary Oleskey, MD)...36

PROCEDURES & SKILLS
Section editor Aubrey Yurie Ferguson, MD

1. Foreign Body Removal (Tianci Liu, MD)..39
2. Laceration Repair & Wound Management (Tianci Liu, MD).................41
3. Lumbar Puncture (James H. Williams, MD).......................................44
4. Procedural Sedation & Analgesia (Gabriel H. Campion, MD)...............47

CARDIOVASCULAR
Section editor Lilly Bellman, MD

1. Approach to Pediatric EKG Interpretation (Yang Ding, MD).................51
2. Arrythmias (Yang Ding, MD)...53
3. Congenital Heart Disease (Andrew Thorne, MD)................................56
4. Infective Endocarditis (Brandon J. Wang, MD)..................................63
5. Pericarditis & Myocarditis (Cindy D. Chang, MD)...............................65

DERMATOLOGY
Section editor Patricia Padlipsky, MD, MS
1. Bacterial Infections (Michael T. Jordan, MD) 69
2. Dermatitis (Gwendolyn Hooley, MD; Daniel J. Brownstein) 72
3. Drug Rashes (Michael T. Jordan, MD) 74
4. Fungal Infections (Michael T. Jordan, MD) 76
5. Infestations & Ticks (Alison Rosser, MD) 78
6. Viral Exanthems (Michael T. Jordan, MD) 80
7. Vascular Lesions (Adam Garibay, MD) 84
8. Urticaria & Anaphylaxis (Zachary Oleskey, MD) 86

EAR-NOSE-THROAT
Section editor William White, MD, MA
1. Ear & Nose (Alexander M. Garrett, MD) 89
2. Laryngotracheal Pathology & Complications (Alexander M. Garrett, MD) ... 94
3. Throat & Neck (Alexander M. Garrett, MD) 99

ENDOCRINOLOGY
Section editor Ryan Pedigo, MD
1. Glucose Metabolism (Cindy D. Chang, MD) 105
2. Adrenal Insufficiency (Elizabeth Scott, MD) 110
3. Thyroid Disorders (Elizabeth Scott, MD) 112

ENVIRONMENTAL
Section editor Sheetal Khiyani, MD, MS
1. Bites & Envenomations (Shane Zeshonski, MD) 115
2. Hyperthermia (Fardis Tavangary, DO) 121
3. Hypothermia (Fardis Tavangary, DO) 123
4. Submersion Injuries (Shane Zeshonski, MD) 125

GASTROENTEROLOGY
Section editor Ilene Claudius, MD
1. Acute Gastroenteritis (Nathan Jasperse, MD, MBA) 127
2. Appendicitis (Ronald Luu, MD) 129
3. Biliary Pathology (Nathan Jasperse, MD, MBA) 130
4. Bowel Obstruction (Moira Smith, MD, MPH) 132
5. Constipation (Aixin Chen, MD) 134
6. Enteral Feeding Tube Complications (Jake Toy, DO) 136
7. Gastrointestinal Bleeding (Sophia Fornbacher, MD) 138
8. Inflammatory Bowel Disease (Sophia Fornbacher, MD) 142
9. Intussusception (Sarah J. Zyzanski, MD) 142
10. Pyloric Stenosis (Ronald Luu, MD) 145

GENETICS/METABOLISM
Section editor Aubrey Yurie Ferguson, MD
1. Common Syndromes (Jonathan S. Warren, MD) 147
2. Inborn Errors of Metabolism (Jonathan S. Warren, MD) 150

GENITOURINARY
Section editor Supriya Sharma, MD
1. Female-Specific Pathology (Alexa Golden, MD)........................155
2. Male-Specific Pathology (Alexa Golden, MD)......................... 160

HEMATOLOGY/ONCOLOGY
Section editor Raymen Rammy Assaf, MD, MPH, MIA
1. Anemia (Karin Collins, MD) 165
2. Bleeding Disorders (Karin Collins, MD)..............................167
3. Immune Thrombocytopenia (ITP) (Nicole V. Bahrami, MD) 170
4. Oncologic Emergencies (Andres Park, MD) 171
5. Sickle Cell Disease (Andres Park, MD) 175

INFECTIOUS DISEASES
Section editor Nicole Titze, MD
1. Fever of Unknown Origin (Kyle McLain, MD) 179
2. Infectious Mononucleosis (Andrew Pham, MD) 181
3. Influenza-Like Illness (Kyle McLain, MD)............................183
4. Meningitis & Encephalitis (James H. Williams, MD)....................184
5. Meningococcemia (James H. Williams, MD) 188
6. COVID-19 & MIS-C (Richmond M. Castillo, MD, MA, MS) 190

NEONATAL
Section editor Kelly D. Young, MD, MS
1. Abdominal Pathology (Nadia Faiq, MD) 193
2. Brief Resolved Unexplained Event [BRUE] (Melanie Pham, MD).........198
3. Crying Infant (Alexander M. Garrett, MD)............................199
4. Febrile Infant and Neonate (Jijoe Joseph, MD, MBA) 201
5. Jaundiced Neonate (Andrew Thorne, MD)............................ 204
5. Neonatal Emergencies [THE MISFITS] (Tiffany J. Au, MD) 207
6. Normal Feeding, Elimination & Growth
   (Jessica L. Chow, MD, MPH; Kenneth Kim)........................... 211
7. Post-NICU Premature Baby (Jessica L. Chow, MD, MPH) 213
8. Skin Findings (Hoang Xuan Pham, MD) 216
9. Umbilical Cord Issues (Nadia Faiq, MD) 218

NEUROLOGY
Section editor Adedamola Ogunniyi, MD
1. Ataxia & Paralysis (Frederick N. Milgrim, MD) 221
2. Headache (Hoang Xuan Pham, MD)... 223
3. Seizures (Melanie Pham, MD).. 225
4. Stroke (Adam Garibay, MD).. 227
5. Ventriculoperitoneal Shunt Complications (Melanie Pham, MD) 229

OPHTHALMOLOGY
Section editor Mohsen Saidinejad, MD, MS, MBA
1. Preseptal & Orbital Cellulitis (Gabriel H. Campion, MD) 231
2. Red Eye (Gabriel H. Campion, MD).. 234

ORTHOPEDICS
Section editor Tabitha Cheng, MD
1. Back Pain & Discitis (Alex Bonilla, MD).. 239
2. Limp (Gwendolyn Hooley, MD)...241
3. Nursemaid's Elbow (Nicole V. Bahrami, MD) 243
4. Orthopedic Infections (Hannah M. Carr, MD) 244
5. Osgood-Schlatter, Sever, Pelvic Avulsions (Hannah M. Carr, MD)....... 247

PSYCHIATRY
Section editor William White, MD, MA
1. Autistic Child in the ED (Katherine L. Dickerson, MD, PhD)............... 249
2. Behavior (Heather Jones, DO) 250
3. Depression and Suicidal Ideation (Ngoc Bui, MD)........................... 252
4. Eating Disorders (Brandon J. Wang, MD)....................................... 253
5. Managing the Agitated Child (Brandon J. Wang, MD) 255

PULMONARY
Section editor Manpreet Singh, MD, MBE
1. Asthma (Andrew Thorne, MD).. 257
2. Bronchiolitis (Kendra R. Campbell, MD) 260
3. Cough (Jonathan S. Warren, MD) 262
4. Cystic Fibrosis (CF) (Sydney Beck, MD) 264
5. Pneumonia (Kendra R. Campbell, MD) 267
6. Spontaneous Pneumothorax (PTX) & Pneumomediastinum
   (Kendra R. Campbell, MD)...271
7. E-Cigarette or Vaping Associated Lung Injury (EVALI/VALI)
   (Kendra R. Campbell, MD)... 273

RENAL & URINARY SYSTEM
Section editor Katie Rebillot, DO
1. Fluid and Electrolyte Disturbances (Sophia Fornbacher, MD) 275
2. Hematuria (Ryan Gleber, MD) 279
3. Hemolytic Uremic Syndrome (Sarah J. Zyzanski, MD) 283
4. Hypertension (Ahmed Farhat, MD) 285
5. Nephrotic and Nephritic Syndromes (Ahmed Farhat, MD) 287
6. UTI and Pyelonephritis (Ryan Gleber, MD) 289

RHEUMATOLOGY & VASCULITIDES
Section editor Shirley Tung, MD
1. Acute Rheumatic Fever (Adam F. Barnes, MD) 293
2. Henoch-Schonlein Purpura (Sarah J. Zyzanski, MD) 295
3. Juvenile Idiopathic Arthritis (Adam F. Barnes, MD) 296
4. Kawasaki Disease (Sarah J. Zyzanski, MD) 298
5. Systemic Lupus Erythematosus [SLE] (Andrew Pham, MD) 300

TOXICOLOGY
Section editor David Tanen, MD
1. Caustic Exposures (Sydney Beck, MD) 303
2. Common Pediatric Ingestions (Michael Ghermezi, MD) 305
3. Gases (Gabriel H. Campion, MD) 312
4. Methemoglobinemia (Michael Ghermezi, MD) 314
5. One Pill Can Kill (Tiffany J. Au, MD) 316
6. Recreational Drugs (Gabriel H. Campion, MD) 320

TRAUMA
Section editor David B. Burbulys, MD
1. Abdominal Trauma (Elise Molnar, MD) 325
2. Burns (Elise Molnar, MD) 328
3. Electrical Injury (Aixin Chen, MD) 331
4. Extremity Trauma (Ahra Cho, MD, MBA) 333
5. Head and Neck Trauma (Elise Molnar, MD; Alexander M. Garrett, MD) . . . 338
6. Non-Accidental Trauma (Supriya Sharma, MD) 344
7. Spinal Trauma (Michelle S. Davis, MD, MA; Sriram Venkatesan) 348
8. Thoracic Trauma (Suresh K. Pavuluri, MD, MPH) 351

INDEX 354

Section I
Quick Reference

1 ▶ Normal Vital Signs by Age

Age	Heart Rate (per min)	Respiratory Rate (per min)	Systolic BP (mm Hg)
Newborn	70-190	40-60	60-70
0-3 months	100-160	30-50	65-85
3-6 months	100-150	20-30	70-100
6-12 months	90-130	20-30	70-100
1-3 years	80-125	20-30	80-110
3-6 years	70-115	20-30	80-110
6-12 years	60-100	18-25	90-120
> 12 years	60-100	14-20	110-120

2 ▶ Weight by Age

Digit	Left Hand (age in yrs)	Right Hand (weight in kg)
First	1	10
Second	3	15
Third	5	20
Fourth	7	25
Fifth	9	30

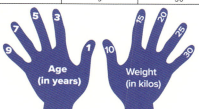

3 ▶ Pediatric GCS

Sign	Pediatric Glasgow Coma Scale Score	Score
Eye Opening	Spontaneous	4
	To sound	3
	To pressure	2
	No response	1
	Non-testable	NT
Verbal Response	Coos, babbles (oriented)	5
	Irritable cry (confused)	4
	Cries to pain (inappropriate)	3
	Moans to pain (incomprehensible)	2
	No response	1
	Non-testable	NT
Motor Response	Moves spontaneously (obeys commands)	6
	Withdraws to touch (localizes pain)	5
	Withdraws to pain	4
	Abnormal flexion	3
	Abnormal extension	2
	No response	1
	Non-testable	NT

4 ▶ Equipment Sizing

Neonatal Airway Equipment					
Weight (g)	Gestational Age (weeks)	Cuffless ETT Size (mm)	Depth (cm) at lip Weight (kg) + 6	Blade (Miller)	LMA
<1000	< 28	2.5	6-7	00	0.5-1*
1000-2000	28-34	3.0	7-8	0	0.5-1
2000-3000	34-38	3.5	8-9	0	1
> 3000	> 38	3.5-4 (if LGA)	9-10	0-1	1

* Size 1 LMA has been used in as small as 800 g
LGA = Large for gestational age

Pediatric Airway Equipment

Age	Weight (kg)	Cuffless ETT Size (mm)	Cuffed ETT Size (mm)	Depth (cm) at lip	Blade			Glidescope	LMA
					Miller	Wis-Hip	Mac		
Neonate	2.5-4	3.5		Weight (kg) + 6	0-1			1	1
6 mo	6-7.5	3.5	3.0	10-11	1			2	1.5
1 yr	10	4	3.5	12	1	1-1.5		2	2
2-3 yr	12-15		4.0-4.5	13-14	2	1.5	2	3	2
4-6 yr	16-20		4.5-5.0	15-16	2	1.5	2	3	2.5
7-9 yr	22-26		5.0-5.5	16-18	2		2	3	2.5-3
10-12 yr	28-32		6.0-6.5	18-19	2		3	3-4	3
13-15 yr	34-38		6.5-7.0	19-20	2		3	3-4	3
16-18 yr	>40		7.0-8.0	21-24	2		3	3-4	4

Cuffless ETT = $(Age / 4) + 4$
Cuffed ETT = $(Age / 4) + 3.5$ (typically used in > 1 mo old)
Laryngeal Mask Airway = $[Weight (kg) / 20] + 1$
ETT placement depth
- Uncuffed ETT size $\times 3$ = cm at the lips
- Neonate: estimated Wt (kg) + 6 cm at lips

Other Equipment

Age	Central Line	Chest Tube	NG/OG tube & Foley
Neonate	3 Fr	10-12 Fr	5-8 Fr
6 mo	3-4 Fr	12-18 Fr	8 Fr
1 yr	4-5 Fr	16-20 Fr	10 Fr
2-3 yr	4-5 Fr	16-24 Fr	10-12 Fr
4-6 yr	5 Fr	20-28 Fr	10-12 Fr
7-12 yr	5-7 Fr	20-32 Fr	10-16 Fr

Tube, Tape, Tap (Approximate)
$2 \times$ ETT size (uncuffed) = NG/OG tube & Foley size
$3 \times$ ETT size (uncuffed) = Depth of ETT, taped at lip
$4 \times$ ETT size (uncuffed) = Chest tube size

5 ▶ Common Pediatric Medication Dosages

AIRWAY (Rapid Sequence Intubation & Post-Sedation Medications)

Induction	Dose (IV)	Comment
Etomidate	0.3 mg/kg (max 20 mg)	Preferred: hemodynamic instability, TBI Avoid: septic shock, possible adrenal suppression
Ketamine	1-2 mg/kg 3-7 mg/kg IM	Preferred: bronchospasm, septic shock unless contraindicated
Propofol	1-2 mg/kg	Use if hemodynamically stable, status epilepticus
Midazolam	0.2-0.3 mg/kg (max 10 mg)	Use if hemodynamically stable, status epilepticus
Fentanyl	1-3 mcg/kg (max 100 mcg)	Given over 30-60 sec ↓ dose if in shock Limited evidence: some recommend in cardiogenic shock or if on pressors

Paralytics	Dose (IV)	Comment
Rocuronium	0.6-1.2 mg/kg	Duration 30-45 min For immediate reversal: sugammadex 16 mg/kg
Succinylcholine	Infant: 2-3 mg/kg Child: 1-2 mg/kg Teen: 1-1.5 mg/kg 4-5 mg/kg IM Max: 150 mg/dose	Avoid if concern for rhabdomyolysis, burns > 48-72 hrs, skeletal muscle or neuromuscular disease, CKD/hyperkalemia, malignant hyperthermia

Post-intubation	Dose	Comment
Dexmedetomidine	0.2-0.5 mcg/kg/hr • Can cause bradycardia and hypotension • PICU input for higher doses	
Fentanyl	Bolus: 0.5-2 mcg/kg Continuous: 1-2 mcg/kg/hr Max 200 mcg/hr	
Midazolam	Bolus: 0.05-0.2 mg/kg over 2-3 min Continuous: 0.06-0.12 mg/kg/hour or 1-2 mcg/kg/min	
Propofol	50-100 mcg/kg/min (max 300 mcg/kg/min)	

RESUSCITATION

Fluid Management & Blood Products

- Bolus
  - 10-20 mL/kg
- Maintenance fluids infusion rate mL/hr (4-2-1 method)
  - First 10 kg body weight: 4 mL/kg/hr
  - Second 10 kg body weight: add 2 mL/kg/hr
  - Every kg > 20 kg body weight: add 1 mL/kg/hr
  - Generally D5 NS with 20 mEq/L K⁺ (normal renal function, + urine output)
    - Do not use 1/4NS at any age, even neonate

Blood Products	Dose
PRBC, Platelets, Fresh Frozen Plasma	10 mL/kg
Cryoprecipitate	1-2 units/kg

Resuscitation	Dose (IV/IO)	Comment
Adenosine	• 1st dose: 0.1 mg/kg (max 6 mg) • 2nd dose: 0.2 mg/kg (max 12 mg)	Rapid push and immediate saline flush
Amiodarone	5 mg/kg (max 300 mg)	• Run over 20-60 min for SVT, VT w/ pulse • Bolus if cardiac arrest • May repeat up to 15 mg/kg/day (max total dose 2.2 g)
Atropine	• 0.02 mg/kg (max 0.5 mg prepubertal, 1 mg pubertal) • ETT: 0.04-0.06 mg/kg	May repeat q3-5min (max total dose 1 mg child, 3 mg teen)
Calcium chloride 10%	20 mg/kg	Repeat PRN
Calcium gluconate	60 mg/kg	Repeat PRN
Dextrose	2-4 mL/kg of D25 5-10 mL/kg of D10 2 mL/kg of D10 (neonate)	Recheck in 15 min, redose as necessary
Insulin regular	0.1 U/kg (max 10 U) IV	For hyperkalemia Give with dextrose: 5 g (50 mL of D10) for every 1U of insulin

Resuscitation	Dose (IV/IO)	Comment
Epinephrine	**Arrest or symptomatic bradycardia:** • 0.01 mg/kg (0.1 mL/kg of 0.1 mg/mL concentration) every 3-5 min, max 1 mg/dose • ETT: 0.1 mg/kg (0.1 mL/kg of 1 mg/mL concentration) every 3-5 min, max 2.5 mg/dose **Neonate specific:** • 0.01-0.03 mg/kg (0.1-0.3 mL/kg of 0.1 mg/mL concentration) every 3-5 min • ETT: 0.05-0.1 mg/kg of (0.5-1 mL/kg of 0.1 mg/mL concentration) every 3-5 min	
Hydrocortisone	2 mg/kg (max 100 mg)	Consider for refractory shock, adrenal insufficiency
Lidocaine	• Bolus: 1-1.5 mg/kg (max cumulative dose 3 mg/kg) • Maintenance: 20-50 mcg/kg/min	For VF/pulseless VT, wide-complex tachycardia with a pulse
Magnesium	25-50 mg/kg (max 2 g)	Bolus if pulseless VT Run over 20 min if VT with pulses or status asthmaticus
Procainamide	15 mg/kg (max 500 mg)	Run over 30-60 min
Sodium bicarbonate	1 mEq/kg	For severe metabolic acidosis or hyperkalemia

Seizures	Dose	Comments
Lorazepam	0.05-0.1 mg/kg (max 4 mg) IV/IO/IM	
Midazolam	• 0.1 mg/kg (max 5 mg) IV, IO • 0.2 mg/kg (max 10 mg) IN, IM, buccal	
Diazepam	0.5 mg/kg 2-5 yr, 0.3 mg/kg 6-11 yr, 0.2 mg/kg ≥ 12 yr (max 20 mg) PR	

Toxicology	Dose	Comments
Flumazenil	0.01 mg/kg (max 0.2 mg)	Benzodiazepine reversal
Naloxone	0.1 mg/kg IV/IM/SQ/IN (max 2 mg), may repeat every 2-3 min	Opiate reversal

Respiratory	Dose
Albuterol	• 0.15-0.3 mg/kg (min 2.5 mg, max 10 mg) every 20 min — Often, 2.5 mg for < 20 kg, 5 mg for > 20 kg every 20 min • MDI 4-8 puffs q20min with spacer • Severe exacerbations: continuous nebulization 0.5 mg/kg/hr (max 20 mg/hr)
Dexamethasone	**Asthma** 0.3-0.6 mg/kg (max 16 mg) PO, IV, IM, 2nd dose in 36-48 hrs **Croup** 0.3-0.6 mg/kg (max 10 mg) PO/IV/IM
Epinephrine	**Anaphylaxis** • 0.15 mg IM autoinjector < 10-30 kg, 0.3 mg IM autoinjector ≥ 30 kg • 0.01 mg/kg IM (0.01 mL/kg of 1 mg/mL concentration), max 0.3 mg • 0.01 mg/kg IV/IO (0.1 mL/kg of 0.1 mg/mL concentration), max 1 mg **Asthma** • 0.01 mg/kg IM (0.01 mL/kg of 1 mg/mL concentration) every 5-15 min (max 0.3 mg prepubertal, 0.5 mg pubertal) **Croup** • Racemic epinephrine 2.25% (0.5 mL in 2.5 mL saline) nebulized over 15 min, or 3 mg (3 mL of 1 mg/mL concentration) in 3 mL saline every 1-2 hrs, for stridor at rest
Ipratropium bromide	• Nebulized 0.25-0.5 mg every 20 min × 3 — Often 0.25 mg for < 20 kg, 0.5 mg > 20 kg • MDI 4-8 puffs every 20 min with spacer
Methylprednisolone	1-2 mg/kg (max 125 mg) IV
Terbutaline	• 10 mcg/kg SQ, IV (max 400 mcg), may repeat every 20 min • Continuous infusion 0.3-0.5 mcg/kg/min, titrate to max 3 mcg/kg/min

Intracranial Hypertension	Dose (IV/IO)	Comment
Mannitol	0.25-1 g/kg usually (max 2 g/kg) over 20-30 min	Cerebral edema/DKA, TBI, ↑ICP
Sodium chloride 3%	2.5-5 mL/kg bolus over 10-15 min	Cerebral edema/DKA, TBI, ↑ICP

COMMON VASOPRESSORS

Vasopressors	Mechanism	Effects	Dose	Uses
Epinephrine	α1, α2, β1, β2 agonist	↑ HR ↑SVR ↑CO	Start at 0.1-1 mcg/kg/min and titrate to effect	Cardiogenic, anaphylactic, and septic shock (cold)
Norepinephrine	α1 >> β1, β2 agonist	Vasoconstriction ↑SVR ↑CO	Start at 0.05-1 mcg/kg/min and titrate to effect	Cardiogenic and septic shock
Dopamine	Low doses: Dopamine (DA) agonist	↑CO mild↑SVR	DA effects primarily: 1-5 mcg/kg/min Inotropic β: 5-10 mcg/kg/min Vasoconstrictive α: 10-20 mcg/kg/min	Cardiogenic, septic, neurogenic shock
	High doses	↑↑SVR ↑CO		
Dobutamine	Primarily β1, β2 agonist	↑CO ↓SVR	Start at 2-20 mcg/kg/min and titrate to effect	Cardiogenic and septic shock

*For others, refer to "PALS: Shock chapter"

OTHER CARDIAC MEDICATIONS

Drugs	Dose (IV)	Maximum Dose	Comment
Prostaglandin E1	0.05 mcg/kg/min, titrate to effect	0.1 mcg/kg/min	• Life-saving medication in ddCHD • Consider empiric treatment in < 1 mo with shock or cyanosis + failed hyperoxia test
Esmolol	• Bolus: 100-500 mcg/kg over 1 min • Maintenance: 100-500 mcg/kg/min		Can either start maintenance only, or bolus and then maintenance
Furosemide	0.5-1 mg/kg	20-40 mg	
Labetalol	Bolus 0.2-1 mg/kg	40 mg	Caution in asthma
	Maintenance 0.25-3 mg/kg/hr	3 mg/kg/hr	
Nicardipine	Bolus 30 mcg/kg	2 mg	
	Maintenance 0.5-1 mcg/kg/min	4-5 mcg/kg/min	

Antiepileptics
- See Seizures chapter

Overdose Antidotes
- See Toxicology section

Procedural Sedation
- See Procedural Sedation and Analgesia chapter

OTHER MEDICATIONS: ANALGESIA, ANTIPYRETICS, ANTIEMETIC, ALLERGY

Analgesia & Antipyretics	Dose	Comment
Acetaminophen	15 mg/kg PO/IV every 4 hrs	Max 650 mg-1 g/dose. Do not exceed 75 mg/kg/day
Ibuprofen	10 mg/kg PO/IV every 6 hrs	Max 400 mg/dose for antipyretic/analgesic. Max 800 mg/dose for anti-inflammatory
Ketorolac	0.5 mg/kg IV/IM	Max 30 mg/dose
Morphine	Age < 6 mo • PO: 0.1 mg/kg every 3-4 hrs • IV/SQ: 0.03 mg/kg every 2-4 hrs Age > 6 mo • PO: 0.2-0.5 mg/kg (max 15-20 mg) every 3-4 hrs • IV/SQ: 0.05-0.2 mg/kg (max 4 mg) every 2-4 hrs, may repeat PRN *Use lower doses if opioid naive*	
Fentanyl	IN: If > 10 kg, 1.5 mcg/kg (max 100 mcg) IV: 1-2 mcg/kg (max 50-100 mcg) every 2-4 hrs infants, every 30-60 min older	
Hydrocodone & Acetaminophen	PO/elixir: < 50 kg 0.1-0.2 mg/kg every 4-6 hrs > 50 kg: 5-10 mg every 4-6 hrs	• Doses are based on hydrocodone • Careful when combining with other acetaminophen products, do not exceed 75 mg/kg/day acetaminophen
Oxycodone	Age < 6 mo: 0.025-0.05 mg/kg PO every 4-6 hrs Age > 6 mo • < 50 kg: 0.2 mg/kg (max 5-10 mg) PO every 4-6 hrs • > 50 kg: 5-10 mg PO every 4-6 hrs	

Gastrointestinal	Dose	Comment
Aluminum hydroxide & magnesium hydroxide	0.5-1 mL/kg (max 20 mL) PO four times daily	
Famotidine	0.25 mg/kg PO/IV two times daily (max 40 mg/day)	
Ondansetron	Age > 6 mo: 0.15 mg/kg (max 8 mg) PO/IV	
Metoclopramide	0.1-0.2 mg/kg (max 10 mg) PO/IV	
Polyethylene glycol 3350	Age > 6 mo: 1 g/kg (max 17 g) PO mixed with 8 oz fluids daily	

Allergy	Dose	Comment
Diphenhydramine	1 mg/kg (max 50 mg) PO/IV/IM every 6 hrs	
Cetirizine	≥ 6 mos to < 2 yrs: 2.5 mg PO daily 2-5 yrs: 2.5-5 mg PO daily > 5 yrs: 5-10 mg PO daily	≥ 6 mos to ≤ 5 yrs: 2.5 mg IV once daily 6 to 11 yrs: 5-10 mg IV once daily ≥ 12 yrs: 10 mg IV once daily
Loratadine	≥ 2 to < 6 years: 5 mg daily PO ≥ 6 years: 10 mg daily PO	

COMMON PEDIATRIC ANTIBIOTICS

- Dosing and duration of treatment are variable based on diagnosis

Antibiotics	Dose	Comment
Amoxicillin	• High dose: 45 mg/kg (max 1-2 g) PO two times daily • Low dose: 22.5 mg/kg (max 1-2 g) PO two times daily	• High dose for otitis media, pneumonia, sinusitis • Range of treatment 5-10 days depending on diagnosis
Ampicillin-sulbactam	50 mg/kg (max 2 g) IV every 6 hrs	
Amoxicillin-clavulanate	High dose • Use 600 mg/5 mL concentration • 45 mg/kg PO two times daily Low dose: 22.5 mg/kg PO two times daily	Dosing based on amoxicillin component 600 mg/5 mL has less clavulanate = ↓ diarrhea Max usually 875 mg/dose
Azithromycin	Day 1: 10 mg/kg (max 500 mg) PO once daily Day 2-5: 5 mg/kg (max 250 mg) PO once daily	AOM, atypical pneumonia

Antibiotics	Dose	Comment
Cefdinir	7 mg/kg (max 300 mg) PO two times daily or 14 mg/kg (max 600 mg) once daily	May color stool red or magenta
Cefepime	50 mg/kg (max 2 g) IV every 12 hrs (or every 8 hrs for pseudomonas)	• Dose depends on diagnosis • Higher dose for epiglottitis, bacterial tracheitis, meningitis, penicillin-resistant pneumococcal pneumonia
Cefotaxime	50-100 mg/kg (max 2 g) IV every 8 hrs	
Ceftriaxone	50-100 mg/kg (max 2-4 g) IV once daily	
Cephalexin	15-25 mg/kg (max 500 mg) PO	Given 3-4 times daily Use the higher dose for severe infection
Clindamycin	10 mg/kg (max 600 mg) PO/IV every 8 hrs	Higher doses used in severe infections
Gentamicin	2.5 mg/kg IV every 8-12 hrs depending on age	
Metronidazole	10 mg/kg (max 500 mg) PO/IV every 8 hrs	
TMP-SMX	5 mg/kg (max 160 mg) PO two times daily	Dosing based on TMP component
Vancomycin	15 mg/kg (max 1 g) IV every 6-8 hrs	

6 ▶ Ventilator Settings

VENTILATOR

- Neonates often use pressure-controlled
  - Initial Peak Insp Pressure (PIP) 16-25 cm H2O, Pressure Support (PS) 6-10 cm H2O
  - Avoid peak pressure > 30 cm H2O
- Circuit (3 sizes): use neonatal for ETT ≤ 4.0, else pediatric, use adult once tidal volume ≥ 300mL

STANDARD SETTINGS

- FiO2 100% and wean
- Tidal volume 5-8 mL/kg ideal body weight
- PEEP 4-5 cm H2O
- Rate: neonate 25-35, infant 20-30, child 15-25, adolescent/adult 12-20
- I-time: neonate 0.5 sec, toddler/child 0.7 sec, adolescent/adult 0.8-1 sec
- Flow trigger: infant 0.25-0.5 L/min, child/adult 0.8-2 L/min

SITUATION SPECIFIC

- ARDS: ↓ tidal volume 3-6 mL/kg, ↑ PEEP 8-10 or higher
- Obstructive disease (asthma): ↓ tidal volume as tolerated, ↓ PEEP 3-4 (decrease to 0 if significant gas trapping) to avoid barotrauma
  — Rate: set to avoid "breath-stacking" aka "auto-PEEP" = ventilator breath begins before complete exhalation
    - Rate = 60 / (time in sec to completely exhale)
      - Rate may be as low as 6-10
    - Maintain I:E ratio 1:3 to 1:5
- Acidosis (DKA, salicylate toxicity)
  — Hyperventilate to match pre-intubation rate and ETCO2
    - Do not take away patient's respiratory compensation
- Single ventricle lesions
  — 3 stage repair: Norwood, Glenn, Fontan
  — After 2nd stage, patient dependent on passive venous return for pulmonary blood flow (Glenn via SVC, Fontan via SVC & IVC)
    - Avoid mechanical ventilation if possible as PPV → ↓ venous return
  — After Glenn, keep PaCO2 40-45 to avoid decreased cerebral perfusion

TROUBLESHOOTING

- Can't oxygenate: O2 connected; inadequate FiO2, PEEP, or I-time; breath-stacking
- Can't ventilate: inadequate tidal volume, insp:exp (I:E) ratio too high, breath-stacking, air leak, large dead space

POST-INTUBATION COMPLICATIONS

D	Displacement of tube	Check connections, tube depth
O	Obstruction of tube	Suction tube
P	Pneumothorax (high risk of barotrauma in mechanically ventilated asthmatic)	• Diagnose with POCUS or CXR • Tube thoracostomy
E	Equipment failure	Disconnect from ventilator and use BMV
S	Stacked breaths (aka auto-PEEP): incomplete exhalation → hyperinflation, can ↓ preload → hypotension	• Disconnect and physically compress chest to promote exhalation • Reduce ventilator rate to allow complete exhalation

7 ▶ Immunizations

SIMPLIFIED IMMUNIZATION SCHEDULE

	Birth	1 mo	2 mo	4 mo	6 mo	12-15 mo	4-6 yr	11-12 yr	16 yr
HepB	#1	#2-----	------>		#3				
Rota			#1	#2	#3*				
DTaP			#1	#2	#3		#4	#5 Tdap	
Hib			#1	#2	#3*	#3 or 4			
PCV			#1	#2	#3	#4			
IPV			#1	#2	#3				
MMR						#1	#2		
Vari						#1	#2		
HepA						#1	#2 min 6 months after #1		
HPV								#1, #2, 6 months later	
Men								#1	#2
Men B									#1, #2
Flu					Start, annually henceforward				

* Whether this dose needed depends on specific vaccine product

RELEVANT TO ED CARE

- Schedule
  - Primary series except MMR, varicella, given at 2, 4, 6 months of age
  - There are no "9 month shots," but there is a 9mo well child check-up
  - MMR, Varicella = the 2 live virus vaccines, given at 12-15mo old
- Implications for febrile child work-up
  - Pneumococcal vaccine 80-90% efficacy against most serotypes 4 wks after 1 dose
  - Hib efficacy against invasive disease after 1 dose 59%, 2 doses 92%
  - Herd immunity also against both diseases
    - Adequately vaccinated well-appearing child low risk for occult bacteremia
  - Ask if vaccines given in last 2 weeks and which ones
- Pertussis immunization after 3 doses 85% protective, after 5 doses 89%
  - Can have pertussis even if fully immunized
  - Give Tdap tetanus booster to adolescents / adults to boost waning pertussis immunity to protect at-risk contacts

- MMR high efficacy but can still get disease, usually milder
  - Least protective against mumps
- Varicella 1-3% breakthrough disease per year in vaccinated
  - Mild: low/no fever, ≤ 50 lesions, may not have vesicles, transmissible
- Common adverse reactions
  - DTaP: fever within first 48 hrs
    - Higher fever or > 48 hrs post-vaccine = look for other fever source
  - DTaP: 2-3% entire limb swelling, especially after dose #4 or #5
  - Rotavirus very small increased risk of intussusception
  - MMR & varicella → fever, rash 1-2 *weeks* post-vaccine, ↑ febrile seizures
- Tetanus prophylaxis

Immunization / Wound Hx	Tetanus Immunization	Tetanus Immune Globulin
< 3 doses or unknown Clean, minor wound	< 7 yr: DTaP 7-11 yr: Tdap > 11 yr: Tdap or dT	No
≥ 3 doses Clean, minor wound	Only if ≥ 10 years since last booster	No
< 3 doses or unknown Contaminated or high risk wound	< 7 yr: DTaP 7-11 yr: Tdap > 11 yr: Tdap or dT	250u IM (regardless of age or weight); give at different site from vaccine
≥ 3 doses Contaminated or high risk wound	Only if ≥ 5 years since last booster	No

8 ▶ Developmental Milestones

Milestones development is variable from child to child. These are only guidelines.

Age	Gross motor	Fine Motor	Personal-Social	Language
2 wk	• Moves head side to side	• Hands fisted	• Regards face	• Alerts to bell
2-4mo	• Lifts shoulder while prone	• Tracks past midline	• Social smiles	• Coos/localizes sound
4-6mo	• Lifts up on hands • May roll front to back • No head lag	• Reaches for objects • Raking grasp	• Looks at hand • Begins to work towards toy	• Laughs and squeals • Copies facial expressions

Age	Gross motor	Fine Motor	Personal-Social	Language
6 - 9mo	• Sits alone/tripod position • (Upright by 8 mo) • Rolls over both ways • Puts weight on both legs	• Transfers object from hand to hand • Brings things to mouth	• Feeds self • Recognizes strangers • Holds bottle • Responds to others emotions	• Babbles • Responds to sounds by making sounds
9-12mo	• Pulls to stand • Gets into sitting position • Crawls • Cruises	• Beginning of pincer grasp • Bangs 2 block together	• Plays pat-a-cake • Waves bye-bye • Stranger anxiety • Points	• Says mama and dada nonspecific • 2-syllable sounds
12-15mo	• Walks • Stoops and stands	• Puts block in cup	• Plays peek a boo • Drinks from cup	• Says mama/dada specifically • Says 1-2 other words
15-18mo	• Walks backwards	• Scribbles • Stacks 2 blocks	• Uses spoon/fork	• Says 3-6 words • Follows commands
18-24mo	• Runs • Kicks a ball	• Stacks 4 blocks • Start to show handedness	• Remove clothes • Feeds doll	• Says at least 6 words
2 yrs	• Walks up and down stairs • Throws overhand (2.5 yrs)	• Copies line	• Brushes teeth/washes hands • Dresses self	• Puts 2 words together • Knows body parts, concept of "today"
3 yrs	• Alternates feet with steps • Broad jump	• Wiggles thumb • Preference for left / right hand	• Uses spoon well	• Names pictures • 75% intelligible to strangers • Understands "tomorrow" and "yesterday"
4 yrs	• Balances well on each foot • Hops on one foot	• Draws person with 3 parts	• Dresses and brushes teeth without help	• Names colors/understands adjectives • 100% intelligible by strangers
5 yrs	• Skips • Walks heel-to-toe	• Copies a square	• Follow rules	• Counts • Understands opposites

Developmental Milestones

9 ▶ Teeth Chart

Upper Teeth	Primary Erupt	Primary Shed	Permanent Erupt
Central incisor	8-12 mos	6-7 yrs	7-8 yrs
Lateral incisor	9-13 mos	7-8 yrs	8-9 yrs
Cuspid (canine)	16-22 mos	10-12 yrs	11-12 yrs
First bicuspid			10-11 yrs
Second bicuspid			10-12 yrs
First molar	13-19 mos	9-11 yrs	6-7 yrs
Second molar	25-33 mos	10-12 yrs	12-13 yrs
Third molar (wisdom)			17-21 yrs

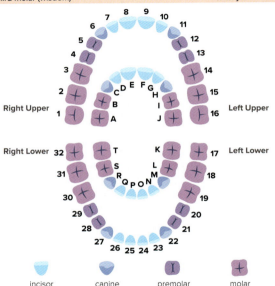

Lower Teeth	Primary Erupt	Primary Shed	Permanent Erupt
Third molar (wisdom)			17-21 yrs
Second molar	23-31 mos	10-12 yrs	12-13 yrs
First molar	14-18 mos	9-11 yrs	6-7 yrs
Second bicuspid			10-12 yrs
First bicuspid			10-11 yrs
Cuspid (canine)	17-23 mos	9-12 yrs	11-12 yrs
Lateral incisor	10-16 mos	7-8 yrs	8-9 yrs
Central incisor	6-10 mos	6-7 yrs	7-8 yrs

10 ▶ Return to School

Symptom / Disease	Return Recommendations
Common cold without fever	No exclusion necessary (follow infection control: hand hygiene, cough into elbow)
Febrile viral illness	Exclude until fever and significant symptoms have resolved
Conjunctivitis	Contagious until symptoms resolve; exclude only if cannot adhere to appropriate hand hygiene
Skin / soft tissue infection	Exclude only if open/draining lesion that cannot be kept covered
Vomiting ≥ 2 times in 24 hrs	Exclude until vomiting resolves or vomiting diagnosed as due to non-infectious cause and can maintain hydration
Diarrhea	Exclude only if stools cannot be contained in diaper, until frequency < (usual + 2) / day
Salmonella typhi or paratyphi	Exclude until meets criteria for diarrhea AND 3 consecutive cultures collected > 48 hrs after antibiotic therapy completed negative
Shiga-toxin producing *E. Coli* (STEC) or *E. Coli O157:H7*	Exclude until meets criteria for diarrhea AND 2 consecutive cultures collected > 48 hrs after antibiotic therapy completed negative
Shigella	Exclude until meets criteria for diarrhea, treatment complete, and ≥ 1 post-treatment culture negative
C. difficile	Same as diarrhea criteria above, no need for test of cure
COVID-19	Exclude until 10 days since symptoms first appeared (or positive test) AND afebrile × 24 hrs (without antipyretics) AND symptoms improving
Oral viral stomatitis	Exclude until afebrile; exclude if cannot contain drool
Rash w/o fever or behavior change	No exclusion
Group A Strep pharyngitis	Afebrile, at least 12 hrs after antibiotics started
Erythema infectiosum (parvovirus B19)	Once rash appears, no longer contagious
Pertussis	Exclude until complete 5 days of antibiotics (or 21 days after cough onset)
Hepatitis A	Exclude until 1 week after illness onset

Symptom / Disease	Return Recommendations
Herpes labialis, herpetic whitlow	Exclude if cannot keep sores covered / primary infection with extensive mouth sores
Head lice	May return once treatment completed (no-nit school policies are not recommended)
Tinea capitis/corporis	May return once therapy started, with instructions to not share potential fomites
Scabies	May return once treatment completed (next day)
Tuberculosis	Children < 10 yr cannot transmit, older children require clearance by public health
Mycoplasma pneumoniae	Exclude until respiratory symptoms resolved; antibiotic initiation does not reduce contagion
Measles	Exclude until 4 days after rash onset
Mumps	Exclude until 5 days after parotid gland swelling onset
Rubella	Exclude until 7 days after rash onset
Varicella	Exclude until all lesions crusted over and/or no new lesions × 24 hours
CMV, HIV, HBV, HCV	No exclusion from school Consult AAP Red Book for more extensive guidelines regarding school and sports participation

11 ▶ Tips & Tricks for Examining Children

DON'T BE SCARY
- Get down to same level as child
- Keep facial expressions and voice light
- Helpful to have toys/distractors
- Relate to child; know the current popular TV show characters

"DOORWAY EVALUATION"
- Before young child notices you, observe from doorway
  — Mental status, interaction with others, playfulness
  — Respiratory work of breathing
  — Skin signs / pallor

PALS TICLS
Tone
Interactions
Consolability
Look or gaze
Speech or cry

ORDER OF EXAM MATTERS
- If child is quiet, listen right away before crying starts
  - Lung exam from back before child sees you
  - Heart exam
- Leave noxious exams (ears, oropharynx) for last
- Have light ready to look at oropharynx if child cries with mouth open

SPECIFIC EXAM SITES
- Head
  - Examine fontanelles and measure head circumference in infants
  - Posterior fontanelle closes in first few months of life
  - Anterior fontanelle closes by 9-18 months
- Eyes
  - Check red reflexes in infants
    - Leukocoria (white pupillary reflex) concerning for retinoblastoma
- Ears
  - If needed, have caretaker immobilize child
    - Child seated on caretaker lap, legs/torso facing to side
    - Child's legs can be trapped between caretaker's legs
    - Child's arm closest to caretaker wrapped around caretaker
    - Caretaker hugging child and anchoring head against caretaker chest
  - Grasp pinna and pull up, back, and slightly out to straighten canal
    - For infants, sometimes pulling back and down improves view
  - Aim otoscope anteriorly
    - Use small ~2.75 mm specula in < 12 mo
    - Start with larger ~4.25 mm specula ≥ 12 mo
- Oropharynx
  - Take advantage of any time mouth is widely open to examine
    - Child may cry with ear exam and open mouth; have otoscope light ready
  - The "dentist chair" position
    - Child on caretaker's lap, face-to-face and legs wrapped around caretaker
    - Caretaker leans child backward on their lap with head hanging off caretaker's knees slightly
    - Mouth will naturally open
- Lymphadenopathy
  - Small mobile rubbery "shotty" adenopathy common anterior and posterior cervical, sometimes occipital also

- Lungs
  - Download free virtual candle app onto phone for child to "blow" out
    - Or, use a hand (yours, caretaker's) as "candles" and put fingers down as they blow them out; put more fingers up and ask to "blow harder"
  - If crying, listen between cries
  - To differentiate transmitted upper airway sounds from nasal congestion with lower airway rhonchi, pinch the nose closed briefly to encourage mouth breathing
- Heart
  - Calm anxious child with pacifier (+/- dipped in sucrose solution) to ↓ tachycardia
  - Still's murmur very common in children, benign
    - Systolic "musical" or vibratory low-pitched murmur at left lower sternal border
- Abdomen
  - Start just above pelvic bones and work up to appreciate hepatomegaly
    - One of the best signs of CHF in pediatrics (don't see ankle edema or JVD as in adults)
  - Have caretaker palpate child to assess tenderness
  - For ticklish child, place child's own hand on abdomen and yours on top to palpate
  - Examine the umbilical stump in newborns
  - Examine gastrostomy tube site if present
- Genitourinary
  - Familiarize with Tanner staging
  - Always examine when complaint is abdominal pain
  - Female
    - Positions to evaluate hymen
      - Sitting on caretaker in lithotomy position, caretaker helps open legs
      - Knee-chest position facing prone
    - Hymen estrogenized in toddler years and after puberty
      - Thin, friable in years between
  - Male
    - Warm hands prior to examining testes
    - May need to "milk" testis down inguinal canal to ascertain descent
- Neurologic
  - Move toy around to assess extraocular muscles
  - Assess muscular tone and look for spontaneous movement all 4 extremities
  - Observe gait — have child walk/run to caretaker

Section II
Resuscitation

1 ▶ PALS: Dysrhythmias

BACKGROUND
- Pediatric sudden cardiac arrest (SCA), sudden cardiac death (SCD) are rare
- Infants ↑ SCD (11.2 per 100,000) relative to older (1.2-2.2 per 100,000)
- Survival from out of hospital cardiac arrest: 2-3% in infants, 9% in older
- Asystole most common pediatric arrest rhythm, then PEA, bradycardia
  — V-fib, V-tach uncommon

BASICS OF PALS/BLS
- Initial: compressions–airway–breathing (C-A-B) sequence
- Compression:ventilation ratios
  — 1-rescuer 30:2
  — 2-rescuer 15:2 pre-pubertal, 30:2 pubertal
- Location: over sternum, between nipples
  — Two-thumb encircling technique for infants
  — Heel of one hand for 1-8 yrs
  — Heels of both hands for > 8 yrs
- Rate 100-120/min
- Depth 1.5 inches in infants, 2 inches in children
- Allow chest to completely recoil between compressions
- Never stop CPR for > 10 sec; avoid excessive ventilation
- Monitor ETCO2 to assess effectiveness and detect ROSC

INITIAL STEPS FOR DYSRHYTHMIA MANAGEMENT
- Maintain airway, place head into sniffing position
- PPV if needed, ensure adequate oxygenation
- Attach SpO2, ETCO2, blood pressure, cardiac monitors
- IV/IO access
- EKG if stable

CONSIDER AND TREAT REVERSIBLE CAUSES: H'S AND T'S

Cause	Initial Treatment
Hypovolemia	20 mL/kg IVF bolus NS
Hypoxia	Maintain airway, supplemental O2
Hydrogen (acidemia)	Ventilate, sodium bicarbonate
Hyper/hypokalemia	Calcium, insulin/dextrose, sodium bicarbonate/K^+ binders
Hypothermia	Active warming measures
Hypoglycemia	Dextrose
Toxins	Toxin specific, supportive care
Tamponade	Pericardiocentesis
Tension PTX	Needle decompression
Thrombosis (PE)	Fibrinolytics, anticoagulation
Thrombosis (MI)	Aspirin, percutaneous coronary intervention

- Mnemonic for 6H's ASHOCK: Acid, Sugar, Hypovolemia, Oxygen, Cold, K^+

PULSELESS ARREST

Asystole/PEA
- Initiate high-quality CPR
- Perform pulse/rhythm checks every 2 min
- Epinephrine IV/IO 0.01 mg/kg (max 1 mg) of 0.1 mg/mL every 3-5 min
- Consider H's and T's

Ventricular Fibrillation/Pulseless Ventricular Tachycardia
- Defibrillate immediately at 2 J/kg and continue CPR for 2 min
- Perform pulse/rhythm checks every 2 min
- ↑ to 4 J/kg for second defibrillation
- Continue CPR, give epinephrine IV/IO (0.01 mg/kg of 0.1 mg/mL) every every 3-5 min
- Can ↑ up to 10 J/kg (max 200 J biphasic, 360 J monophasic) for subsequent defibrillations
- Continue CPR, give amiodarone 5 mg/kg (max 300 mg) IV/IO or lidocaine 1-1.5 mg/kg IV/IO (may repeat 0.5-0.75 mg/kg, max total 3 mg/kg)
    — May repeat amiodarone up to 15 mg/kg total (max 2.2 g)
- MNEMONIC: 2,4,6,8 who do we defibrillate

Symptomatic Bradycardia

- HR too slow → insufficient blood flow to the brain (varies by age)
- Definition: bradycardia for age + symptoms
  - Fatigue, weakness, dizziness, confusion, (near)-syncope, SOB, DOE
- Most common cause: hypoxia
  - BMV with 100% oxygen
- *Persistent HR < 60 bpm with poor perfusion*
  - Initiate CPR and reassess every 2 min
  - Epinephrine 0.01 mg/kg (max 1 mg) of 0.1 mg/mL IV/IO
  - Consider atropine 0.02 mg/kg (max 0.5 mg pre-pubertal, 1 mg pubertal) IV/IO if suspect ↑ vagal tone, AV block, sick sinus syndrome, cholinergic toxicity
    - May repeat PRN to max total 1 mg child, 3 mg adolescent
  - Consider reversible causes: H's and T's, ↑ ICP
  - Consider transcutaneous/transvenous pacing if refractory to medications

Tachycardia

- SVT
  - Ddx sinus tachycardia: absent p waves, minimal rate variability
  - Determine whether patient hemodynamically stable
  - *Stable:* vagal maneuvers (Valsalva or blow into a syringe for older children; apply bagged ice water to face for infants)
    - If vagal maneuvers fail, adenosine 0.1 mg/kg (max 6 mg) IV
      - Push rapidly through IV (antecubital or above) using 3-way stop cock, with all ports open, immediately followed by a flush
    - If no response, double adenosine to 0.2 mg/kg (max 12 mg) IV
    - Avoid verapamil in < 1 yr
    - Refractory: consult pediatric cardiologist
  - *Unstable:* immediate cardioversion 0.5-1 J/kg (consider sedation/analgesia)
    - If IV access readily available, reasonable to give adenosine while preparing for cardioversion (do not delay)
    - May ↑ to 2 J/kg if first cardioversion attempt unsuccessful
  - Disposition
    - Most can be discharged with pediatric cardiologist referral
    - Admit
      - Unstable SVT
      - Difficult to convert
      - Consider for nonverbal patients

- Wide complex tachycardia with a pulse
  — Determine whether patient hemodynamically stable
  — *Stable:* consult cardiologist
    - Consider aberrant SVT if regular, monomorphic - treat as above
    - Pubertal: consider procainamide 15 mg/kg (max 500 mg) or amiodarone 5 mg/kg (max 300 mg) IV/IO over 30-60 min, or lidocaine 1-1.5 mg/kg IV/IO (may repeat 0.5-0.75 mg/kg, max total 3 mg/kg)
  — *Unstable:* assume VT, immediate synchronized cardioversion as above
    - Consult cardiologist
  — Disposition: admit to monitored bed

POST-RESUSCITATION

- Optimize oxygenation and ventilation
  — Titrate oxygen to SpO2 goal 94%-99%
  — Consider placing advanced airway if not already done
  — Avoid severe hyper/hypocapnia; maintain PaCO2 35-50 mmHg depending on underlying condition
- Assess and treat persistent shock
  — Maintain euvolemia with 10-20 mL/kg isotonic fluid boluses PRN
  — Consider inotropes/vasopressors in fluid-refractory shock
- Avoid hyperthermia: antipyretics, cooling blankets
- Avoid hypoglycemia: monitor glucose levels, supplement PRN

DISPOSITION

- Admit patient with ROSC to PICU for close monitoring
- Standardized guidelines for termination of resuscitation do not exist
    — Individualized by considering specific clinical situation, family wishes

BEWARE

(!) Initiate CPR in children with persistent symptomatic bradycardia (HR < 60 bpm) despite adequate oxygenation

2 ▶ Neonatal Resuscitation

BACKGROUND
- In U.S., ~10% newborns require some assistance at birth
- ~1% require substantial resuscitative efforts

EQUIPMENT

Weight (g)	Gestational Age (weeks)	Cuffless ETT Size (mm)	Depth (cm) at lip Weight (kg) + 6	Blade (Miller)	LMA
< 1000	< 28	2.5	6-7	00	0.5-1*
1000-2000	28-34	3.0	7-8	0	0.5-1
2000-3000	34-38	3.5	8-9	0	1
> 3000	> 38	3.5-4 (if LGA)	9-10	0-1	1

* Size 1 LMA has been used in as small as 800 g
LGA = Large for gestational age

ASSESSMENT
- Apgar score
  — Standard assessment of newborn immediately after birth
  — Based on color, muscle tone, HR, respiratory effort, reflex irritability
    - Score 0, 1, or 2 given for each category, max total 10
  — Measured at 1 min and 5 min
    - If 5 min score < 7, measure additional scores at 5 min intervals up to 20 min
  — Not used to determine need for resuscitation or guide resuscitation efforts
- Premature infant's weight: up to 28 weeks gestational age (GA)
  — Add 2 numbers from GA, multiply that sum by 100 = weight in grams
    - Example: 26 wk premature infant: $(2 + 6) \times 100$ = ~800 g
- Preductal SpO2 monitor on right hand to assess hypoxemia

Targeted Preductal SpO2 After Birth	
1 min	60-65%
2 min	65-70%
3 min	70-75%
4 min	75-80%
5 min	80-85%
10 min	85-90%

- Immediately after delivery, dry and warm all newborns: skin-to-skin contact, lamp, overbed warmer, bed with radiant warmer, incubators

- Full-term infants with good muscle tone and strong cry: dry and place on mom for skin-to-skin contact
- Infants not requiring resuscitation: delay cord clamping 30-60 sec (after initial assessment)

ALGORITHM FOR RESUSCITATION

- *Initial steps*: If premature, poor tone, apnea, gasping, or not crying:
  — Dry and place supine under radiant heat source
  — Open airway by placing head into sniffing position
  — Clear secretions PRN; suction mouth then nose
    - Avoid deep suctioning (can cause reflex bradycardia from vagal nerve stimulation)
  — Stimulate (flick sole of foot) if respirations inadequate after suctioning
  — Attach SpO2 (right hand) and cardiac monitors
- *HR > 100 bpm with normal respirations:* give supplemental O2 PRN; observe
- *Labored breathing or persistent cyanosis with HR > 100 bpm:* reposition airway, suction mouth then nose
  — Give supplemental O2 to targeted preductal SpO2; consider CPAP
- *Apneic or gasping with HR < 100 bpm:*
  — Provide PPV (40-60 breaths per min); reassess HR after 30 sec of PPV
- *Persistent HR < 100 bpm:* continue PPV, assess chest wall motion to ensure adequate ventilation
  — Perform corrective actions for inadequate ventilation (reposition airway, suction, adjust mask, ensure seal)
  — Perform ET intubation or laryngeal mask if needed
- *HR < 60 bpm*
  — Perform ET intubation, give 100% O2
  — Initiate chest compressions using two-thumb technique
    - Compression: ventilation ratio 3:1, 120 events/min
  — Obtain vascular access via UVC (preferred), IV, or IO
  — Reassess HR after 60sec of chest compressions and PPV
    - Via 3-lead EKG preferably
- *Persistent HR < 60 bpm*
  — Epinephrine IV 0.01-0.03mg/kg of 0.1 mg/mL every 3-5 min
    - If vascular access not obtained, epinephrine via ETT 0.05-0.1 mg/kg of 0.1 mg/mL concentration
      - Absorption variable
      - Repeat dose once vascular access established

- Volume expansion
  - Maternal hemorrhage ↑ risk neonatal hypovolemia
  - 10 mL/kg NS, Ringer's lactate, or Rh-negative type O blood
  - Caution in premature infants: ↑ risk intraventricular hemorrhage
- Consider pneumothorax
- Glucose monitoring if undergoing resuscitation or signs of hypoglycemia
  - Maintain normoglycemia (> 50 mg/dL) by giving 2 mL/kg of D10W IV PRN
- Meconium aspiration: ETT suctioning no longer recommended
- Temperature regulation: goal 36.5-37.5°C
  - If concern for hypoxic ischemic encephalopathy (HIE), consider therapeutic hypothermia (33-35°C)
    - Do not start during resuscitation; will → bradycardia, ROSC less likely
- Stopping resuscitation: reasonable to stop if no pulse after 10 min

POST-RESUSCITATION CARE

- Avoid hypoglycemia; start patient on D10W maintenance

Umbilical Line Placement (refer to Vascular Access Chapter)

BEWARE

- Preparation and training key for neonatal resuscitation
- Focus is primarily on respiratory management with PPV, not cardiac
- Initiate compressions if HR < 60 bpm after 30 seconds of PPV
- Caution with IVF in premature infants

3 ▶ PALS: Shock

BACKGROUND

- Definition: physiologic state defined by circulatory collapse resulting in insufficient oxygen and nutrient delivery to meet cellular metabolic requirements
- Pathophysiology: changes in cardiac preload, afterload, contractility, and obstruction of circulatory blood flow

TYPES OF SHOCK

- **Distributive**
  - Etiology: ↓ vascular tone, loss of blood vessel integrity → inappropriate distribution of blood volume → ↓ preload
  - Normal or ↑ cardiac output (CO) with ↓ systemic vascular resistance (SVR)
  - Causes: sepsis (infection), anaphylaxis, neurogenic

- **Hypovolemic**
  - **Etiology**: volume depletion → ↓ preload and stroke volume (SV) → compensatory tachycardia
  - Most common cause of pediatric shock
  - ↓ preload, ↓ SV, ↑ SVR
  - **Causes**: acute hemorrhage, dehydration/hypovolemia due to osmotic diuresis (DKA, GI losses (vomiting/diarrhea), or insensible losses (burns)
- **Cardiogenic**
  - **Etiology**: poor myocardial contractility → cardiac dysfunction with ↓ SV, CO
  - Classically causes ↓ CO and ↑ SVR
  - **Causes**: myocarditis, arrhythmia, cardiomyopathy, infarction, poisoning, drug toxicity
- **Obstructive**
  - **Etiology**: compromised CO due to obstruction to blood flow
  - Compensatory mechanisms → tachycardia, ↑ SVR
  - **Causes**: tension pneumothorax, tamponade, aortic coarctation, massive pulmonary embolism, ductal dependent heart lesions, congenital heart disease

EVALUATION

- Early recognition key to preventing morbidity and mortality
- **High Yield History**
  - Vomiting, diarrhea, PO intake, urine output, diabetes, blood loss
  - Fever, immunodeficiency, sickle cell
  - Trauma
    - Hemorrhage, pneumothorax, tamponade, spinal cord injury (neurogenic)
  - Allergen exposure (insect sting, food)
  - Congenital heart disease, cardiomyopathy, URI symptoms
  - Toxin exposure
  - Risk for adrenal insufficiency (adrenal disease, chronic steroids)
- **Exam**
  - Vitals
    - Tachycardia, pallor = shock until proven otherwise
    - ↑ capillary refill time (CRT) often first sign
    - Hypotension: often a late finding in children
      - Neonate < 60
      - 1 mo-10 yr < 70 + 2(age in yrs)
      - 10 yr < 90

- **Distributive**: fever, urticaria, angioedema, signs of infection, spine trauma
- **Hypovolemic**: dry cracked lips, sunken orbits/fontanel, skin tenting, crying without tears, pallor, active bleeding, signs of trauma
- **Cardiogenic**: palpable liver, pulmonary rales, cardiac murmur/gallop, edema, elevated JVD
- **Obstructive**: highly variable depending on site of obstruction, absent lung sounds on one side of the chest, elevated JVD, muffled heart sounds, enlarged liver, cyanosis
- **Neurogenic**: spinal trauma, focal weakness, hypotension + bradycardia
- **Diagnostics**
  - POC GLC, CBC, CMP, LFTs, UA, blood gas, lactate
  - Specific labs by type of shock
    - Blood, CSF, sputum, urine cultures
    - PT, PTT/INR, DIC panel
    - BNP/troponin
  - Imaging (CXR, CT) PRN
    - POCUS RUSH Exam (Rapid Ultrasound for Shock and Hypotension)
  - EKG

MANAGEMENT

- Early, aggressive intervention crucial
  - Restore oxygen delivery to tissues by optimizing blood oxygen content
  - Improve tissue perfusion by improving CO volume and distribution
- ABCs, 2 large-bore IV/IO, O2
- **Distributive**
  - **Anaphylaxis**: IM or IV epinephrine, fluid bolus(es), steroids, antihistamines, albuterol, airway control, remove offending agent
  - **Sepsis**: early antibiotics, fluid bolus(es) with frequent reassessment, vasopressors (epinephrine first line for cold shock, norepinephrine for warm shock)
    - Consider stress dose steroids if refractory to above
  - **Neurogenic**: vasopressors, avoid hypotension/hypoxia, neurosurgical consult
    - Steroids no longer recommended
- **Hypovolemic**
  - **Hemorrhage**: stop the bleed, fluids/blood products
    - PRBC (females get O neg , males get O pos), 10 mL/kg
  - **Dehydration**: fluid bolus(es), control losses, electrolyte repletion, antiemetics PRN, burn management
    - If not improving after 3 boluses, consider alternate diagnosis

- **Cardiogenic**
  - Worsening hypoxia, tachypnea, tachycardia with IVF = suspect cardiogenic cause
    - Fluid bolus 5-10 mL/kg NS with frequent reassessment
  - Arrhythmia control (see PALS: Dysrhythmias chapter)
  - Ionotropic and contractility support (see below)
  - Drug reversal if suspected toxicity (glucagon, calcium, consider insulin for beta blocker or calcium channel blocker, Digoxin Immune Fab for cardiac glycosides)
- **Obstructive**
  - Key is reversal of obstruction
    - Pulmonary embolism: thrombolysis, thrombectomy, anticoagulation
    - Tamponade: pericardiocentesis, pericardial window
    - Tension pneumothorax: needle decompression, tube thoracostomy
    - Ductal-dependent heart lesions: prostaglandin E1
  - Supportive care: fluids, vasopressors

Vasopressors	Mechanism	Effects	Dose	Uses
Epinephrine	α1, α2, β1, β2 agonist	↑ HR ↑SVR ↑CO	Start at 0.1-1 mcg/kg/min and titrate to effect	Cardiogenic, anaphylactic, and septic shock (cold)
Norepinephrine	α1 >> β1, β2 agonist	Vasoconstriction ↑SVR ↑CO	Start at 0.05-1 mcg/kg/min and titrate to effect	Cardiogenic and septic shock
Dopamine	Low doses: Dopamine agonist (DA)	↑CO mild ↑SVR	DA effects primarily: 1-5 mcg/kg/min Inotropic β: 5-10 mcg/kg/min	Cardiogenic, septic, neurogenic shock
	High doses	↑↑SVR ↑CO	Vasoconstrictive α: 10-20 mcg/kg/min	
Dobutamine	Primarily β1, β2 agonist	↑CO ↓SVR	Start at 2-20 mcg/kg/min and titrate to effect	Cardiogenic and septic shock
Vasopressin	Vasopressin agonist	↑SVR ↓CO	Start at 0.01-0.04 milliunits/kg/min	Septic shock
Phenylephrine	α1 agonist	↑SVR	5-20 mcg/kg bolus, then 0.1-0.5 mcg/kg/min	Septic shock
Milrinone	Activates cAMP by inhibiting phosphodiesterase	↑CO ↓SVR (vasodilate pulmonary and arterial blood vessels)	50 mcg/kg/min loading dose over 10-60 min Maintenance 0.25-0.75 mcg/kg/min	Cardiogenic shock

DISPOSITION

- Admission to PICU
- If surgical emergency causing shock, early surgical consultation because operative intervention key

BEWARE

- ⚠ Early recognition and treatment necessary to prevent poor outcomes
- ⚠ Overaggressive fluid resuscitation in cardiogenic shock can be harmful
- ⚠ Hypotension is an ominous, late sign

4 ▶ Airway Management

BACKGROUND

- **Pediatric airway differences**
  — Smaller airway diameter, shorter length
  — Large head and occiput
  — Large tongue relative to oropharynx size
  — Floppy, narrow, curved epiglottis (omega shaped)
  — Superior larynx and anterior vocal cords
  — Cricoid is narrowest point vs. vocal cords in adults
  — Small cricoid cartilage
  — Large adenoids and tonsils
  — Low gastroesophageal sphincter tone
  — Smaller lung volumes
  — ↑ metabolism and oxygen consumption
  — At 8-10 yrs, airway more similar to adult airway

EVALUATION

- **Recognizing potential difficult airway**
  — Congenital syndromes with associated facial malformations
  — Obesity
  — Short neck
  — Known head / neck tumors
  — Facial or oropharyngeal swelling
    - Orofacial burns
    - Chemical inhalations
    - Allergic reactions

- Laryngomalacia or tracheal stenosis
- Head and neck infections (epiglottitis, bacterial tracheitis, PTA, RPA, Ludwig's angina)
- Head and neck trauma
- Active vomiting
- Known prior challenging intubations
- Recent extubation

MANAGEMENT

- **Oxygenating spontaneously breathing child**
  - Blow-by O2: variable FiO2 delivery, likely < 40% FiO2
  - Nasal cannula: up to 24-40% FiO2
  - Venturi-mask: depending on valve attachment, up to 60% FiO2
  - Simple face mask: 40-60% FiO2
  - Non-rebreather face mask: 60-90% FiO2
  - High flow nasal cannula (HFO2): 21-100% FiO2
    - Flow rate 1-2 L/kg/min
  - CPAP/BiPAP: 21-100% FiO2
    - Also provides inspiratory +/– expiratory pressure support
- **Managing the pediatric airway**
  - Determine the level of support required, simple maneuvers to advanced
  - Airway repositioning
    - Chin lift/head tilt
    - Place towel roll under shoulders (infant relatively large head)
    - Removing obstructing devices from mouth
      - Retainers, mouth guards, pacifiers
    - Consider side or prone positioning to improve oxygenation
  - Provide oxygen as above
  - Airway adjuncts
    - Nasopharyngeal airway
      - Size = length from nares to tragus
      - Place with beveled side facing nasal septum
      - Contraindications: concern for basilar skull fracture, midface trauma, bleeding disorder
    - Oropharyngeal airway
      - Patient must not have a gag reflex
      - Size = length from corner of mouth to angle of mandible

- Bag-mask ventilation (BMV)
  - Often bridge to more invasive strategies or as temporary support in reversible airway event (oversedation, post-ictal state)
  - Can use in combination with airway adjuncts
  - Bag/mask size determined by patient size and age
    - Mask: bridge of nose to cleft of chin
  - Bag types
    - Self-inflating: does not require a pressurized oxygen source
      - Allows for high inflation pressures
      - Does not deliver blow-by oxygen or CPAP
      - Can deliver PEEP with additional separate valve
    - Flow-inflating: flimsier bag, requires pressurized oxygen source for bag filling
      - Can deliver blow-by oxygen, CPAP and PEEP
      - Allows visualization of spontaneous ventilation
      - Often used in neonates
- Supraglottic devices can be airway rescue device if failed intubation or in patient unable to oxygenate or ventilate with BMV
  - Laryngeal Mask Airway (LMA), King Airway (for adolescents)
  - Connect to BMV or ventilator
  - Size based on patient's weight
- Endotracheal intubation (ETI)
  - Common indications: cannot oxygenate or ventilate otherwise, airway protection, expected course, GCS ≤ 8
  - ETT size based on age, calculate using following formula:
    - Age (yrs) / 4 + 3.5 (cuffed tube)
      - Cuffed tubes now preferred over uncuffed tubes in > 1 mo
    - Age (yrs) / 4 + 4 (uncuffed tube)
    - May also use length-based tape to size
    - Have tubes one size above and below available
  - Calculate tube placement depth
    - Uncuffed ETT size $\times$ 3 = cm at the lips
    - Neonate: estimated wt (kg) + 6 cm at the lips
  - Laryngoscope blade size: Miller (straight) or Macintosh (curved)
    - 00: premature neonate
    - 0: neonate
    - 1: neonate - 2 yrs
    - 2: 2 yrs
    - 3: 3rd grade (8 yrs)

- Needle cricothyrotomy
  - Emergent last-ditch intervention for pediatric patients (< 8-12 yrs) unable to oxygenate or ventilate via other means
  - Prep and drape. Place large bore 14-18G angiocath through cricothyroid membrane, remove needle
  - Attach 3-0 ETT adapter directly to angiocath, or 3mL syringe to angiocath and 7-0 ETT adapter to syringe
  - Attach BMV to ETT adapter
  - Secure by suturing to neck
- Cricothyrotomy
  - Definitive surgical rescue airway for > 8-12 yrs

- **Approach to Endotracheal Intubation**
  - RSI with sedative and paralytic medications allows for quickest and safest mode of ED intubation
  - Patient assessment, resuscitation
    - Assess difficult airway risk factors
    - Resuscitate to intubate: consider fluid bolus to counteract RSI medication hypotensive effects
  - Preparation
    - Laryngoscope, ETTs, ETT stylet
    - Suction
    - Airway adjuncts, BMV
    - Medications
      - Sedative, paralytic, post-intubation sedation infusions
    - Oxygen source, preoxygenation equipment
    - Rescue devices for difficult airway (bougie, LMA, airway adjuncts, video laryngoscope, fiberoptic scope)
    - If anticipate difficult airway, call anesthesia for back-up
  - Premedication (optional)
    - Consider atropine to reduce oral secretions, blunt bradycardic response
      - Infants or repeat dose succinylcholine
    - Consider lidocaine in head trauma to blunt ↑ ICP during laryngoscopy
    - Falling out of favor, often no longer routinely used
  - Preoxygenation
    - Allows for longer apneic period during intubation
    - Nasal cannula or non-rebreather face mask
    - Leave nasal cannula or HFNC in place during ETI
      - 5 L/min infant, 10 L/min child, 15 L/min adolescent

- Induction
    - Etomidate 0.3 mg/kg IV, avoid if suspect sepsis, adrenal insufficiency
        - Hemodynamically neutral
    - Ketamine 1-2 mg/kg IV, may cause: increased secretions, hypertension, ↑ ICP, laryngospasm
        - Preferred for asthmatics (bronchodilating), septic shock
    - Propofol 1-2 mg/kg IV, may cause transient hypotension
    - Midazolam 0.2-0.3 mg/kg +/– fentanyl 1-3 mcg/kg IV
- Paralysis
    - Commonly rocuronium 0.6-1.2 mg/kg IV or succinylcholine 1-1.5 mg/kg IV
    - Avoid succinylcholine: suspected renal failure, hyperkalemia, neuromuscular disease, burn/trauma > 24-72 hrs ago, malignant hyperthermia
    - Succinylcholine shorter onset, duration of action (onset 30 sec, duration 5-7 min) vs. Rocuronium (onset 45-60 sec, duration 30-45 min)
- Intubation
    - Sniffing position key for success; towel roll under shoulders PRN
    - Keep laryngoscope blade midline, lift (airway anterior in kids)
    - Assistant may pull corner of mouth outwards to give more room
    - Cricoid pressure no longer routinely recommended
- Confirm successful placement
    - Color change capnography
    - End tical CO2
    - Bilateral lung sounds (listen in axillae)
    - No lung sounds over stomach
    - POCUS, CXR
- Post-intubation checklist
    - See Ventilator Settings chapter
    - Post-intubation sedation infusions and plan for ongoing sedation
    - Propofol 50-100 mcg/kg/min, titrate up PRN
        - Risk propofol infusion syndrome if given > 48 hrs
    - Midazolam 0.06-0.12 mg/kg/hr +/– fentanyl 1-2 mcg/kg/hr
    - Dexmedetomidine 0.2-0.5 mcg/kg/hr

BEWARE

(!) Anticipate and plan for potential difficult airway
- Consider calling anesthesia if anticipate difficulty

(!) Don't use a neonatal BMV in children

(!) Prolonged BMV may distend infant's stomach; NGT/OGT placement PRN

5 ▶ Vascular Access

GENERAL PRINCIPLES
- Emergency resuscitations: pursue IV and IO access simultaneously
- Less emergent: consider US-guided IV prior to IO access
- Larger bore, shorter length catheters = highest flow rates

PERIPHERAL VENOUS
- 22-24 G catheters newborns/infants; 18-20 G older kids
- Sites
  - Extremities: cephalic, basilic, median cubital, dorsal hand, great saphenous, dorsal arch of foot
  - Other: external jugular, scalp (consider rubber band around head at forehead level as tourniquet)
- Tips for success
  - Difficult IV: transillumination, near-infrared light devices, US-guided
  - Distraction/ pain reduction: EMLA, vapo-coolant spray, needle-free lidocaine delivery (J-Tip), breastfeeding, sucrose solutions
- Complications: infiltration, hematoma, cellulitis, thrombosis, phlebitis, arterial puncture, placement failure

INTRAOSSEOUS
- Sites: proximal tibia, distal femur most common
- Technique
  - Prep skin sterilely, push needle tip through the skin until bone contact
  - Push/twist/drill through cortex at perpendicular angle until feel a give → stop
  - May be able to aspirate marrow and blood
    - However, lack of marrow aspirate does NOT = incorrect placement
  - Inject small volume of saline prior to use: ensure no leaking or swelling of surrounding soft tissues (extravasation)
- Contraindications: underlying fracture, overlying cellulitis / burn, previous attempt on same bone, osteomyelitis
- Complications: extravasation, slow infusion rate, needle displacement, fracture, compartment syndrome, osteomyelitis, skin infection, fat embolism
- Can withdraw from IO and send labs
  - May be inaccurate: PaO2, WBC, K$^+$, AST/ALT, iCa2+
- May stay in place and be used up to 24 hrs

Infant

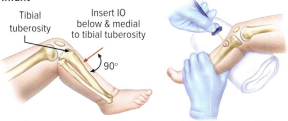

Child/Adolescent

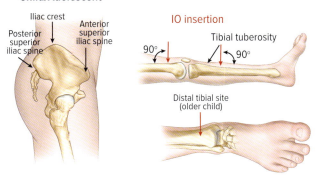

CENTRAL VENOUS CATHETER

- Choose size based on patient age and weight

Pediatric Central Line Sizes				
Age (yrs)	0-6 mo	6 mo-3 yr	4-10 yr	≥11 yr
Catheter	3-4 F	4-5 F	5 F	7 F
Optimal insertion depth (cm) = 1.7 + [(0.07 × height (cm) for patients 40-140 cm]				

- Sites: internal jugular, subclavian vein, femoral vein
- Placed sterilely under US guidance using Seldinger technique

- Confirm correct placement with CXR for high lines (line terminates at junction of SVC and right atrium), KUB for femoral lines (line terminates below diaphragm)
  — Can also consider US to confirm placement
- Complications: inadvertent arterial puncture, catheter malposition, hematoma, bleeding, pneumothorax, infection, thrombosis, surrounding structure damage

UMBILICAL VENOUS CATHETER (UVC)

- For emergency resuscitation of a neonate < 10 days old
- Equipment: antiseptic solution, sterile gloves/drapes, UVC (3.5F for < 1500 g, 5F for > 1500 g), three-way stopcock, umbilical tape or nylon suture, scalpel, small curved hemostats, forceps, adhesive tape and/or wound dressing
- Technique
  — Flush UVC, attach to syringe
  — Scrub umbilical stump with antiseptic
  — Tie off umbilical stump base with suture or umbilical tape
  — Apply upward traction using forceps and cut cord 2 cm from base
  — Identify single thin-walled vein and dilate with hemostat
  — Advance UVC into vein while withdrawing until blood returns
  — For resuscitation use, place and advance UVC only until free flow of blood
  — Advance additional 1-2 cm (no > 4-5 cm total in full term infant) and secure line
- Complications: air embolism, infection, thromboembolism, hemorrhage, vessel perforation, hepatic necrosis

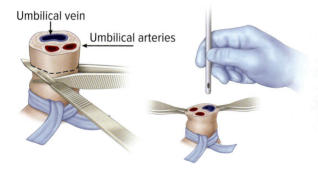

Section III
Procedures and Skills

1 ▶ Foreign Body Removal

EXTERNAL AUDITORY CANAL

- **Presentation:** ↓ hearing, otalgia, otorrhea, bleeding
  - Can include organic material (leaves, insects, food, etc.), inorganic material (beads, rocks, dirt, toys)
- **Complications:** otitis externa, cellulitis, TM perforation, vertigo, ossicular disruption, tissue necrosis, facial nerve paralysis
- **Preprocedural considerations**
  - Do not irrigate if concern for TM perforation, tympanostomy tube present, button battery (liquefactive necrosis risk), matter that may expand (eg, beans)
- **Methods**
  - May need procedural sedation
  - Insects
    - Ensure no TM perforation
    - Mineral oil or viscous lidocaine (provides analgesia and kills insect) in ear canal
  - Irrigation: 20-60 mL of body temperature sterile water using a shortened 14/16G angiocatheter
  - Mechanical: alligator/Hartman forceps, cerumen curette, right angle hook
  - Consider topical skin adhesive on swab stick for visible, round, or fragile objects
  - Magnet (metallic objects)
  - Suction: Schuknecht/Frazier suction
- Consult ENT if button battery, penetrating FB, large object causing high tension against canal, FB too close to TM
- Post-procedure: Otic antibiotic drops if signs of trauma

INTRANASAL

- **Presentation:** pain, epistaxis, unilateral (malodorous) nasal discharge, dysosmia, halitosis
- **Complications:** dislodgement into airway, barotrauma (mother's kiss), tissue necrosis (large objects with high tension, button batteries, magnets in each nares), sinusitis (prolonged FB blocking ostia)
- **Preprocedural considerations:** 0.5% phenylephrine or lidocaine with epinephrine topical to reduce swelling
- **Methods**
  - Mother's kiss: occlude contralateral naris, form seal around patient's mouth, exhale quickly into patient's mouth (may use bag mask valve)
  - Katz extractor or 5-6 French Foley catheter: Insert past FB, inflate balloon, remove
  - Suction
  - Alligator forceps, cerumen curette, right angle hook
- Consult ENT if button battery, magnets in both nares, deep objects near cribriform plate/nasopharyngeal space
- Post-procedure: Prophylactic antibiotics against sinusitis if prolonged duration

PINNA

- **Presentation:** due to ear piercings
- **Complications:** perichondritis, chondritis, poor cosmetic outcome
- **Preprocedural considerations**
  - Aseptic preparation
  - Auricular block vs. local anesthetic infiltration
- **Method**
  - Grasp visible portion with mosquito hemostat while applying direct pressure against ear
  - Clamp another hemostat to other portion
  - If entire earring is embedded, make a small incision to the *posterior* pinna and grasp object using hemostat
- Consult ENT if perichondritis or chondritis
- Post-procedure: Antibiotic ointment & healing by secondary intention

BEWARE

! Always check both ears and nostrils — may have multiple FB
! Refer to ENT if unable to remove and symptoms mild
! Consider X-ray to rule out button battery; requires emergent consult

2 ▶ Laceration Repair and Wound Management

PREPROCEDURAL CONSIDERATIONS

- **High Yield History**
  - Event, timing, contamination
  - Tetanus immunization status
  - Prior scarring, caretaker/patient preference re: plastic surgeon if available
- **Exam**
  - Length: document in cm
  - Location, shape (V-shape, stellate, etc.), depth, multi-layer
    - Check for galea involvement on scalp
- **Diagnostics**
  - XR if possible FB or fracture
  - US may locate radiolucent FB
- **Types of closure**
  - Primary closure: clean wounds, well-approximated edges, < 12 hrs old
    - Contraindications
      - Overlying skin infection, laceration > 12 hrs old unless face/scalp
      - Most bite & puncture wounds (depends on location & offender)
  - Secondary closure: wounds with significant skin tension from tissue loss, puncture wounds
    - Allow wound to fill in on own ("by secondary intention")
  - Tertiary closure aka delayed primary closure: contaminated wound, > 12 hrs old (24 hrs face/scalp)
    - Irrigate, ABx, perform closure 4-5 days later
- **Wound preparation**
  - Explore, evaluate for FB
  - High pressure irrigation with water or saline, debridement PRN
    - Running tap water over wound acceptable irrigation
- **Analgesia/anxiolysis**
  - LET (lidocaine, epinephrine, tetracaine) gel over open wounds (nonintact skin) 20-30 min
    - EMLA is not used for open lacerated skin

- Local anesthetic infiltration
    - Infiltrate warmed anesthetic with small (27-30 gauge) needle, slowly, from wound inner edge to minimize pain
        - Buffering 1 part bicarb: 10 parts lidocaine with epinephrine reduces pain of infiltration
    - Maximum doses

Anesthetic	Max Dose (≤ 70 kg)	Absolute Max (> 70 kg)
Bupivacaine	2.5 mg/kg	175 mg
Bupivacaine w/epi	3 mg/kg	225 mg
Lidocaine	5 mg/kg	350 mg
Lidocaine w/epi	7 mg/kg	490

- Consider intranasal midazolam 0.3 mg/kg, max 10 mg, max volume 1 mL per nostril
- Regional blocks with lidocaine, bupivacaine, or mix
    - Avoids distorting tissue architecture: vermillion border, external ear

TECHNIQUES

- **Tissue adhesive**
    - Indications: small linear lacerations with minimal tension, especially face
    - Contraindications
        - Near eyes, eyebrow, mucosal surface, hands, feet, joints, axillae, perineum
        - Bites, punctures, crush wounds
        - Contaminated wound, infected surface
    - Equal strength to 5-0 nylon
    - Technique: dry site, approximate wound edges, apply in one continuous stroke over top (not inside wound)
- **Butterfly bandages**
    - Indications: small lacerations, minimal tension, multiple parallel lacerations
    - Technique: apply perpendicular to wound, use benzoin adhesive on ends
        - Sometimes combined with tissue adhesive
- **Staples**
    - Indications: scalp lacerations
    - Technique: approximate wound edges, apply using wound stapler
        - Repair actively bleeding vessels with figure of 8 first
        - Repair galea with absorbable sutures prior to scalp closure

- **Hair apposition technique**
  - Indications: scalp lacerations
  - Technique: carefully separate hair on each side of wound, take thin strand from each side and twist to bring wound edges together, apply drop of tissue adhesive over twist
- **Suturing**
  - Indications: depth/wound tension not amenable to above techniques
  - Techniques
    - Simple interrupted
    - Horizontal mattress: reduces tension
    - Vertical mattress: everts edges for improved cosmesis
    - Corner: V-shaped wound
    - Deep dermal: reduces tension
    - Figure of eight: actively bleeding vessel
    - Purse string for stellate lacerations

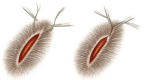
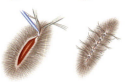

Suture	Absorbable?	Time to 50% strength	Full absorption	Common uses
Polyglactin	Yes	21 days	56-70 days	Deep dermal sutures
Polyglactin irradiated	Yes	5 days	42 days	Mucosal surfaces, trunk, extremities
Fast absorbing plain gut	Yes	7 days	21-42 days	Facial laceration
Nylon	No	> 10 years	n/a	Skin sutures (simple interrupted, mattress)
Polypropylene	No	Indefinite	n/a	Skin sutures esp. near dark hair (suture is blue)

Body site	Common closure	Suture removal
Scalp	Staples, Hair apposition technique, Sutures 4-0 or 5-0 nylon, polypropylene	7-10 days
Face	Tissue adhesive, Suture 5-0 fast absorbing plain gut or 5-0 or 6-0 nylon	3-5 days (nylon)
Extremities, Trunk	Tissue adhesive, Suture 4-0 or 5-0 nylon	7-10 days
Crossing joints	Suture 4-0 nylon	14 days
Mucosa	Suture 4-0 polyglactin irradiated	N/A

POST-PROCEDURE

- Dressing
  - Secure dressing (wicking gauze wrap for young child) +/– antibiotic ointment
    - Do not apply ointments to wounds closed with tissue adhesive
  - Splint wound overlying joint
- Tetanus update per Immunizations chapter
- Prophylactic antibiotics (3-5 days) only if bite, contamination, high risk for infection, full-thickness intraoral
  - Cephalexin 25 mg/kg (max 500 mg) PO two times daily OR
  - Clindamycin 10 mg/kg (max 600 mg) PO three times daily
  - Amoxicillin-clavulanate 22.5 mg/kg (max 875 mg) PO two times daily for bites
- Aftercare education/follow-up
  - Nonabsorbable suture & staple removal
    - Face: 3-5 days
    - Scalp, arms, trunk: 7-10 days
    - Legs: 10 days
    - Over joint: 14 days
- Sun protection to minimize scar discoloration
- 48-72 hr wound check for high-risk wounds

TRICKS OF THE TRADE

- To avoid getting tissue adhesive in eye for lacerations near eye: gauze over eye, Tegaderm over gauze with hole cut out for laceration
- C-collar and papoose/wrap to immobilize young children

BEWARE

! Consult surgeon if open fracture, involves joint space, tendon, nerve, blood vessel, lacrimal duct, tarsal plate, parotid duct, or cosmetically complex closure

3 ▶ Lumbar Puncture (LP)

PREPROCEDURAL CONSIDERATIONS

- Spinal cord ends at L3 at birth, L2 in adulthood
  - LP performed at L3-L4/L4-L5 in older children/adults
    - L4-L5/L5-S1 in infants/young children
  - Iliac crests at level of L4 vertebral body

- Continuous monitoring (risk of hypoxia/apnea in neonates)
- May need anxiolysis with midazolam (IN, IV) or procedural sedation

INDICATIONS
- Suspected CNS infection
- Suspected subarachnoid hemorrhage
- Diagnosis/treatment of idiopathic intracranial hypertension
- Diagnosis of neurologic disease (Guillain-Barré, MS, etc.)

CONTRAINDICATIONS
- Elevated ICP
- CNS space-occupying lesion
- Coagulopathy
  - Platelets < 50,000
  - INR > 1.4
  - Anticoagulants, hemophilia
- Skin infection near puncture site
- Abnormal spinal anatomy
- Physiologically unstable

PREPARATION
- Resuscitate before LP
- Empiric antibiotics if meningitis suspected; perform LP within 1 hr
- Neuroimaging before LP if signs of ↑ ICP, focal neurologic findings, AMS, immunocompromised

EQUIPMENT
- Skin cleanser (mild agent for neonates - chlorhexidine)
- Sterile drape, gloves, cap, mask
- Anesthetic
  - EMLA
  - Injected 1% lidocaine
- 22-gauge spinal needle with stylet
  - < 2 yrs: 1.5 inches
  - 2-12 yrs: 2.5 inches
  - > 12 yrs: 3.5 inches
  - Obese adolescent may require 5 inches

- Manometer/stopcock if measuring opening pressure
- 4 numbered collection tubes
- Gauze, bandage

TECHNIQUE

- Upright seated or lateral recumbent position
  - Lateral recumbent allows opening pressure measurement
- Assistant holds child to minimize movement
- Identify site, sterile prep, drape patient
- Needle bevel toward patient's side
- Needle insertion depth estimate in cm: 10[wt (kg) / ht (cm)] + 1
- Collect 1-2 mL of CSF per tube (20 drops = 1 mL)
- Stylet in place when needle inserted/removed (potential for epidermoid cyst if removed when passing dermis)
- Send CSF for cell count, culture/gram stain, protein, glucose, +/– pathogen PCR panel

TROUBLESHOOTING

- Bony resistance: withdraw to skin, redirect cephalad ("toward umbilicus")
- No CSF
  - Reconfirm landmarks, patient position
  - Interspace above/below
  - Rotate needle 90° if slow flow
- Traumatic tap
  - May hit venous plexus
  - New needle, reconfirm landmarks, ensure midline
  - Correction formula may be used: 1000 RBCs per 1 WBC

COMPLICATIONS

- Headache most common
  - Prevent with smaller needle, atraumatic needle
  - Bedrest does not decrease
  - Oral analgesics, caffeine
  - Definitive treatment is blood patch
- Spinal hematoma
- Infection
- Cerebral herniation extremely rare

BEWARE

- ❗ Neck hyperflexion does NOT improve success
  - Hyperflexed neonates may become apneic or hypoxic
- ❗ Never use a syringe to withdraw CSF

4 ▶ Procedural Sedation & Analgesia

DEFINITIONS

- Analgesia: pain relief
- Sedation continuum
  - Minimal sedation/anxiolysis: responds normally to verbal commands
  - Moderate sedation: depressed consciousness, responds purposefully to verbal commands, maintains own airway
  - Deep sedation: depressed consciousness, responds to painful stimuli, cannot be easily aroused, may require assistance maintaining airway
    - Propofol, opiate + benzodiazepine
  - General anesthesia: unconscious, not arousable
    - Not appropriate for ED
  - Dissociation: trance-like state with analgesia, followed by amnesia
    - Ketamine

INDICATIONS

- Facilitate performance of painful procedures or procedures requiring no motion

CONTRAINDICATIONS

- Difficult airway anticipated - consider procedure in OR
- Unstable patient
- Prolonged procedure inappropriate for ED

PREPROCEDURAL CONSIDERATIONS

- PMH: cardiopulmonary disease, seizures, prior sedations, sleep apnea, prior difficult airway swallowing problems, atlantoaxial instability
  - Obesity is an independent risk factor for adverse events
    - Use ideal body weight for dosing
- Allergies

- Medications
- Last oral intake
- Airway assessment: Mallampati score, mouth opening, neck mobility
- Equipment preparation (SOAP ME)
    - **S**uction catheters (appropriately sized, connected & tested)
    - **O**xygen (tank full, appropriate size mask & bag)
    - **A**irway equipment and backups (NP/OP airways, bougie, LMAs, video laryngoscope, tubes & blades)
    - **M**edications: RSI, reversal agents, resuscitation
    - **M**onitors (cardiopulmonary, pulse oximetry, EtCO2)
    - **E**quipment needed for procedure

AGENTS

- Nonpharmacologic
    - Sugar solution in infants
    - Vapocoolants
    - Visual or vibratory distractions
- Pharmacologic

Commonly Used Agents for Pediatric Procedural Sedation					
Medication	Route	Dose	Frequency	Onset	Duration
Analgesia					
Fentanyl	IV (slow push)	Initial: 0.5-1 mcg/kg/dose (max single dose: 50 mcg) Repeat doses: 50% of initial dose	once, then every 3-5 min	1-2 min	30-60 min
	Nasal	Initial: 1-2 mcg/kg (max single dose: 100 mcg) Repeat doses: 0.3-0.5 mcg/kg/dose (max total dose: 3 mcg/kg)	once, then every 5 min	5-10 min	30-60 min
Morphine	IV	< 6 mos: 0.025-0.03 mg/kg/dose ≥ 6 mos: 0.05-0.1 mg/kg/dose (max single dose: 4 mg)	once, then every 2-4 hrs	5-10 min	3-5 hrs

Sedative/Anxiolytic					
Midazolam	IV	< 6 yrs: 0.05-0.1 mg/kg (max total dose: 6 mg) ≥ 6 yrs: 0.025-0.05 mg/kg (max total dose: 10 mg)	once, then every 10-15 min	3-5 min	1-2 hrs
	PO	< 6 yrs: 0.5-1 mg/kg/dose ≥ 6 yrs: 0.25-0.5 mg/kg/dose (max single dose: 20 mg)	once	10-20 min	1-3 hrs
	IM	0.1-0.15 mg/kg/dose (max total dose: 10 mg)	once	5-15 min	1-6 hrs
	Nasal	0.2-0.3 mg/kg/dose (max total dose: 10 mg)	once	5-10 min	30-60 min
Sedative/Hypnotic					
Ketamine	IV (slow push)	Initial: 1-2 mg/kg/dose Repeat doses: 0.5-1 mg/kg/dose	once, then every 5-15 min	1 min	5-10 min
	IM	Initial: 4-5 mg/kg/dose Repeat doses: 2-4 mg/kg/dose	once, then every 15-30 min	5-10 min	15-30 min
Propofol	IV (slow push)	Initial: 1-2 mg/kg/dose Repeat doses: 0.5 mg/kg/dose	once, then every 3-5 min	< 1 min	1-3 min
	Infusion	75-150 mcg/kg/min	continuous	< 1 min	3-5 min after discontinuing
Nitrous oxide	Inhaled	1:1 oxygen: nitrous oxide	continuous	30-60 min	5 min after discontinuing
Dexmedetomidine	Infusion	0.2-1 mcg/kg/hr	continuous	30-60 min	1-4 hrs after discontinuing
Etomidate	IV (slow push)	Initial: 0.1-0.2 mg/kg/dose Repeat doses: 0.1 mg/kg/dose (max total dose: 0.4 mg/kg)	once, then every 3-5 min	< 1 min	2-10 min

COMPLICATIONS

- Prolonged vs. insufficient sedation
  — Many children enter deeper sedation level than intended
- Hypoxia → reposition airway, supplemental oxygen
- Bradypnea or apnea → assist ventilation
- Transient hypotension → IV fluids, pressors if needed
- Laryngospasm → pressure at laryngospasm notch (Larson's maneuver), BMV

POST-PROCEDURE

- Recovery
  — Keep on monitors
  — Visually monitor until rousable, responding appropriately, protecting airway
- Discharge criteria
  — Normal VS, return to pre-sedation mental state, able to sit up & maintain head control without assistance (especially young children in car seats), ambulatory
- Patient education
  — Possible drowsiness over next day: avoid driving, operating machinery, biking/skateboarding, contact sports
- No routine follow-up needed

Section IV
Cardiovascular

1 ▶ Approach to Pediatric EKG Interpretation

SYSTEMATIC APPROACH

- Always use an age-based reference
- **ID, calibration:** ensure correct patient, note voltage benchmark, leads
  - Full standard (normal) vs. half-standard (50% reduction) vs. mixed (reduction precordial leads only)
    - Double voltage in mm when half standard
  - V3R and V4R: right-sided often used in young child, CHD

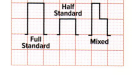

- **Rate:** varies with age
- **Rhythm**
  - Normal sinus rhythm requires:
    - 1:1 ratio of P-waves:QRS with constant PR interval
    - Normal P-wave axis (positive in I, II, aVF; negative in aVR)
  - Sinus arrhythmia (HR variation through respiratory cycle) common
- **Axis:** varies with age
  - Neonates right ventricular dominant (high pulmonary pressures in utero)
    - Can have right axis deviation to +180
    - Axis gradually normalizes ~ 6 months of age
  - Extreme superior axis -90 to -180 suggests AV Canal
- **Intervals**
  - **PR and QRS** vary with age
    - Shorter in younger children (less myocardial mass)
    - If very short PR (< 100 msec), evaluate for delta wave = pre-excitation
    - 1st degree AV block common, benign

- **QT interval:** evaluate in leads II, V5-6
  - QT varies inversely with heart rate (HR), should be corrected (QTc)
    - Bazett formula: QTc = QT / √ RR
  - Normal: 0.44 seconds < 1 week old, 0.45 seconds all males > 1 week old and prepubertal females, 0.46 seconds pubertal females and older
  - Visual estimation: normal QTc if < ½ RR interval (unless HR < 60)
- **Voltages**
  - **Atrial:** evaluate p wave amplitude in leads II and V1
    - Tall P-waves > 3 mm = right atrial enlargement
    - Wide P-waves > 2 mm (0.08 sec) for infants, > 2.5 mm (0.10 sec) for children = left atrial enlargement
  - **Ventricular:** evaluate QRS amplitude in precordial leads
    - QRS voltages exaggerated due to small chest walls
      - Vary with age
    - Right ventricular hypertrophy
      - R in V1 or S in V6 > 98th percentile for age
      - Upright T-wave in V1 age ~7 days to adolescence
      - Q-wave present in V1
    - Left ventricular hypertrophy
      - S in V1 or R in V6 > 98th percentile for age
      - Left axis deviation for age
      - Q-wave > 5 mm and tall T-waves in V5 or V6
- **Repolarization, Ischemia**
  - **Juvenile T-wave pattern**
    - First week of life, T-waves upright in most leads
    - Beyond 1st week, T-waves inverted in V1 to V2/V3
    - Typically resolves in adolescence; "juvenile T-wave pattern" may persist into young adulthood
  - **ST segment:** normally isoelectric compared to TP segment
    - Elevation/depression > 1 mm limb leads, > 2 mm precordial leads concerning for ischemia
  - **J point:** junction between QRS/ST segment
    - Benign Early Repolarization: J point elevation with upsloping ST
      - Common in adolescents, young adults
  - **Q waves**
    - Normal: inferior (II, III, aVF) and left precordial (V4-V6) leads if < 5 mm (or 25% of QRS amplitude) and < 40 msec
    - Q waves up to 8 mm in lead III normal age 0-3 yrs

AGE-BASED NORMALS

Age	Axis	PR (sec)	QRS (sec) 98th%	R in V1 98th%	S in V1 98th%	R in V6 98th%	S in V6 98th%
0-7 days	30-180	0.08-0.12	0.07	25.5	18.8	11.8	9.6
1-3 wks	30-180	0.08-0.12	0.07	20.8	10.8	16.4	9.8
1-6 mo	10-125	0.08-0.13	0.07	19	15	22	8.3
6-12 mo	10-125	0.10-0.14	0.07	20.3	18.1	22.7	7.2
1-3 yrs	10-125	0.10-0.14	0.07	18	21	23.3	6
4-5 yrs	0-110	0.11-0.15	0.08	16	22.5	25	4.7
6-8 yrs	-15-110	0.12-0.16	0.08	13	24.5	26	3.9
9-11 yrs	-15-110	0.12-0.17	0.09	12.1	25.4	25.4	3.9
12-16 yrs	-15-110	0.12-0.17	0.10	9.9	21.2	23	3.7
> 16 yrs	-15-110	0.12-0.20	0.10	9	20	20	3.7

Adapted from Harriet Lane Handbook, 22nd edition

2 ▶ Arrhythmias

BACKGROUND

- **Bradyarrhythmias:** sinus or AV node problem
  - **Sinus bradycardia:** normal sinus P-waves/conduction but heart rate below normal
    - Benign if stable, well-perfused
    - Hypoxia #1 cause in children when unstable
    - Hypothermia can also cause bradycardia
  - **Sick sinus syndrome:** sinus node dysfunction → chronotropic incompetence
    - HR not meeting body's metabolic demands
    - EKG: variable
      - Sinus bradycardia
      - Long sinus pauses (> 3 sec)
      - Tachy-brady syndrome (bradycardia alternating with paroxysmal SVT)
  - **AV blocks:** abnormal conduction at or below AV node
    - Causes and management similar to adults
    - **1st degree, 2nd degree Mobitz Type I:** typically benign
    - **2nd degree Mobitz Type II, 3rd degree:** may require pacing
      - Lyme disease can present as 3rd degree block
- **Tachyarrhythmias**
  - **Sinus tachycardia:** search for underlying cause (pain, fever, infection, anxiety, anemia toxicologic)

- **Supraventricular:** most common tachyarrhythmia in structurally normal hearts
    - Fixed high HR, no p waves
    - Re-entrant circuits: 90% of pediatric SVT
        - AV node reentrant tachycardia most common
            - *Functional* re-entry circuit
        - AV reentrant tachycardia
            - *Anatomic* accessory pathway
            - Orthodromic: anterograde conduction through AV node, retrograde through accessory, narrow complex
            - Antidromic (opposite), wide complex
- **Abnormal atrial automaticity:** AFib, AFlutter, and ectopic atrial tachycardia
    - Rare in structurally normal pediatric hearts
- **Ventricular tachycardias (VT, VFib):** abnormal ventricular automaticity
    - Structural causes (CHD/cardiomyopathies, post-MI, peri/myocarditis)
    - Medications (anti-arrhythmics, inotropes)
    - Electrolyte disturbance
    - Misplaced IV/device in ventricle
    - Fascicular VT = Verapamil-sensitive VT
- **Sudden Cardiac Death (SCD) etiologies:** red flags on EKG (syncope patients screen)
    - **Brugada Syndrome:** sodium channelopathy
        - Classic EKG: "coved" ST elevation in V1/V2 (Type 1) or "saddleback" ST elevation (Type 2); RSR' pattern that looks similar to RBBB
        - Normal EKG does NOT rule out
    - **HOCM:** hypertrophic obstructive cardiomyopathy
        - Inherited ventricular and septal hypertrophy causing dynamic LV outflow tract obstruction
        - EKG: LVH, nonspecific ST/T wave changes, "dagger" Q waves > 3 mm deep and/or > 40 msec in duration in inferior/lateral leads
    - **Long QT Syndrome:** potassium channelopathy, risk for Torsades
        - Subtypes with different classic syncope triggers (swimming, exercise, loud noise, sleep)
    - **WPW:** accessory conduction pathway
        - Upsloping delta wave before QRS (pre-excitation)
        - Risk for AVRT and AFib/Flutter
        - Avoid AV nodal blocking agents (beta-blockers, calcium channel blockers, digoxin, amiodarone)

- **Arrhythmogenic RV Cardiomyopathy/Dysplasia (ARVC/ARVD):** inherited disorder of pathologic RV myocardium replacement by fibrous fatty tissue
    - Second most common cause of SCD in young people after HOCM
    - EKG: epsilon waves: small positive deflection/notch between the end of the QRS complex and onset of the T-wave in leads V1–V3
- **Catecholaminergic polymorphic VT (CPVT):** Ca channelopathy
    - Normal EKG at rest, but polymorphic VT on stress test

EVALUATION

- **High Yield History**
    - Nonspecific in infants (fussiness/irritability, poor feeding, BRUE)
    - Older children: palpitations, chest pain, exercise intolerance, syncope
    - Red flags: chest pain or syncope with exertion, family history of SCD, classic sudden syncope trigger (loud noise, strong emotion, exercise)
    - Ingestions, medications, supplements
- **Exam**
    - Determine hemodynamic stability
        - Perfusion, mental status, presence/quality of peripheral pulses
    - Cardiac auscultation: regular/irregular rhythm, gallops or murmurs
        - Sinus arrhythmia (HR variation with respiratory cycle) common, normal
        - Murmur that increases with valsalva concerning for HOCM
    - Thoracotomy scars
    - Signs of CHF: crackles, hepatomegaly, edema
- **Diagnostics**
    - Labs
        - POC GLC, BMP, Mg, Phos, CBC
        - Troponin, BNP
        - Consider toxicology labs or drug levels
    - Imaging
        - CXR: cardiomegaly, pulmonary edema
        - POCUS and/or formal echocardiogram: global function, pericardial effusion
    - EKG: 12-lead, ideally during symptomatic period
    - Continuous EKG strip during medical interventions to assess response to therapy

MANAGEMENT

- See Resuscitation section (PALS: Dysrhythmias)
- ABCs, apply defibrillation pads
  — IV fluid bolus for poor perfusion
    - Caution if signs of CHF/myocarditis
- Supportive care and identify and treat reversible causes
- Cardiology consultation
  — Red flags on history, even if patient is now stable/asymptomatic
  — Concerning EKG findings
  — Any medical intervention, especially if not responding

DISPOSITION

- Ongoing resuscitation/symptoms: PICU
- Resolved with interventions: Cardiology consult
- Concerning red flags on history/workup: Cardiology consult, outpatient follow-up
  — No exertion until follow-up

BEWARE

- ❗ Children with arrhythmias may present as syncope, BRUE, fussy baby
  — Watch for subtle EKG findings
- ❗ Normal EKG does NOT rule out all causes of SCD

3 ▶ Congenital Heart Disease

BACKGROUND

- CHD = most common major congenital abnormality, affecting ~ 1/100 children
- Critical CHD (cCHD): subset requiring surgical repair in the 1st year of life ~1/1000
- Ductal dependent lesions (ddCHD) require a PDA to supply pulmonary or systemic circulation
  — Emergent intervention necessary for survival
  — Presents in first days to weeks of life
- Age of presentation
  — Infants < 1 mo have ddCHD until proven otherwise
  — Patients > 1 mo often present in respiratory distress, cyanosis, or CHF from shunting lesions

- CHD presents variably in 3 main categories

Presentation	Shock (gray)	Cyanosis (blue)	Respiratory distress (pink)
Physiology	Usually ddCHD, left obstructive lesion with ductal-dependent systemic circulation	• ddCHD, right obstructive lesion with ductal-dependent pulmonary flow • Cyanotic CHD with R→L shunt, CHF • Hypercyanotic episode, Eisenmenger syndrome	L→R shunt causing pulmonary overcirculation, CHF
Age	Presents < 1 month old	Newborn ddCHD, cyanotic CHD Older: Hypercyanotic, Eisenmenger syndrome	Often presents 1-6 months of age
Lesions	Critical AS, HLHS, ALCAPA with MI	• Pulm atresia, tricuspid atresia, Ebstein anomaly, TGA w/o VSD, severe TOF • TAPVR, truncus arteriosus, TOF, TGA with VSD	VSD, PDA, AV canal, PAPVR, "pink" ToF, ALCAPA with recurrent ischemia
Presenting symptoms	Lethargy/altered mental status, poor feeding, pallor/ashen, weak pulses, delayed cap refill, hypotension	Cyanosis Subset with signs of CHF	Irritability, sweating, feeding difficulty, failure to thrive, tachypnea, increased work of breathing, rales, hepatomegaly
DDx	Sepsis, other causes of shock, respiratory infection, metabolic abnormality, methemoglobinemia, abdominal catastrophe, anemia, polycythemia, toxidrome, myocarditis, pericarditis		
Diagnosis	Empiric PGE1 begun prior to confirming diagnosis with echocardiogram	Low SpO2 Failed hyperoxia test CXR: ddCHD - dark lung fields, R → L shunt with CHF — wet lungs	Elevated BNP CXR: pulmonary edema EKG: chamber hypertrophy

- *Understanding physiologic categories and their emergent management is more important than memorizing specific lesions*

EVALUATION

- **High Yield History**
  — Onset
    - Rapid decompensation
      - ddCHD with closing ductus
      - Post-op patient → concern for shunt occlusion
    - CHF presents more gradually
  — Growth and feeding: failure to thrive, feeding difficulty, sweating, long feeds
  — Family history (CHD often hereditary)
  — Known CHD: anatomy, stage and dates of operative repair
- **Exam**
  — General appearance: mental status, pink/blue/gray, dysmorphic features
    - CHD associated with many genetic syndromes
  — Vital signs: tachycardia, hyper/hypotension, hypoxia, tachypnea
  — Cyanosis: visible when ≥ 5 g/dL Hgb deoxygenated (may not see if anemic)
    - Central cyanosis on exam (inside the mouth, not just lips)
  — Cardiac: murmurs (diastolic always abnormal), gallops
    - *Absence of murmur does NOT rule out CHD*
  — Lungs: quiet tachypnea (tachypnea with normal work of breathing), respiratory effort, crackles/rales, cardiac wheezing
  — Abdomen: hepatomegaly (start palpating in pelvis)
  — Extremities: pulses, clubbing, edema (uncommon in children)
    - Upper vs. lower extremity pulses: delayed, absent, or weaker femoral pulses concerning for CoA
- **Diagnostics**
  — Bedside tests
    - 4 limb BP: > 20 mmHg difference between right upper and lower extremities concerning for CoA
    - Pre (right upper extremity) and postductal (lower extremity) SpO2 difference of 3% (shunting across ductus), RUE *and* LE < 95%, or any limb < 90% is concerning
    - Hyperoxia test: failure of SpO2 to improve with 100% FiO2 concerning for cyanotic CHD (mixing or R→L shunt)
      - ABG traditional but difficult to obtain
  — Labs: POC GLC, CBC, CMP, BNP, troponin, ABG
    - BNP most useful in respiratory distress presentation

- Pediatric data sparse with varying cutoffs suggesting CHD
    - BNP > 40 pg/mL (child-adolescent)
    - BNP > 170 pg/mL (1st week of life)
- CXR: pulmonary edema, cardiomegaly, stereotypical cardiac silhouette, alternative diagnoses
- EKG: chamber enlargement, axis deviation, dysrhythmia, characteristic patterns
- Echocardiography: definitive diagnosis; evaluate heart anatomy, flow, estimated pressures
    - Consider POCUS for global function, chamber enlargement, wrong number chambers, large wall defects, lungs for B-lines

MANAGEMENT — GENERAL

- Supportive care measures (O2, PPV, fluids) can alter physiology by changing the balance of pulmonary and systemic blood flow and through other complex cardiopulmonary interactions
    - *Use each with caution and reassess frequently*
- Supplemental O2
    - Potent pulmonary vasodilator (↓ PVR)
    - Initial presentation, unknown lesion, goal SpO2 > 85%
        - Indicative of balanced pulmonary and systemic flows when abnormal connections of the usually in-parallel circulatory systems
    - Known lesion: goal = baseline SpO2
- Advanced respiratory support
    - PPV can ↑ squeeze but ↓ preload and cardiac output
        - Helpful in pulmonary edema
        - Can worsen obstructive lesions
    - RSI medications: be prepared as apnea and hemodynamic changes can cause decompensation, cardiac arrest
        - Rocuronium: paralytic of choice
        - Etomidate: hemodynamically neutral
        - Ketamine: generally avoid
            - ↑ SVR helpful for hemodynamic support but risks decompensation in left obstructive lesions
        - Atropine at bedside for bradycardia not rapidly improved with PPV
- Fluids: small boluses of 5-10 mL/kg NS for dehydration, poor perfusion
    - Frequent reassessment for hepatomegaly, crackles, HR changes

> **PGE1:** life-saving medication in ddCHD
> - Give empirically in infants < 1 mo with shock or cyanosis + failed hyperoxia test
>   — Do not wait for confirmatory echocardiogram
> - IV infusion at 0.05 mcg/kg/min, titrated to effect (max 0.1 mcg/kg/min)
>   — Monitor perfusion, SpO2, BP
> - Needs dedicated IV line; don't interrupt infusion
> - Side effects: flushing, tachycardia, hypotension, fever, jitteriness, seizure, apnea (~10%)
>   — Prophylactic intubation controversial; consider if long transport

- Diuretics: use when signs of CHF
  — Furosemide 0.5-1 mg/kg IV (max 20-40 mg)
- Vasoactives: severe shock
  — Epinephrine 0.1 mcg/kg/min IV
  — Additional vasoactives in consultation with cardiologist or intensivist
- Empiric broad spectrum antibiotics in shock, given DDx of sepsis
- Early consult: pediatric cardiology and PICU

Management by Presentation	Shock	Cyanosis + poor pulm flow	Cyanosis + CHF	CHF
Resuscitation goal	Improve systemic circulation	Improve pulm blood flow (↓PVR)	Reduce shunting, mobilize fluid	↓Pulm over-circulation, mobilize fluid
O2	Cautious	Helpful	Cautious Consider NIPPV	Cautious Consider NIPPV
IV Fluid	Bolus 10 mL/kg	Cautious	Cautious	Minimize
PGE-1	Yes < 1 mo	Yes < 1 mo	< 1 mo consider	No
Others	Antibiotics Vasoactives	Antibiotics Vasoactives iNO	Antibiotics Diuretics	Diuretics

KNOWN CHD OR POST-OPERATION

- **Background**
  — Determine if ED presentation is due to common childhood illness, worsening or change in underlying CHD, or post-op complication
  — Common childhood respiratory and GI infections can precipitate decompensation

- DDx cardiac complication: pericarditis (postpericardiotomy syndrome 2-3 weeks post-op), stenosis, thromboembolic events, CHF, arrhythmias, ischemia, endocarditis
- **High Yield History**
  - Surgical history and timing, residual lesions (review latest echo report), chest pain, syncope, medication adherence, URI, or AGE symptoms

Red Flags on History & Exam
- History of pulmonary hypertension
- Single ventricle physiology
- Syncope
- Decreased exercise/activity tolerance
- Tachycardia
- Arrhythmia
- Change in baseline SpO2
- Poor perfusion or pulses
- Signs of CHF
- Absence of murmur in child with surgical shunt → shunt occlusion

- **Diagnostics**
  - Labs: low threshold for CBC, CMP, BCx if febrile, BNP, Mg
  - EKG (compare to prior)
  - CXR
  - POCUS (general squeeze, effusion), echocardiogram
- **Management**
  - Treat underlying illness (with awareness of physiologic effects of interventions)
    - Special case: single ventricle s/p Glenn or Fontan are volume dependent

Single Ventricle Repair Stage	I: Norwood	II: Glenn	III: Fontan
Description	Neonate, shunt between aorta & right pulm artery (BT shunt) or RV and PA (Sano)	4-6 mo old, BT shunt or Sano removed, connect SVC to RA	2-5 yr old, IVC to RPA, connection between LA and RA closed (no more mixing)
Expected SpO2	75-85%	75-85%	92-98%
Need to balance pulm/syst circulation, O2 may cause problems	Yes	No	No

Single Ventricle Repair Stage	I: Norwood	II: Glenn	III: Fontan
Passive venous return to pulm circulation, try to avoid PPV and hypovolemia = ↓ venous return	No	Yes, SVC return only	Yes, SVC and IVC return
Mechanical ventilation	O2 to keep SpO2 75-80% only	Keep PaCO2 40-45, higher tidal volume, lower rate (maximize e-time)	Higher tidal volume, lower rate (maximize e-time)

— Early cardiology consult
  - Notify pediatric cardiothoracic surgeon if suspect post-op complication

HYPERCYANOTIC EPISODE

- **Background**
  — Classically uncorrected TOF patients (but can occur any right obstructive lesion)
  — Acute cyanosis (shunting) and acidosis triggered by abrupt ↑PVR
    - Common triggers: agitation, dehydration, illness, crying, defecation
  — Most common in young infants
- **High Yield History:** appropriate lesion, sudden onset cyanosis, irritability, crying
- **Exam:** severe cyanosis, decreased or absent murmur, hyperpnea
- **Diagnostics:** clinical diagnosis, pulse oximetry
- **Management**
  — Simple: calming (↓PVR), knee to chest position (↑SVR), O2 (↓PVR)
  — Pharmacologic: opiate treats pain, possibly relaxes pulmonary resistance
    - Morphine 0.1 mg/kg IV (max 4 mg) or fentanyl 1 mcg/kg IV (max 50 mcg) or 2 mcg/kg IN (max 100 mcg)
  — Adjuncts: 10 mL/kg NS bolus, ketamine 1.5 mg/kg IV (max 100 mg) esmolol 0.1 mg/kg IV, phenylephrine 5-20 mcg/kg IV if above failing
    - Consult cardiologist when starting additional meds

4 ▶ Infective Endocarditis (IE)

BACKGROUND
- Epidemiology
  - Rare, prevalence increasing due to improving CHD survival, high mortality
  - 90% are CHD patients, especially complex surgical palliations
  - 10% have structurally normal heart
    - Risk factors (central venous catheter)
    - More often in infants
- Common pathogens: *Viridans streptococci, Staph aureus*, *Enterococcus* spp, HACEK organisms, *Candida* spp.
- Subacute: indolent course, nonspecific symptoms, classic textbook findings uncommon
- Acute: sudden onset, less common, fulminant sepsis

EVALUATION
- **High Yield History**
  - Risk factors: CHD (surgeries, transcatheter device procedures, timing), previous IE, CVC, rheumatic heart disease, poor oral health, dental procedure
  - Fever (prolonged), fatigue, myalgias, arthralgias, arthritis, rashes, weight loss, neurologic (seizures, focal deficit from emboli)
  - Infants: poor feeding, respiratory distress, apnea
- **Exam**
  - Toxic appearance in acute endocarditis
  - Pulse oximetry/hypoxia: change from baseline
  - Cardiac
    - New/changed murmur
    - Tachycardia
    - CHF: respiratory distress, crackles, edema, hepatomegaly
  - Skin: perfusion, classic skin lesions rare in infants and children (petechiae, Roth spots, Janeway lesions, Osler nodules)
  - Complete neurologic exam
- **Diagnostics**
  - Labs: blood cultures from 3 venipuncture sites (within 1st hr if unstable, within first 24 hrs otherwise, prioritize aerobic), CBC, CMP, ESR, CRP, UA, UCx
  - Echocardiogram: vegetations, regurgitant jets
    - May require transesophageal

- Modified Duke Criteria: 2 major, 1 major + 3 minor, or 5 minor
  - Suspect if 1 major, 1 minor

Major	Minor
• 2 positive blood cultures with typical IE organism • 3 or majority of ≥ 4 positive blood cultures for other organisms consistent with IE (common skin contaminants) • Single positive culture for *Coxiella burnetti* or IgG titer > 1:800 • Echocardiogram positive • New valvular regurgitation	• Predisposing condition (CHD, IV drug use) • Fever ≥ 38°C • Vascular phenomena seen in IE (arterial emboli, pulmonary infarcts, mycotic aneurysm, ICH, conjunctival hemorrhages, Janeway lesions) • Immunologic phenomena (glomerulonephritis, Roth spots, Osler nodes, rheumatoid factor positive) • Microbiologic evidence by serology or blood cultures not meeting major criteria

MANAGEMENT

- Acute IE suspected and unstable: start empiric antibiotics
  - Native valves or "late" (> 1 yr after surgery) prosthetic valve
    - Ampicillin/sulbactam 50 mg/kg (max 2 g) IV every 6 hrs AND gentamicin 2.5 mg/kg IV every 8 hrs
    - Vancomycin 15 mg/kg IV (max 1 g) every 6 hrs
  - "Early" (< 1 yr) prosthetic valve
    - Vancomycin + gentamicin (as above) + cefepime 50 mg/kg (max 2 g) IV every 8 hrs
- Subacute IE suspected + stable: consider waiting for cultures and sensitivities
- Consult ID, Cardiology

DISPOSITION

- Admit; PICU in acute cases

BEWARE

- ❗ Consider IE with unexplained, prolonged fever + history of CHD, CVC, prior IE
- ❗ Septic emboli can cause multisystem involvement: stroke, pneumonia, pulmonary embolism, osteomyelitis, glomerulonephritis
- ❗ Heart disease patients may need antibiotic prophylaxis prior to dental procedures

4 ▶ Pericarditis & Myocarditis

I. PERICARDITIS

BACKGROUND

- Inflammation of the pericardial sac
- Common causes: idiopathic, viral (Coxsackie group B, EBV, adenovirus, influenza, mumps), bacterial (*S. aureus, H. influenzae, N. meningitidis, S. pneumoniae, M. tuberculosis* in developing world), post-surgical, autoimmune, neoplastic, uremia, trauma, drugs
- May lead to pericardial effusion; rarely cardiac tamponade

EVALUATION

- **High Yield History**
  - Recent viral prodrome
  - Chest pain, relieved in sitting position, worse with coughing
- **Exam**
  - May be anxious and refuse to lay down
  - Tachycardia, tachypnea, friction rub, pulsus paradoxus
  - Beck's triad: JVD, muffled heart sounds, hypotension
  - Constrictive pericarditis may present with ascites and hepatomegaly
- **Diagnostics**
  - Labs
    - Leukocytosis and elevated ESR/CRP may be present
    - CMP, blood cultures, ABG if concern for sepsis or possible purulent pericarditis
  - CXR normal, unless large pericardial effusion present
  - POCUS and/or echocardiogram
    - Assess for pericardial effusion, signs of tamponade
    - Contractility normal; if not, suspect myocarditis
  - EKG: diffuse ST-segment elevation in precordial leads, PR depression, diffuse T-wave inversions
    - Findings not always present

MANAGEMENT

- Careful fluid resuscitation
- NSAIDs
  - Ibuprofen 10 mg/kg (max 600 mg) PO every 6 hrs

- Steroids not indicated initially unless autoimmune disease
- Empiric antimicrobial coverage for MRSA, if concern for purulent pericarditis (more ill appearing, febrile)
- Cardiology (and/or cardiothoracic surgery) consult for emergent pericardiocentesis if impending cardiac tamponade

II. MYOCARDITIS

BACKGROUND
- Inflammation of the myocardium
- Most common cause: viral (Coxsackie group B, parvovirus B19, HHV-6, adenovirus, HIV)
- Other causes: bacterial, Lyme disease, Chagas disease (*T. cruzi*), drugs
- Rare in children, easily misdiagnosed as viral syndrome, bronchiolitis, pneumonia, gastroenteritis
- Most common etiology of heart failure in previously healthy children
  — Up to 20% may require heart transplantation
- Cause of sudden cardiac death in infants
- Consider myocarditis in the persistently tachycardic child with viral illness-like symptoms despite defervescence

EVALUATION
- **High Yield History**
  — Nonspecific viral prodrome of 1-2 weeks of fever, respiratory symptoms (rhinorrhea, cough, SOB), GI symptoms (abdominal pain, vomiting, poor PO intake), malaise
  — Heart failure symptoms: difficulty feeding, SOB at rest, exercise intolerance, tachypnea, syncope
  — Chest pain less common
- **Exam**
  — Hypoperfusion (lethargy, pallor, mottling, decreased capillary refill)
  — Tachycardia, S3 or S4 gallops, peripheral edema
  — Retractions, rales, tachypnea
  — Hepatomegaly (start in pelvis and palpate upwards)

- **Diagnostics**
  — Labs: CBC, CMP, lactate, ESR/CRP, troponin, BNP
    - Troponin < C.01 ng/mL has a high negative predictive value
  — CXR: cardiomegaly, pulmonary edema, occasional pleural effusions
  — POCUS and/or echocardiogram: impaired LV function, +/– pericardial effusion
  — EKG: sinus tachycardia (most common finding), low voltage, non-specific ST or T wave abnormalities, atrial or ventricular dysrhythmias, SVT or ventricular arrhythmias
  — Definitive diagnosis made as inpatient with endomyocardial biopsy (gold standard, rarely used), or more commonly cardiac MRI

Lab Pattern
↑ Troponin
↑ BNP
↑ Lactate
↑ ESR/CRP
↑ AST/ALT

MANAGEMENT

- Careful fluid resuscitation
- Respiratory support: start non-invasive, but mechanical ventilation may be needed
- Decompensated heart failure
  — Diuretics: furosemide 0.5-1 mg/kg (max 20-40 mg) IV
  — Inotropes: epinephrine 0.1 mcg/kg/min IV or dopamine 5-10 mcg/kg/min IV (max 20 mcg/kg/min)
- Arrhythmia
  — SVT or ventricular arrhythmia with hemodynamic instability
    - Cardioversion 0.5-1 J/kg (max 2 J/kg)
  — Hemodynamically stable
    - See PALS: Dysrhythmias chapter
  — Complete heart block → may need transcutaneous/transvenous pacing
- *Give heart failure and antidysrhythmic agents in consultation with pediatric cardiologist*
- ECMO may be needed for fulminant myocarditis

DISPOSITION

- Pericarditis: dependent on severity
- Fulminant myocarditis: PICU, preferably with ECMO capabilities

BEWARE

- ❗ Maintain a high index of suspicion in the tachycardic, ill-appearing child with non-specific respiratory / GI symptoms
- ❗ Consider myocarditis and heart failure if a child's respiratory status worsens after receiving fluids
- ❗ Acute fulminant myocarditis patients may present in cardiogenic shock, can be difficult to differentiate from septic shock or dehydration
- ❗ Give empiric broad spectrum antibiotics and cardiovascular support until definitive diagnosis

Section V
Dermatology

1 ▶ Bacterial Infections

IMPETIGO

- Background
  - Contagious superficial infection; spreads by autoinoculation
  - Most common 2-5 yrs
  - *S. aureus* (MRSA rare), *Streptococcus pyogenes* in non-bullous

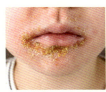
Nonbullous Impetigo

- Exam
  - Non-bullous: erythematous papules/pustules → vesicles rupture releasing yellow/cloudy fluid → dries, crusts → "honey-colored" lesions with erythematous base
    - Face, hands, neck, extremities
  - Bullous: thin-walled fluid-filled (clear-yellowish or cloudy) bullae, typically < 3 cm; rupture in 1-3 days → shallow, shiny, scaling erosions over erythematous base
    - Intertriginous areas, diaper region, face, extremities
  - Ecthyma: ulcerative lesions extend deep into dermis
    - "Punched-out" ulcers with overlying crusts, raised violaceous borders

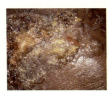
Impetigo

- Management
  - Localized: mupirocin 2% three times daily for 5 days or retapamulin two times daily for 5 days
  - Widespread or ecthyma: cephalexin 25 mg/kg (max 500 mg) PO three times daily or dicloxacillin 6.25 mg/kg (max 250 mg) PO four times daily for 7 days
  - Return to school/daycare 24 hrs after initiating therapy

CELLULITIS/ERYSIPELAS/LYMPHANGITIS

- Background
  - Erysipelas: dermis, *Streptococci*
  - Cellulitis: deeper subcutaneous tissues, *S. aureus*, GABHS
  - Lymphangitis: seen with either, *Streptococci*
- Exam
  - Erysipelas: raised area of shiny erythema with well-demarcated border, tenderness, warmth; lower extremities, face, scalp, hands
    - Peau d'orange appearance
  - Cellulitis: blanching erythema with ill-defined borders, +/− edema, tenderness, warmth
  - Lymphangitis: streaking linear erythema of lymphatic channels, tender, warm
- Management
  - Cephalexin 25 mg/kg (max 500 mg) PO three times daily for 7 days

FOLLICULITIS/FURUNCLES/CARBUNCLES/ABSCESS

- *S. Aureus*: most common, ↑MRSA in abscesses
- Folliculitis: hair follicle inflammation
  - Painless, small, yellow/white pustules, develop in crops, hair shaft protruding from center
- Furuncle: folliculitis → perifollicular tissue involvement, can → cellulitis, abscess
  - Tender, erythematous, fluctuant nodules, hair follicle at center; +/− purulent discharge
- Carbuncle: multiple coalescing furuncles
  - Aggregate of furuncles, multiple tender nodules & drainage points, often neck, back
    - ↑risk diabetes mellitus, immunocompromised
- Abscess: painful fluctuant mass +/− erythema, edema, often central pustule
  - Ultrasound helpful to delineate size
  - +/− wound culture
- Management
  - Folliculitis: warm compresses, topical antibiotics as above, oral antihistamines
  - Large furuncles, all carbuncles, abscesses → incision + drainage
    - Needle aspiration if very small
    - Wound packing or loop drain for larger abscesses
  - Antibiotics: Cephalexin as above if widespread, cellulitis; otherwise I&D alone may suffice
    - Significant purulence = cover MRSA
      - Clindamycin 10 mg/kg (max 600 mg) PO three times daily for 7 days or TMP/SMX 5 mg/kg (max 160 mg) PO two times daily for 7 days

SCARLET FEVER

- GABHS throat, perianal, or wound infection
- History: fever, sore throat, headaches, abdominal pain, minor wounds
- Exam
  - Fine, erythematous, maculopapular "sandpaper" rash starts neck/axillae/groin, spreads to trunk
  - ↑ in flexural creases (Pastia lines)
  - Circumoral pallor
  - "Strawberry" tongue
  - Desquamation palms, soles
- Diagnostics: rapid strep +/− throat, perianal, wound culture
- Management: Bicillin LA (< 27 kg: 600,000U; ≥ 27 kg: 1.2 millionU IM) once OR
  - Penicillin VK (≤ 27 kg: 250 mg; > 27 kg: 500 mg PO two to three times daily) or amoxicillin 25 mg/kg (max 1 g) PO two times daily for 10 days
- Return to school after 24 hrs ABx, fever resolution

STAPHYLOCOCCAL SCALDED SKIN SYNDROME (SSSS)

- Background: caused by *S. Aureus* exfoliative toxin (A or B)
  - Most common: neonates, young children
- Evaluation
  - History
    - Prodrome: fever, malaise, lethargy, irritability, poor feeding
    - Rash rapid progression over 48 hrs

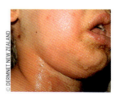

Staphylococcal Scalded Skin Syndrome (SSSS)

  - Exam: painful patches of erythematous skin (resembles sunburn), large superficial bullae, skin often appears wrinkled, can wax and wane
    - Thick crusting, fissuring around mouth, nose, eyes (dried oatmeal appearance)
    - Minor friction → sloughing (Nikolsky sign), leaving denuded, tender skin
    - Most obvious flexural creases, skin folds
    - Can occur anywhere EXCEPT mucous membranes
- Management
  - Penicillinase-resistant penicillins first-line
    - Oxacillin 25-37.5 mg/kg (max 3 g) IV every 6 hrs or nafcillin 50 mg/kg (max 3 g) IV every 6 hrs
    - Alternatives: first or second-generation cephalosporin, vancomycin
    - Consider adding MRSA coverage, clindamycin for toxin

- Dress denuded skin with saline soaked gauze
  - Avoid betadine, sulfadiazine; can be absorbed → toxicity
- Admit ICU or transfer to burn center

BEWARE

- ❗ Ill-appearing, crepitus on exam, skip lesions = consider necrotizing soft tissue infection
- ❗ Impetigo can mimic cigarette burns
- ❗ May be difficult to appreciate in dark-skinned patients

2 ▶ Dermatitis

ATOPIC DERMATITIS

- High Yield History
  - Family history atopy, seasonal/food allergies, asthma
  - Onset often infancy → improvement late childhood
  - Triggers: excessive baths, heat, allergens
  - Pruritus (infants → fussiness)
- Exam
  - Dry skin, erythematous papules/plaques, excoriations, +/− weeping vesicles
  - Infants: face/scalp or diffuse, spares diaper area
  - Children: symmetric in flexural areas + neck
  - Dyshidrotic eczema: vesicular/bullous on palms/soles
- Management
  - Minimize triggers, irritants, activities that dry skin (excess bathing)
  - Emollients/moisturizers
  - Antihistamines PRN pruritus
  - Topical steroids for active inflammation, low potency for face, genitals
  - Antibiotic vs. antiviral for superinfection (impetigo, HSV)

ALLERGIC (ACD) AND IRRITANT (ICD) CONTACT DERMATITIS

- High Yield History
  - ACD: delayed reaction from physical contact with allergen (plant, perfume, topical antibiotic such as bacitracin)

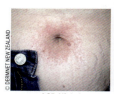

ACD Nickel

- ICD: physical/chemical/mechanical agents causing direct irritation (diaper, soap, thumb-sucking, lip-licking, frequent water exposure)
- Nickel common allergen and irritant
- Exam
    - Odd, asymmetric distribution depending on areas of contact (differentiate from atopic)
    - ACD: erythema, edema, weeping vesicles/bullae, pruritus → generalized dermatitis if prolonged exposure (autoeczematization)
    - ICD: dry, cracked, macular erythema, burning (itchiness < ACD)
- Management
    - ACD: identify / avoid allergen, topical steroids × 2-3 wks, antihistamines PRN pruritus
    - ICD: topical moisturizers, ↓ skin-drying activities
    - May require systemic steroids, topical calcineurin inhibitors

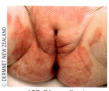

ICD Diaper Rash

DIAPER DERMATITIS

- High Yield History
    - Diaper change frequency (urine/feces exposure irritates), recent change diaper or wipe brand, heat, irritability/crying with urination/defecation
    - \> 72 hrs = possible *Candida*
- Exam
    - Irritant: erythema/scaling, spares folds
    - Candidal: "beefy red" erythema, sharply demarcated, scaling, satellite lesions
        - Intertriginous areas, may be superimposed on irritant dermatitis
        - Check for oral thrush
- DDx
    - Langerhans cell histiocytosis, acrodermatitis enteropathica
    - Consider nutritional, immunodeficiency if severe/unresponsive to treatment
- Management
    - Prevention: frequent diaper changes, gentle cleansing, air drying, avoid talcum powder & cloth diapers
    - Irritant: barrier cream (zinc oxide/petrolatum), +/− low potency topical steroids
    - Candidal: topical nystatin or clotrimazole four times daily
    - Do NOT use combination steroid/anti-candidal products with high potency steroids

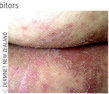

Candidal Diaper Rash

SEBORRHEIC DERMATITIS

- High Yield History
  - 2-6 wks (cradle cap) or adolescence
  - Scalp, face, eyebrows, perineum, intertriginous areas
- Exam: greasy yellow scales, painless, nonpruritic
- Management: frequently self resolves
  - Infants: topical oil w/ combing, non-prescription shampoos
  - Older: antifungal, anti-dandruff, ketoconazole shampoos
    - Topical steroids for non-scalp locations

Cradle Cap

PHYTOPHOTODERMATITIS

- High Yield History: sunlight + either citrus fruits (limes), carrots, celery, or parsley exposure = phototoxic rash
- Exam: papular → vesicular/bullous, linear streaky lesions
  - Inflamed/hyperpigmented in sun-exposed areas
  - May have form of handprint (lime juice on close contact's hand)
- Management: remove offending agent, self-limited (may take weeks)
  - Topical steroids, oral analgesics if severe

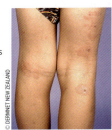

Phytophotodermatitis

BEWARE

- Look for signs of superinfections
- Eczema herpeticum: vesicle clusters → hemorrhagic crusts, punched-out erosions
- Phytophotodermatitis = child abuse mimic (handprint, dripped boiling water appearances)

3 ▶ Drug Rashes

ANTIBIOTIC ALLERGY

- Beta-lactams most common
- Immediate urticaria: minutes to 6 hrs after antibiotic use
- Delayed: > 6 hrs to 8 wks, even if ABx discontinued
  - Nonspecific morbilliform/maculopapular rash
- Management: discontinue antibiotic, supportive
- Amoxicillin can cause morbilliform/maculopapular copper colored rash in patient with EBV

DRUG REACTION WITH EOSINOPHILIA AND SYSTEMIC SYMPTOMS (DRESS)

- Extensive skin rash + organ involvement (liver most common, myocarditis, thyroid), lymphadenopathy, eosinophilia, atypical lymphocytosis, 1-8 wks after medication initiation
  - 10% mortality
- History: recent anticonvulsants (most common), antibiotics (TMP-SMX), allopurinol, etc.
  - Fever (90%), pulmonary symptoms (30%): SOB, cough
- Exam: facial edema (70%); erythematous, maculopapular rash progressing to coalescing erythema, spreads caudally, mild mucosal involvement (up to 50%)
  - Can have purpura, plaques, pustules, target-like lesions
  - May be pruritic; lasts weeks to months
  - Cardiac (up to 20%): hypotension (LV dysfunction), tachycardia
  - Cervical lymphadenopathy
- Diagnostics: CBC, BMP, LFTs, lipase, PT/INR, PTT, ESR/CRP, UA, troponin, TSH, EKG, echo
- Management: discontinue offending agent, antihistamines + topical steroids for mild, systemic corticosteroids × wks if organ involvement + consider IVIG
- Disposition: Admit
- BEWARE: DRESS flare 3-4 wks after onset

ERYTHEMA MULTIFORME (EM) MINOR AND MAJOR

- Majority due to HSV 1, 50% follow herpes labialis
  - Other common: mycoplasma, NSAIDs, anticonvulsants, antibiotics
- History: no prodrome, abrupt onset, not painful or pruritic, lasts 1-4 wks
- Exam: targetoid lesions may → bullous or edematous, < 2% TBSA, symmetric, fixed, classically extensor surfaces
  - EM minor: acral, skin only
  - EM major: EM minor + mucosal involvement, < 10% TBSA
- Management: antihistamines, skin care, resolves 2-3 wks
  - +/– prophylactic acyclovir if recurrent
  - EM major consider systemic corticosteroids
- Disposition: EM major admit (consider ICU, similar to SJS)
- BEWARE: Recurrence common, oral corticosteroids = prolonged course, more frequent episodes

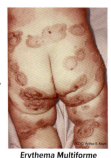

Erythema Multiforme

STEVENS-JOHNSON SYNDROME (SJS) AND TOXIC EPIDERMAL NECROLYSIS (TEN)

- Severe mucocutaneous reactions with epidermal necrosis
  - Mucous membranes (usually ≥ 2 sites: eye, mouth, genitals) affected in > 90%
- SJS > TEN in children
- History: fever, flu-like symptoms (malaise, myalgia, arthralgias) 1-3 days before rash
  - Rash 7-21 days after medication / infection exposure
    - Sulfonamides, penicillins, anticonvulsants, NSAIDS, allopurinol
    - Mycoplasma (most common infectious trigger), HSV
  - Dysuria, photophobia
- Exam
  - SJS: < 10% TBSA, targetoid lesions with dusky erythematous macules and bullae, prominent mucosal involvement
    - Usually begins on face, upper trunk; +Nikolsky sign
  - TEN: > 30% TBSA, less mucosal/more skin involvement than SJS
  - Fever, purulent conjunctivitis, photophobia, lymphadenopathy hepatosplenomegaly, mouth/genital sores
- Diagnostics: CBC, BMP, LFTs, lipase, PT/INR, PTT, UA, blood + skin cultures
  - Anemia, lymphopenia common
  - Neutropenia (⅓ patients) → poor prognosis
- Management: discontinue all medications given in past 2 mos, skin care similar to burn
  - Questionable evidence: IV corticosteroids, IVIG
- Disposition: ICU or burn center
- BEWARE: 5-35% mortality

4 ▶ Fungal Infections

TINEA CORPORIS "RINGWORM"

- Pre-pubertal, warm climates, fitted clothing, pruritic
- Asymmetrical sharply-demarcated plaques, clear center and scaly/vesicular/papular/pustular border, trunk and extremities
- Tinea cruris intertriginous perineum (commonly near scrotum, upper thigh)
  - ↑ obese adolescent males

TINEA PEDIS "ATHLETE'S FOOT"
- Adolescents, most common interdigital, pruritic, exposure to public sites (showers, gyms, locker rooms)

TINEA CAPITIS
- Highest in Black population, M > F
- Scalp scaling with patchy alopecia, single or multiple, black dots (ends of broken hairs), +/− pustules
- Complication: kerion = fungal abscess

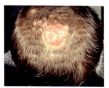
Kerion

TINEA VERSICOLOR
- *Malassezia furfur*, normal skin flora, high sun exposure
- Hyper- or hypo- pigmented elliptical or oval scaling macules and patches with thin scaly plaques/papules over trunk and arms, occasionally neck, face

MANAGEMENT
- Tinea corporis, pedis, cruris: topical allylamine (terbinafine) or imidazole (clotrimazole) two times daily × 2-3 wks, absorbent antifungal powders containing aluminum chloride
  - Keep affected areas dry, avoid tight-fitting clothing
- Tinea capitis: oral antifungal medication to penetrate hair follicle, griseofulvin ultramicrosize for > 2 yrs 10-15 mg/kg (max 750 mg) PO daily for 6-8 weeks or terbinafine for > 4 yrs 10-20 kg: 62.5 mg; 20-40 kg: 125 mg; > 40 kg: 250 mg PO once daily for 4 weeks

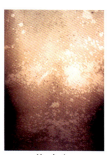
Versicolor

  - Topical antifungals as adjuncts, haircuts unnecessary
- Tinea versicolor: selenium sulfide shampoo, topical allylamine or imidazole creams, oral imidazole or terbinafine if recurrent or topical therapy fails
- Can attend school after treatment initiated

BEWARE
- ! Topical steroids can → worsen / alter infection appearance
- ! Id reactions
  - Widespread hypersensitivity-type papular or vesicular skin reaction (not a drug reaction) after antifungal therapy initiation
  - Responds to topical steroids, oral antihistamines
  - Resolves with treatment of primary infection

5 ▶ Infestations and Ticks

LICE

- School-age; F > M
- Direct head-to-head contact, infested headwear, brushes, jackets
- History: itchy scalp, known exposure
- Exam: nits (nape of neck, behind ears), live louse, posterior auricular nodes
- Management
  - Permethrin 1% (Nix) applied to scalp → wash off after 10 min
    - Reapplication in 1 wk increases cure rate
    - Recommend nit combing afterwards
  - Spinosad 0.9% topical suspension ≥ 4 yrs applied similarly
    - Once only, no nit combing
  - Malathion 1% topical shampoo (prescription) for > 6 yrs
- Prevention
  - Decontaminate environment
  - Avoid sharing brushes or hats; hair pulled back
- No longer "no nit" policy for return to school

SCABIES

- All ages and socioeconomic classes
- Mites burrow into epidermis, transmitted by close contact
- History: intense itching + rash; affected family members
- Exam
  - Classic-burrows: serpiginous, interdigital folds, wrist, elbows, axilla, genitalia
  - Nodular: 2-5 mm nodules, genitalia/axilla
  - Vesicular: infant scalp, head, palms, soles
  - Crusted: "Norwegian," severe, infant/immunocompromised
- Management
  - 5% permethrin (> 2 mo)
    - Apply entire body once, wash off in 8-14 hrs
    - ↑ pruritus after, antihistamines PRN
  - Treat entire household, wash clothing/bedding in hot water

LYME DISEASE

- Often under-reported; New England, Mid-Atlantic, Midwest U.S.
- History: travel, outdoors/hiking
  - Fever, myalgias/arthralgias, lethargy, headache, stiff neck, burning/itching rash
- Exam
  - Examine skin for tick
  - Early localized
    - Erythema migrans (EM) commonly axilla, inguinal, popliteal fossa, belt line, up to 20 cm diameter
      - Warm ↑ over days-weeks, central clearing (bull's eye)
    - Lymphadenopathy
  - Early disseminated (wks-mos after tick bite), may be first manifestation
    - Multiple EM
    - Cardiac, neurologic, ocular involvement
  - Late disseminated: arthritis, neurologic (encephalopathy)
- Diagnosis
  - Early localized: clinical diagnosis
  - Early and late disseminated: ELISA, Western blot confirmation, PCR
- Management
  - Remove tick
  - Consider ID consult
  - Antibiotics: (early disease × 14-21 days; late disease × 28 days)
    - Doxycycline (≥ 8 yrs) 2.2 mg/kg (max 100 mg) PO two times daily or
    - Amoxicillin (< 8 yrs) 17 mg/kg (max 500 mg) PO three times daily or
    - Cefuroxime 15 mg/kg (max 500 mg) PO two times daily
    - IV ceftriaxone: meningitis, carditis, encephalitis
- Disposition: admit meningitis, carditis, encephalitis
- Prevention: DEET spray, long clothes, skin inspection after outdoors

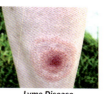

Lyme Disease

ROCKY MOUNTAIN SPOTTED FEVER

- Mild to fulminant, potentially fatal
- Most common rickettsial infection in U.S.
- Symptomatic 2-14 days (most 5-7 days) after tick bite
- History
  - Known tick bite or exposure where ticks common in last 14 days
  - Headache, fever, malaise, nausea/vomiting, myalgias, arthralgias
  - Rash (80-90%)
  - +/– severe abdominal pain
- Exam
  - Blanching erythematous maculopapular rash, becomes petechial
    - Starts wrists/ankles, spreads to trunk
    - Palms/soles later
  - Pedal edema (children)
  - Conjunctival erythema
  - Confusion, meningismus
  - Late disease: AMS, seizures, CN palsies
- Diagnosis: presumptive
  - May have hyponatremia, thrombocytopenia, ↑AST/ALT and bilirubin, azotemia, ↑ PT/PTT, CSF: pleocytosis and ↑ protein
  - Serology or PCR
- Management
  - Doxycycline 2.2 mg/kg (max 100 mg) PO two times daily (even age < 8 yrs) until 3 days afebrile
  - Treat empirically within 5 days of symptom onset
- Prevention: skin inspection, tick removal
- Admit for antibiotics, close monitoring

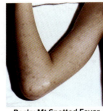

Rocky Mt Spotted Fever

6 ▶ Viral Exanthem

NONSPECIFIC VIRAL EXANTHEM

- Nonspecific, most benign, self-limited
- History: fever, URI/GI symptoms
- Exam: blanchable erythematous macules/papules, diffuse, nonpruritic, no desquamation

HAND-FOOT-MOUTH, HERPANGINA

- Enteroviruses
- HFMS: vesicles on tongue, hard/soft palate, buccal surface, hands, feet occasionally knees, buttock, trunk
- Herpangina: vesicles on soft palate, anterior tonsillar fossae
- DDx from petechial rashes associated with life threatening infections
- Management: NSAIDs, ensure tolerating PO
- Beware: onychomadesis (nail shedding) may occur 1-2 mos after illness

MEASLES (RUBEOLA)

- Background
  - Small outbreaks U.S., often unvaccinated, immigrants
  - Contact and airborne (in air up to 2hrs after cough/sneeze)
- History: vaccinations, travel/exposure, prodrome high fever, malaise, anorexia → 3C's: cough, coryza, conjunctivitis → rash
- Exam
  - ~48 hrs before rash Koplik spots (blue to erythematous papules with white centers on buccal mucosa) pathognomonic
  - 2-4 days after fever: maculopapular rash on face/head, spreads downwards, often coalesces, resolves same order as appearance → copper-colored macules with desquamation
- Diagnostics: clinical suspicion, must have laboratory confirmation
  - 3 samples best: serum IgM, throat/nasopharyngeal PCR, Urine PCR
- Management
  - Antipyretics, fluids, treat superinfections (pneumonia, otitis)
  - Ribavirin: severely ill, immunocompromised
  - Vitamin A if from area of vitamin A deficiency or where fatality rate > 1%
  - Reportable disease
- Disposition: isolation, infective 4 days prior to symptoms to 4 days after rash onset
- BEWARE: subacute sclerosing panencephalitis 7-10 yrs after measles diagnosis

RUBELLA (GERMAN MEASLES)

- Outbreaks in unvaccinated, rare in U.S., 50% asymptomatic
  - Contact or droplet transmission
- History: vaccinations, prodrome: low grade fever, malaise, URI symptoms, lymphadenopathy, arthralgias; pruritic rash 2-5 days after prodrome

- Exam: erythematous macules/papules, may coalesce, commonly face/trunk spreading caudally, resolves 1-3 days
  - Forchheimer spots: erythematous/petechial macules on soft palate
  - Pea-sized postauricular lymphadenopathy
- Diagnostics: difficult clinically, non-specific
  - Throat, nasal, urine specimens for PCR
- Management supportive, reportable disease
- Disposition: contact isolation × 7 days after rash onset, avoid pregnant contacts (congenital rubella syndrome)

FIFTH DISEASE (ERYTHEMA INFECTIOSUM)

- Parvovirus B19, often school-age
- History: fever, headaches, malaise, arthralgias, respiratory symptoms
  - Rash after 2-3 days
- Exam: intense red rash over bilateral cheeks (slapped cheeks)
  - 1-4 days after facial rash → lacy reticular pruritic rash (trunk, extremities), fades over 2-3 wks
  - Sunlight, warm temperatures → rash waxing and waning
- Management: supportive, avoid contact with pregnant (fetal hydrops) and sickle cell / immunocompromised (aplastic crisis), no longer contagious when rash begins

ROSEOLA INFANTUM

- HHV type 6 or 7, often < 3 yrs
- History: fever up to 41°C/105.8°F × 3-5 days, periorbital edema, cervical lymphadenopathy; as defervesce, rash appears, resolves in 1-3 days
- Exam: erythematous blanching macules/papules with peripheral halo
  - Neck/torso before spreading to face, head, extremities
  - Nagayama spots (erythematous papules on soft palate and uvula) in ⅔
  - Often nontoxic, well-appearing
- Management: supportive
- BEWARE: febrile seizures, encephalitis, bulging fontanelle

VARICELLA (CHICKEN POX)

- Contact and airborne
- History: prodrome fever, malaise, myalgia, headache, arthralgia → skin lesions in 24-48 hrs

- Exam: erythematous macules / papules → vesicles → eventually crust
  - "Dewdrop on a rose petal", head / trunk spreads → extremities
  - Appears in crops over 3-4 days, lesions in different stages
- Diagnostics: clinical, –/– cultures
- Management: supportive
  - Consider acyclovir/valacyclovir in immunocompromised
    - Most effective in the first 24 hrs of rash
- Disposition: infectious until all lesions crusted
- BEWARE: secondary infection from *S. aureus* or GABHS, meningoencephalitis, transverse myelitis, Guillain-Barre, shingles/varicella-zoster ophthalmicus later

ECZEMA HERPETICUM

- HSV-1 or 2, ↑ in patients with atopic dermatitis, other dermatitides
- History: fever, malaise → skin barrier breakdown
- Exam: widespread vesicles → can coalesce and crust
  - Areas of active dermatitis, especially head, neck, trunk
- Diagnostics: clinical, +/– HSV wound culture or antigen testing
- Management
  - Mild: acyclovir 20 mg/kg (max 800 mg) PO four times daily for 7 days or valacyclovir
  - Severe or systemic symptoms: acyclovir 10 mg/kg IV every 8 hrs
- Disposition: May require inpatient supportive care if extensive
- BEWARE: keratoconjunctivitis, secondary superinfection (cellulitis, insensible fluid loss)

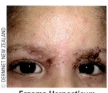

Eczema Herpeticum

MOLLUSCUM CONTAGIOSUM

- Skin-to-skin contact, fomites/sports, especially < 8 yrs, autoinoculation, STI in adults but non-sexually transmitted in children
- Exam: clustered/linear, flesh-colored/pink, often translucent papule, small central umbilication; often axillary, popliteal fossae, groin
- Management: supportive, self-resolves but can take years
  - Consider dermatologist referral if distressing

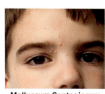

Molluscum Contagiosum

GIANOTTI-CROSTI SYNDROME (PAPULAR ACRODERMATITIS)

- Common 1-6yrs, several etiologies (most common EBV, hepatitis B, vaccinations)
- History: often asymptomatic, or URI symptoms, fever, malaise → rash
- Exam: erythematous, edematous, monomorphous papules/papulovesicles
  — Can coalesce into larger plaques over pressure points
  — Symmetrical; face, buttocks, extensor surfaces; trunk usually spared
- Management: supportive, up to 8-12 wks for resolution
  — If suspect hepatitis/hepatomegaly, check LFTs
- BEWARE: anicteric hepatitis (hepatitis B)

7 ▶ Vascular Lesions

CONGENITAL AND INFANTILE HEMANGIOMAS (CH, IH)

- IH most common benign vascular tumor
  — ~5% of live births, not present at birth
  — White > Non-Hispanic
  — ↑ risk F > M, prematurity, multiple gestations
  — Often involute spontaneously
- CH
  — Rare, fully grown at birth
  — Size ranges from 2-10 cm
  — Some subtypes involute by age 1 yr, others regress but never involute
- **Complications:** infection, bleeding, ulceration, airway compromise, high-output heart failure (HF), consumptive coagulopathy/thrombocytopenia
- **History:** presence at birth; rapidly growing, involuting, bleeding, ulcerations, fevers, ↑ crying (pain), SOB/poor feeding (HF), rash
- **Exam**
  — Hemangioma(s) size/location
  — Tenderness, redness, pus/drainage, induration
  — ↑ work of breathing, retractions, gallop, palpable liver edge (HF)
  — Stridor, hoarse cry (airway impingement)
  — Active bleeding, petechiae
- **Diagnosis:** clinical
  — Lab tests not routinely performed; guided by complication
    - CBC, PT/INR, PTT (bleeding, coagulopathy)
    - BNP, echocardiogram (HF)
    - Wound, blood cultures

- **Management**
  - Ulcerated: topical/oral antibiotics (↑ risk infection), occlusive dressings, analgesia
  - Infected: oral or IV ABx covering skin organisms
  - Bleeding
    - Minor: direct pressure +/– TXA
    - Persistent/major from ulceration (rare): arterial embolization or surgical excision
  - Specialist consultations: Dermatology, Surgery, Ophthalmology, ENT, GI, Cardiology PRN by presenting problem
    - May treat with beta-blockers, intralesional steroids, laser therapy
  - Prevention for rapidly involuting: petrolatum multiple times per day helps prevent ulceration
- **Disposition**
  - Admit: severe bleeding, coagulopathy, HF, infection failing outpatient management or with systemic symptoms, airway concerns, poor feeding
  - Discharge with PCP follow-up
    - Refer to specialist PRN
- Complications as above
- Concerns for liver, airway, or GI tract lesions
- Risk of functional or permanent impairment
  - Eyelid, lip, nose, ears, anal, oral lesions
  - Multiple facial lesions: concern for neural crest derivatives
  - Beard distribution: concern for PHACE syndrome
  - Lumbosacral hemangioma may → myelopathy, spinal bony, genitourinary, or anorectal anomalies
- Very large (> 5 cm)/rapidly growing

PYOGENIC GRANULOMA

- **Epidemiology**
  - Common benign vascular tumor of skin, mucous membranes
  - Rapidly proliferate following minor trauma or infection
    - ~1/3 known preceding lesion
  - ↑ in < 5yrs; F > M
  - Bleed easily with minor trauma
  - No spontaneous involution; recurrence common
- **History:** trauma, preceding lesion, rapid growth, bleeding

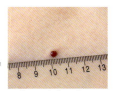

Pyogenic Granuloma

- **Exam**
  - Red, +/− pedunculated nodule, size peaks 1-3 wks after formation at ~0.5-2 cm
  - +/− erosion, crusting, bleeding
  - Commonly: head, gingiva, upper/lower limbs
- **Diagnosis:** clinical
- **Management**
  - Bleeding: direct pressure, consider silver nitrate
- **Disposition:** discharge with PCP follow-up/dermatology referral for excision

8 ▶ Urticaria & Anaphylaxis

BACKGROUND
- Up to 25% lifetime prevalence
- Activation of dermal mast cells triggered by IgE-mediated process
- Chronic > 6 wks vs. acute
- Etiologies
  - Infections (adenoviruses, enteroviruses, HSV-1, influenza, CMV, GABHS, mycoplasma pneumoniae)
    - Infants, young children
  - Food or medications, physical stimuli, insects, autoimmune, idiopathic
    - Older children, adolescents

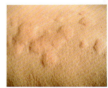
Urticaria

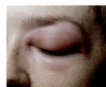
Angioedema

EVALUATION
- History
  - Pruritic, transient, migratory rash
  - Consider possible etiologies; trigger avoidance is key
- Exam: characterized by wheals
  - Raised, well-circumscribed, variable shape/size
    - Found on any skin surface, favors trunk, extremities
    - Often with angioedema
  - Consider anaphylaxis: 2+ of: skin (urticaria, angioedema), respiratory (wheeze, stridor), hypotension, GI (vomiting, diarrhea)
- Diagnostics: clinical diagnosis
  - Consider CBC, ESR/CRP, thyroid/liver function tests in chronic urticaria

- DDx: anaphylaxis, angioedema, erythema multiforme, contact/atopic dermatitis, drug eruptions, HSP, insect bites

MANAGEMENT
- ABCs
- Anaphylaxis
  - Epinephrine 0.15 mg < 30 kg; 0.3mg ≥ 30 kg (or 0.01 mg/kg, max 0.5 mg) IM of 1 mg/mL concentration, repeat PRN
  - PRN H1 and H2 antihistamines, systemic corticosteroids, nebulized albuterol
- Acute urticaria
  - Self-limited; treat with antihistamines, trigger avoidance
  - 2nd generation H1-antihistamines first line (↓sedation, anticholinergic)
    - Cetirizine 2.5mg (≥ 6 mo-2 yrs), 2.5-5 mg (2-5 yrs), 5-10 mg (> 5 yrs) PO once daily
    - Loratadine 5 mg (2-6 yrs), 10 mg (> 6 yrs) PO once daily
    - Fexofenadine 30 mg PO (6-11 yrs) or 60 mg PO (≥ 12 yrs) two times daily
  - 1st generation H1-antihistamines (alternative)
    - Diphenhydramine 1 mg/kg (max 50 mg) PO/IV/IM every 6 hrs
  - Can consider H2-antihistamines (ranitidine/famotidine)
- Chronic urticaria
  - 2nd generation H1-antihistamines
    - May require up to 4x recommended dose
- Consider oral corticosteroids (< 10 days) for acute urticaria, acute episodes of chronic urticaria

DISPOSITION
- Discharge home if anaphylaxis excluded
  - Up to 10 days of H1-antihistamines +/− oral corticosteroids
- Consider admission for anaphylaxis/angioedema or severe symptoms

BEWARE
- Anaphylaxis can have a biphasic course, observe several hours
- Discharge with epinephrine autoinjector

Section VI
Ear, Nose, Throat

1 ▶ Ear and Nose

I. OTITIS EXTERNA

BACKGROUND
- Inflammation of external ear canal, usually bacterial (pseudomonas, staphylococcus)

EVALUATION
- **High Yield History**: water exposure (swimming, hot tubs), traumatic ear cleaning
  — Rapid onset (~48 hrs), otalgia, pruritus, fullness, drainage, +/– impaired hearing
- **Exam**: pain with tragal manipulation, canal edema, otorrhea, debris
  — Rule out concurrent AOM, TM rupture, extensive lymphadenopathy, cellulitis
- **Diagnostics**: +/– POC GLC

MANAGEMENT
- Analgesia
- Clean ear canal with 1:1 dilution of 3% hydrogen peroxide with water if intact TM

Antibiotic	Dosage (duration 7 days)
Ofloxacin 0.3% otic solution	5 drops once daily (10 drops if ≥ 13 yr)
Cipro-dex otic suspension	4 drops two times daily
Cipro-HC otic suspension*	3 drops two times daily
Cortisporin (neomycin/polymyxin B/hydrocortisone)*	3 drops four times daily

*Only use if TM intact

- Place ear wick/ribbon gauze if canal is too edematous for drop placement
- If concurrent otitis media, add oral antibiotics as below

DISPOSITION
- Discharge, follow-up 48-72 hrs

BEWARE
- ❗ Cortisporin is cheaper, but must have intact TM
  — Neomycin is an aminoglycoside and can lead to hearing loss
- ❗ Consider malignant OM especially if DM or immunocompromised. Consider mastoiditis, brain abscess, venous sinus thrombosis if purulent otorrhea with AOM. Consider TBI with skull fracture if persistent clear otorrhea

II. OTITIS MEDIA

BACKGROUND
- Can be viral (5%), bacterial (*S. pneumoniae*, non-typeable *H. influenzae* (NTHi), and *M. catarrhalis*), or noninfectious
- AOM: bacterial infection in middle ear causing inflammation

EVALUATION
- **High Yield History**: recent URI, fever, ear pain/tugging, crying, sleeping changes, prior AOM, last antibiotic use, tobacco exposure
  — Severe symptoms: fever ≥ 39°C, otalgia moderate-severe or > 48 hrs
- **Exam**
  — Remove obstructing cerumen for TM exam with curette or hydrogen peroxide + irrigation
  — TM: bulging, erythematous, opaque (↓ light reflex); otorrhea if TM perforated
  — Pneumatic otoscopy
  — Cerumenolytic + close PCP follow up if unable to evaluate due to cerumen
- **Diagnostics:** Consider CT scan if signs concerning for mastoiditis or other deep infection

MANAGEMENT
- Analgesia
- Antibiotics
  — Amoxicillin (high-dose) 45 mg/kg (max 1500 mg) PO two times daily for 5-7 days
  — Amoxicillin-clavulanate (600 mg/5 mL concentration only) 45 mg/kg (max 2 g) PO two times daily for 5-7 days if had amoxicillin within 30 days, recurrent AOM unresponsive to amoxicillin, or concurrent purulent conjunctivitis (NTHi)
  — Penicillin Allergy
    - Cefdinir 7 mg/kg (max 300 mg) two times daily or 14 mg/kg (max 600 mg) daily for 10 days

- Cefpodoxime 5 mg/kg (max 200 mg) PO two times daily for 10 days
- Cefuroxime 15 mg/kg (max 500 mg) PO two times daily for 10 days
- Ceftriaxone 50 mg/kg (max 1 g) IM/IV daily for 1-3 days
• If < 48 hrs or < 39°C with mild symptoms, consider "wait-and-see prescription" (WASP) to be filled in 2-3 days if not improving
  — Treat all < 6 mos old

DISPOSITION

- Discharge with follow-up in 48-72 hrs

BEWARE

① Complications include mastoiditis, meningitis, hearing loss, brain abscess

III. ACUTE MASTOIDITIS

BACKGROUND

- Purulent infection of the mastoid air cells
- Most common complication of AOM
- Incidence highest in < 2 yr
- Causes: *S. pneumoniae*, *S. pyogenes*, *S. aureus*, NTHi

EVALUATION

- **High Yield History**: recent URI, recent/current AOM
- **Exam**: febrile, irritable, malaise, mastoid tenderness/swelling/erythema, auricular protrusion, abnormal TM, AOM, swelling of external auditory canal
  — Signs of deeper infection: meningismus, CN VI palsy, retro orbital pain, facial nerve paralysis, bezold abscess (under sternocleidomastoid muscle)
- **Diagnostics**
  — Labs: CBC, ESR, CRP
  — Imaging: CT with contrast or MRI to assess for complications

MANAGEMENT

- Antibiotics
  — Vancomycin 15 mg/kg (max 1 g) IV every 6 hrs
  — If recurrent AOM or ABx within 6 months, add *P. aeruginosa* coverage
    - Ceftazidime 50 mg/kg (max 2 g) IV every 8 hrs
    - Cefepime 50 mg/kg (max 2 g) IV every 8 hrs
    - Piperacillin-tazobactam 75 mg/kg (max 4 g) IV every 6 hrs
- ENT consult

DISPOSITION
- Admit

BEWARE
⚠ Complications: periosteal abscess, cranial nerve palsy, brain abscess, lateral sinus thrombosis, meningitis, epidural abscess

IV. EPISTAXIS

BACKGROUND
- Bleeding from the nose, can be anterior or posterior (5-10%)
- Common causes: digital trauma (nose picking), foreign bodies, trauma
- Consider bleeding disorders: Von Willebrand disease, hemophilia, leukemia

EVALUATION
- **High Yield History**: prior epistaxis/gum bleeding, URI, rhinitis, trauma, easy bruising, hemarthrosis, family history of bleeding disorders
  — Persistent/recurrent, unilateral bleed with nasal obstruction may indicate juvenile nasopharyngeal angiofibroma in adolescents
- **Exam**
  — Nasal exam: visible bleeding site, foreign body, mass
  — Oropharynx
    - Lingual and palatal telangiectasias → hereditary hemorrhagic telangiectasias
    - Blood in posterior oropharynx despite anterior compression/packing suggests posterior bleed
- **Diagnostics**: if severe or recurrent, consider
  — Labs: CBC with smear, PT/INR, PTT, TxS
  — Imaging: lateral face XR if concerned for occult foreign body (button battery), CT w/ contrast or MRI if mass seen

MANAGEMENT
- Direct compression
  — Have patient gently blow out clots first
  — Compress nasal alae together with fingers or nasal clip for 15 min
- Topical vasoconstrictors
  — Oxymetazoline 0.05% instill 2 sprays intranasally (max 2 doses/24 hr)
    - Cautious use in children < 6 yrs

- Phenylephrine 0.125% instill 1-2 sprays or 2-3 drops IN every 4 hrs PRN
  - For children ≥ 2 yrs
  - Can dilute phenylephrine 0.25% concentration with an equal volume of sterile saline to make 0.125%
- Can use it on a cotton pledget
- Chemical cautery (silver nitrate) or electrocautery. Area must be dry. Do not do bilateral cautery — risk of nasal septum perforation
- Packing
  - Anterior packing with resorbable or nonresorbable packing material such as polyvinyl acetate sponge or inflatable balloon packing
  - Posterior packing with inflatable tamponade device or Foley catheter
    - Alar necrosis if external nose not protected (with gauze) from clips holding packing in place
  - Packing left in place risks toxic shock syndrome
  - Weigh risks and benefits of prophylactic antibiotics

DISPOSITION

- Most bleeds controlled with compression alone can have routine follow-up
- Anterior packing to be removed in 1-3 days
- Admit with ENT consultation if uncontrolled or posterior bleed
- Consider bleeding disorder workup vs. referral if persistent/recurrent bleeding

BEWARE

⚠ Epistaxis is uncommon < 2 yrs; consider coagulopathy or non-accidental trauma

V. SINUSITIS

BACKGROUND

- May be viral or bacterial, classified by severity and duration of symptoms

EVALUATION

- **High Yield History**: symptoms ≥ 10 days, severe symptoms or high fever (≥ 39°C) AND purulent nasal discharge, facial pain ≥ 3 days, worsening symptoms after initial improvement → all suggest acute bacterial sinusitis
- **Exam**: fever, sinus tenderness, purulent nasal discharge (bacterial)

MANAGEMENT

- Viral: supportive, intranasal saline, nasal bulb suction
- Bacterial
  - Amoxicillin-clavulanate (600 mg/5 mL concentration only) 45 mg/kg (max 875 mg) PO two times daily for 10 days
  - Penicillin allergy or treatment failure
    - Cefdinir 7 mg/kg (max 300 mg) or 14 mg/kg (max 600 mg) PO daily for 10 days
    - Cefpodoxime 5 mg/kg (max 200 mg) PO two times daily for 10 days
    - Levofloxacin 10 mg/kg (max 500 mg/day) 1-2 times daily for 10 days
  - Inpatient
    - Ampicillin-sulbactam 50 mg/kg (max 2 g) IV every 6 hrs
    - Ceftriaxone 25 mg/kg (max 1 g) IV every 12 hrs

DISPOSITION

- Discharge with follow-up in 48-72 hrs
- Admit septic patients or treatment failure
- Consider CT w/contrast for suppurative complications

BEWARE

- For recurrent sinusitis, consider ENT referral
- Complications: facial cellulitis, orbital cellulitis, cavernous sinus thrombosis, meningitis, brain abscess

2 ▶ Laryngotracheal Pathology

I. CROUP

BACKGROUND

- Viral respiratory infection most often caused by *Parainfluenza*
- DDx: foreign body, angioedema/anaphylaxis, bacterial tracheitis, epiglottitis, RPA

EVALUATION

- **High Yield History**: fever, URI symptoms, previous episodes
- **Exam**: barking cough, stridor (at rest vs. when agitated), hoarseness, retractions
  - Impending respiratory failure: AMS, pallor/cyanosis, decreasing retractions, biphasic stridor at rest

- **Diagnostics**
  - Clinical diagnosis, may obtain XR if diagnosis unclear
  - XR neck: "steeple sign", hypopharyngeal distension

MANAGEMENT

- Supportive: avoid causing distress, maintain position of comfort, antipyretics
- Dexamethasone 0.3-0.6 mg/kg (max 10 mg) PO/IV/IM
- Racemic epinephrine 2.25% (0.5 mL in 2.5 mL saline) nebulized over 15 min q1-2hrs PRN
  - For stridor at rest

DISPOSITION

- Admit: requiring > 1 dose of racemic epinephrine, respiratory distress, hypoxia, suspicion for bacterial tracheitis
- Discharge mild croup, post racemic epinephrine × 1 after 3-4hrs observation if no recurrent stridor at rest, normal air entry, normal color, normal mental status

BEWARE

- Agitation may worsen respiratory distress
- Consider bacterial infections (tracheitis, epiglottitis, RPA) if toxic appearing
- Recurrent episodes → ENT consult

II. BACTERIAL TRACHEITIS

BACKGROUND

- Bacterial infection (*S. aureus*, Hib) of larynx/trachea/bronchi, upper airway emergency
- Mortality as high as 20%

EVALUATION

- **High Yield History**: similar to croup, but acutely worsening
- **Exam**: toxic appearing, inspiratory/expiratory stridor, purulent secretions, wheezing if bronchial extension
- **Diagnostics**
  - Clinical diagnosis
  - XR neck: subglottic narrowing ("steeple sign") on AP, "ragged" trachea on lateral

MANAGEMENT

- Vancomycin 15 mg/kg (max 1 g) IV every 6 hrs plus
  — Ceftriaxone 100 mg/kg (max 4 g) first dose, then 50 mg/kg (max 2 g) IV every 12 hrs or ampicillin-sulbactam 50 mg/kg (max 2 g) IV every 6 hrs
- Intubation: prepare for difficult airway, ideally by anesthesia in OR
- ENT consult: bronchoscopy for definitive diagnosis/cultures

DISPOSITION

- PICU once airway protected

BEWARE

- High risk for airway obstruction emergency

III. EPIGLOTTITIS

BACKGROUND

- Bacterial (*S. aureus*, *S. pneumoniae*, GABHS, Hib) infection of the epiglottis and surrounding structures
- Potential airway emergency
- Less common in young children since Hib vaccine

EVALUATION

- **High Yield History**: abrupt onset, high fever, drooling, irritability, voice changes, immunization status, severe sore throat
- **Exam**
  — Child: toxic appearance, tripod positioning, drooling, muffled voice, stridor
    - Do not force exam of posterior pharynx
  — Adolescent: pain out of proportion to throat appearance
- **Diagnostics**
  — Clinical diagnosis: avoid agitation, maintain position of comfort
    - IV to be placed in OR if possible
  — XR lateral neck may show "thumbprint sign" of enlarged epiglottis
    - Should only be performed if it does not cause distress

MANAGEMENT

- Airway management
  — Unstable, young child → intubation
    - Ideally ENT/anesthesia in OR

- Stable, adolescent → ENT evaluation to decide on need for prophylactic intubation
- Antibiotics
  - Ceftriaxone 100 mg/kg (max 4 g) first dose, then 50 mg/kg (max 2 g) IV every 12 hrs
  - If risk factors for MRSA, add vancomycin 15 mg/kg (max 1 g) IV every 6 hrs

DISPOSITION

- Admit PICU vs. OR for airway management

IV. CONGENITAL ANOMALIES

	Laryngomalacia	**Tracheomalacia**
Overview	<ul><li>Congenital supraglottic collapse during inspiration</li><li>Most common cause of neonatal stridor</li><li>Usually resolves by 18 months</li></ul>	<ul><li>Abnormalities of tracheal rings, floppy trachea that collapses during expiration</li><li>Congenital (CHD, masses, genetic syndromes) or acquired (inflammation, infection)</li></ul>
History	Triggered by URI, difficulty feeding, cyanosis, weight loss, irritability	Hx of tracheoesophageal fistula, extrinsic compressive lesions (heart, mediastinal vessels, masses), anomalous arteries. Recurrent respiratory infections, difficulty feeding, cyanosis
Exam	Oxygenation, retractions, inspiratory stridor (worse when supine), weight loss	Wheezing. Intrathoracic defect → airway collapse and biphasic or expiratory stridor (severe if at rest), barky cough, cyanosis, apneic episodes. Extrathoracic lesion → inspiratory stridor
Management	<ul><li>Supportive care, caretaker reassurance and education</li><li>Outpatient ENT</li><li>Admit if failure to thrive, respiratory distress</li><li>Undiagnosed may present as sleep disorder, swallowing problem, gastroesophageal reflux</li></ul>	<ul><li>CXR, lateral neck XR to r/o other causes</li><li>Bronchoscopy for diagnosis</li><li>Admit if failure to thrive, respiratory distress (trial CPAP, +/− bronchodilators/antibiotics)</li><li>Undiagnosed tracheomalacia may present later in life as sleep apnea, exercise intolerance, or frequent infections</li></ul>

V. TRACHEOSTOMY COMPLICATIONS

BACKGROUND
- More tracheostomies (trachs) with improving outcomes for pediatric chronic diseases
- 15-19% will have complications

EVALUATION
- **High Yield History**: timing of / reason for placement
- **Exam**: vital signs, respiratory distress, suction output, bleeding, trach size
- **Diagnostics**: bronchoscopy for bleed

MANAGEMENT
- Dislodgement
  - Can replace with same size trach or ETT if > 7 days from placement
  - If < 7 days, risk of creating false tract due to immature fistula
    - Consult ENT/surgery
- Obstruction
  - Suction
  - Deflate cuff and provide supplemental O2 from above
  - Replace trach or remove trach and intubate from above unless patient had laryngectomy
- Bleed
  - Mild site bleeding: treat with pressure
  - Significant bleed: consider tracheoinnominate artery fistula
    - Life threatening, mortality close to 100%
    - Remove trach, insert finger into ostomy and apply anterior pressure, intubate from above, STAT cardiothoracic-surgery consult, CT angiogram

DISPOSITION
- Admit significant bleeding, secretions → risk of trach obstruction

BEWARE
- Can attempt BMV over stoma with neonatal mask or from above with stoma occluded if tube is dislodged/removed

3 ▶ Throat and Neck

I. ORAL CANDIDIASIS/THRUSH

BACKGROUND
- Oral yeast infection, usually Candida, common in infants

EVALUATION
- **High Yield History**: premature, immune status, asthma/inhaled steroids, antibiotic use
- **Exam**: white coating on tongue and other oral surfaces, tough to scrape off (differentiates from milk)
- **Diagnostics**: HIV and screening labs if pattern of opportunistic infections

MANAGEMENT
- Antifungal
  - Nystatin oral suspension (100,000 U/mL) four times daily for 7-14 days
    - < 30 days old: 0.5 mL each side of mouth
    - > 30 days old: 1 mL each side of mouth
    - Children: 5 mL swish and swallow
  - Fluconazole PO
    - 6 mg/kg (max 200 mg), then 3 mg/kg (max 100 mg) daily for 13 more days
      - Moderate to severe disease in children > 12 mo
      - Refractory thrush or immunocompromised
- Instructions to sterilize bottle nipples, pacifiers, treat nipples of breastfeeding moms if symptomatic

DISPOSITION
- Discharge

BEWARE
- Check for diaper dermatitis in infants

II. PHARYNGITIS

BACKGROUND
- 7.3 million outpatient cases/year
- Most cases are viral; most common bacterial cause is GABHS

EVALUATION
- High Yield History: URI prodrome suggests viral
  — Sexual history, immunocompromised, recent antibiotics
- Exam: assess for red flags; vitals, complete airway assessment, voice changes, stridor, ability to maintain secretions

Diagnosis	Features	Diagnosis/Treatment
Herpetic gingivostomatitis (HSV-1)	Fever, young children, vesicles/ulcers with erythematous base on palate, gingiva, lips Bleeding/inflamed gums, malaise, dehydrated	Pain control, admit if dehydrated or unable to PO Consider acyclovir 20 mg/kg (max 250 mg) PO four times daily for 7 days within 48 hrs of onset if severe or immunocompromised
Herpangina (coxsackie)	Fever, irritability, malaise Papules → vesicles → ulcers in erythematous throat mainly on soft palate, tonsils, uvula Check for rash on hands/feet, dehydration	Pain control, admit if dehydrated or unable to PO
Infectious Mononucleosis (EBV)	Fever, malaise, headache, sore throat, lymphadenopathy, tonsillar exudate, splenomegaly. Complication: splenic rupture	Labs may show lymphocytosis, smear w/ atypical lymphocytes. Heterophile antibody test (high false negative rate) or EBV-specific antibodies. Supportive care. No sports for 4 weeks. ID consult if immunocompromised
Gonorrhea	High risk sexual behavior. Acquired through oral sex, asymptomatic generally. Can have fever, sore throat, lymphadenopathy	NAAT pharyngeal swab or culture for *N. gonorrhoeae* (Thayer-Martin medium). Screen for other STIs

Diagnosis	Features	Diagnosis/Treatment
HIV	High risk sexual behavior. Sore throat with oral mucocutaneous ulcerative lesions on erythematous base	Rapid HIV if high suspicion, screen for other STIs
Streptococcal pharyngitis (GABHS)	Fever, malaise, sore throat, palatal petechiae, tonsillar exudate, lymphadenopathy. Complications: otitis media, abscess, rheumatic fever, glomerulonephritis, scarlet fever, arthritis, toxic shock syndrome, PANDAS	Test for GAS unless the patient has other symptoms suggesting viral illness. Testing < 3 yrs old not recommended. Rapid antigen test followed by throat culture if negative. Benzathine penicillin G 600,000 units IM once for < 27 kg, 1.2 million units IM once for ≥ 27 kg OR amoxicillin 50 mg/kg (max 1 g) PO daily for 10 days

III. DEEP NECK INFECTIONS

- Peritonsillar Abscess
    - Suppurative infection of tissue between palatine tonsil capsule and pharyngeal muscles
    - Suspect with prolonged course of pharyngitis
- Retropharyngeal Abscess
    - Suppurative infection in potential space extending from base of skull to posterior mediastinum between posterior pharyngeal wall and prevertebral fascia
    - URI infection → suppuration of retropharyngeal lymph nodes → abscess; pharyngeal trauma (fishbone, straw); dental procedure
- Polymicrobial; *streptococcus*, *fusobacterium*, *staphylococcus* most common culprits
- If child anxious/toxic appearing, avoid oropharynx exam as can → airway obstruction

	Peritonsillar Abscess	Retropharyngeal Abscess
Age	Adolescents mainly	Usually children < 5 yrs
Symptoms	Fever, sore throat, dysphagia, voice change, drooling	Fever, neck pain, dysphagia, odynophagia, drooling, decreased PO, chest pain and dyspnea if mediastinal extension
Physical Exam	Uvular deviation towards contralateral side, ipsilateral tonsillar bulging, trismus, lymphadenopathy, tender neck mass	Lymphadenopathy, ill, anxious, dysphonia, trismus, limited neck movement or meningismus, stridor

	Peritonsillar Abscess	Retropharyngeal Abscess
Labs/Imaging	Clinical diagnosis. If unclear, may use bedside US (endocavitary probe). CT neck w/ contrast if concern for deep neck abscess, malignancy	Clinical diagnosis. If toxic, respiratory distress → OR for examination/surgery. Consider CBC, BMP, blood culture, rapid strep. XR of lateral neck: prevertebral soft tissue thickening > 7 mm at C2 or > 14 mm at C6, or > ½ width of vertebral body. CXR. CT neck w/ contrast if stable, diagnosis unclear, for better visualization
Treatment	Needle aspiration better tolerated than I&D. Tonsillectomy if deep abscess or airway compromise. Amoxicillin-clavulanate (600 mg/5 mL) 45 mg/kg (max 875 mg) PO two times daily for 10 days or clindamycin 10 mg/kg (max 600 mg) PO three times daily for 10 days	Ampicillin/sulbactam 50 mg/kg (max 2 g) IV every 6 hrs or clindamycin 15 mg/kg (max 900 mg) IV every 8 hrs; if life-threatening, add vancomycin 15 mg/kg (max 1 g) IV every 8 hrs; ENT consult. If intubation is needed → OR/anesthesia ideally, otherwise anticipate difficult airway, careful to not rupture abscess during intubation
Disposition	Home w/ follow-up after I&D if tolerating PO, non-toxic	Admit
Complications	Airway compromise, aspiration pneumonia, carotid artery pseudoaneurysm or rupture, internal jugular vein thrombosis, Lemierre syndrome (jugular vein suppurative thrombophlebitis), mediastinitis	

IV. LYMPHADENITIS

BACKGROUND

- Lymph node inflammation; can be reactionary, primary infection, or malignancy
- Acute
  — Unilateral: *Staphylococcus*, *Streptococcus*, viral, reactive; less likely Kawasaki, autoimmune
  — Bilateral: viral, reactive, EBV, HIV, autoimmune, PFAPA (periodic fever, aphthous stomatitis, pharyngitis, cervical adenitis)
  — Subacute: *Bartonella*, *Toxoplasma*, TB, malignancy

EVALUATION
- **High Yield History**: URI, ENT infection, B symptoms (weight loss, night sweats), fever duration, family history, cat exposure, travel
- **Exam**: location, mobility, firm vs. soft, fluctuance, tenderness, erythema
- **Diagnostics**
  — Consider CBC, BMP, ESR/CRP, PPD, EBV & *Bartonella* titers
  — CXR if malignancy concern
  — Consider US to evaluate for abscess, malignancy

MANAGEMENT
- Observation if mild or reactive
- Primary bacterial lymphadenitis (erythema, tenderness)
  — Amoxicillin-clavulanate (600 mg/5 mL concentration only) 45 mg/kg (max 1500 mg) PO two times daily for 10 days
  — Cephalexin 25 mg/kg (max 500 mg) PO three times daily for 10 days
  — Clindamycin 10 mg/kg (max 600 mg) PO three times daily for 10 days
- Abscess: ENT consult if considering I&D

DISPOSITION
- Discharge, follow-up 24-48 hrs
- ENT consult, admission if severe symptoms
- If concern for malignancy, oncology consult + admission

V. CONGENITAL NECK MASSES

- Common cause of pediatric neck mass
- Patients present when mass is infected
- Congenital abnormalities of head and neck are associated with major nerves and vessels; take care to recognize them and avoid cutting into them

	Branchial Cleft Cysts	**Thyroglossal Duct Cysts**	**Cystic Hygromas (Lymphangiomas)**
Age	Late childhood, early adulthood	Children, adolescents	Newborn, prenatally by US
Origin & Epidemiology	Most common congenital neck lesion, abnormal embryonic neck development. Cysts, sinus tracts, fistulae all possible	Epithelialized cyst formed from embryologic ductal tissue. Can be anywhere from base of tongue to sternal notch	Lymphatic malformations common in the neck. Benign, but can become large. Associated with higher risk of aneuploidy, congenital malformations
History & Exam	Asymptomatic lateral neck mass; if infected can be tender, erythematous. Fever, pain, facial paralysis (CN VII impingement by large 1st arch cysts). Exam may show nodules, sinus openings	URI → infected anterior midline neck lesion (tender, erythematous). Attached to hyoid, moves with swallowing and sticking out tongue	Spongy, mobile, nontender mass in the posterior triangle of the neck, transilluminates. Can suddenly enlarge from infection or hemorrhage → airway compromise
Diagnostics	US. CT neck w/ contrast if unclear dx or if requested for preop planning		US, CT, MRI
Treatment	Antibiotics if lymphadenitis or infected, ENT follow up		Consult ENT; Admit
Complications	Recurrent infections, fistula formation, injury to parotid gland and CN VII (facial paralysis), airway edema, difficulty swallowing, malignancy	Potential for malignant transformation	Airway/neurovascular compromise, hemorrhage, lymphangitis

Section VII
Endocrinology

1 ▶ Glucose Metabolism

I. HYPOGLYCEMIA

BACKGROUND

- Clinical hypoglycemia: plasma glucose (PG) low enough to cause symptoms or signs of impaired brain function
  - ED: initially, before blood draw sent to the lab for plasma glucose results, must act based on point of care glucose (POC GLC) results
- Infants and younger children with PG < 60 mg/dL should be evaluated and treated for hypoglycemia
- *Transitional hypoglycemia*
  - ~30% healthy newborns have PG < 50 mg/dL in the first 24 hrs of life
  - > 24 hrs old, PG should be > 50 mg/dL
  - > 48 hrs old, PG > 60-70 mg/dL is normal and < 50 mg/dL is hypoglycemia similar to older children and adults
- *Neonatal hypoglycemia* is the most common metabolic problem in neonates
  - DDx: at-risk infants of diabetic mothers, small or large for gestational age infants, preterm infants, congenital hyperinsulinism, perinatal stress, hypopituitarism, cortisol or growth hormone deficiencies, intrauterine growth restriction, congenital syndromes (Beckwith-Wiedemann), and inborn errors of metabolism (glucose, glycogen, fatty acids)
- Other causes: poor oral intake, acute diarrhea, infection, malignancy, hypothyroidism, ingestions, iatrogenic
- All acutely ill children should be evaluated for hypoglycemia, especially if ↓ PO intake

EVALUATION

- **High Yield History**
  - Infants: birth weight & history, maternal diabetes, family history
    - Symptoms: lethargy, irritability, ↓ PO intake, seizures

- Older infants/children: recent illness with vomiting and/or diarrhea, ingestions
    - Symptoms: adrenergic symptoms (anxiety, palpitations, tremors, diaphoresis), AMS, seizures, coma, headache
- **Exam**
  - Tachycardia, assess for signs of infection
  - AMS, thorough neurological exam
  - Evidence of hypopituitarism (cleft palate, spina bifida, micropenis, older child with visual disturbances, CNS abnormalities)
  - Signs of adrenal insufficiency (weight loss, hyperpigmentation, abdominal pain)
  - *Beckwith-Wiedemann syndrome* (hemihypertrophy, macroglossia, omphalocele)
- **Diagnostics**
  - Labs
    - POC GLC
    - CBC, CMP, lactate, beta-hydroxybutyrate, ammonia
    - Infection workup if concern for sepsis
    - Urinalysis to assess for ketones
    - If able, save an extra blood tube (3 mL, red top), and first voided urine **prior** to initiating treatment for further metabolic and toxicological evaluations if persistent hypoglycemia is confirmed

MANAGEMENT

- Maintain GLC > 50 mg/dL (neonate < 48 hrs old), > 60 mg/dL (neonate > 48 hrs old, infant, child)
- If alert, able to tolerate PO, and stable, feed patient
- Dextrose
  - Bolus dose: 0.5-1 g/kg, regardless of route of administration
  - For neonates, some recommend 0.2 g/kg to minimize hyperglycemia → increased insulin secretion → reactive hypoglycemia
    - Dextrose 40% oral gel 0.2 g/kg (0.5 mL/kg) buccal can be used
  - If unable to tolerate PO, for dextrose bolus follow "Dextrose 5/2/1 rule or rule of 50s": X mL/kg of DYW gives desired dose of 0.5 g/kg where $X \times Y = 50$

Age	Dose	Bolus (PO/NG/IV/IO)	Maintenance
Neonate	D10W	2 mL/kg	60-80 mL/kg/day (D10W); 80-100 mL/kg/day (D10W) if weight < 1500 g
Infant	D10W	5 mL/kg	D10W at 1.5x maintenance rate
	D25W	2 mL/kg	

Age	Dose	Bolus (PO/NG/IV/IO)	Maintenance
Child	D25W	2 mL/kg	D10W at 1.5x maintenance rate
Adolescent	D25W D50W	2 mL/kg 1 mL/kg	D5W at 1-1.5x maintenance rate

— Use diluted solutions in children as concentrated dextrose can cause vascular injury
— If only have D50W = 1 ampule = 50 mL = 25 grams
  - To make D25W: Discard 25 mL of D50W, add 25 mL sterile water
  - To make D10W: Discard 40 mL of D50W, add 40 mL sterile water
- Glucagon
  — Effective only for (congenital) hyperinsulinism, insulin overdose, sulfonylurea ingestion
  — Consider using IM for severe hypoglycemia if no IV/IO access, no dextrose available, or persistent PG < 50 despite glucose infusion
  — Glucagon at 0.5-1 mg (independent of weight) by IV, IM, or SQ
    - Lower dose 0.03 mg/kg (max 1 mg) IV may lead to less nausea/vomiting
    - Repeat dose in 20 min if no rise in PG
    - Consider drip at 10 mcg/kg/hr if on maximal parenteral glucose infusion and still hypoglycemic

II. DIABETIC KETOACIDOSIS (DKA)

BACKGROUND

- Complication of diabetes, particularly Type 1 DM (T1DM)
  — Many children with new onset diabetes present with DKA
  — Less common in Type 2 DM (T2DM)
- Often precipitated by a stressor such as infection, especially if there is vomiting and diarrhea → dehydration, or medication nonadherence
- In T1DM, cells are unable to take up glucose as an energy source due to insulin deficiency → breakdown of adipose tissue and creation of free fatty acids → converted into ketoacids by the liver → metabolic acidosis
- Cerebral edema occurs in ~1% of children with DKA with mortality of 20-25%
  — In 2018, a large randomized clinical trial by PECARN found that neither the rate nor sodium chloride content of IV fluids significantly impacted the occurrence of cerebral edema nor neurological outcomes of children with DKA
  — Fluids should not be restricted, especially if the child shows signs of dehydration clinically and/or by laboratory markers

EVALUATION

- **High Yield History**: AMS, lethargy, nausea, vomiting, abdominal pain, polyuria, polydipsia
- **Exam**: look for signs of dehydration, concurrent infection
  — Hyperventilation (Kussmaul respirations) often present to compensate for severe metabolic acidosis
  — Drowsiness or lethargy may be present
  — Patient may have odor of ketones
  — *Cerebral edema*: mental status fluctuation, new cranial nerve palsy, posturing, incontinence, vomiting, headache, abnormal respiratory pattern, bradycardia
- **Diagnostics**
  — Labs:
    - CBC, CMP, beta-hydroxybutyrate, VBG, UA, Mg, Phos
    - DKA requires all of the following lab features

Laboratory Features	
Hyperglycemia	Serum GLC > 200 mg/dL
Metabolic Acidosis	Either • Venous pH < 7.3 • Serum bicarbonate < 15 mEq/L
Ketosis	Either • Beta-hydroxybutyrate ≥ 3 mmol/L • Moderate to large urine ketones

  - Children with a venous pH of < 7.2 and/or serum bicarbonate < 10 mEq/L are in moderate-severe DKA
  - Consider obtaining CXR, blood and urine cultures if concern for infection
  - Note: patients on SGLT2 inhibitors may have euglycemic DKA with PG < 250 mg/dL

MANAGEMENT

- *Fluids*: Initiate a 10-20 mL/kg bolus of 0.9% NS or LR solution
  — Second bolus if the patient continues to show signs of inadequate perfusion (poor mentation, urine output, or capillary refill) or hemodynamic compromise
- *Maintenance fluids*: 0.45% or 0.9% NS; add D5W once GLC is 250-300 mg/dL
- *Insulin*: 0.1 U/kg/hr IV infusion, do not give a bolus or SQ insulin
  — Monitor GLC every hour, it should not drop by more than 100 mg/dL/hr

- *Potassium*: use K Phos + either K acetate or KCl (KCl alone can lead to hyperchloremic metabolic acidosis)
  — If normokalemic (3.3-5.3 mEq/L) and voiding (r/o acute renal failure), add 40 mEq/L potassium to maintenance fluids
  — If hyperkalemic (> 5.3 mEq/L), no repletion necessary, continue to monitor
  — If hypokalemic (< 3.3 mEq/L), delay insulin as much as possible until K+ repleted
- *Bicarbonate*: avoid unless severe acidosis or hyperkalemia, impending cardiac arrest or requiring airway intervention
  — Rapidly correcting acidosis → decreased stimulus for hyperventilation → increased CO_2 crossing blood-brain barrier
- *Other electrolytes*: monitor for hypomagnesemia, hypophosphatemia, hypocalcemia q2hrs and replete PRN
- **Cerebral edema**:
  — 1st line: mannitol at 0.5-1 g/kg IV over 10-15 min, q30min PRN
  — 2nd line: hypertonic (3%) saline at 3-5 mL/kg, but may be associated with increased mortality compared to mannitol
  — Avoid hypoxia and hypotension; intubation may be necessary
  — Do NOT delay treatment to obtain CT scan

DISPOSITION

- Hypoglycemia: unless a clear etiology and resolution of hypoglycemia, most require admission for observation
- DKA: Admit to PICU (moderate/severe), or step-down unit (mild)

BEWARE

❗ Hypoglycemia
  — After treatment of hypoglycemia, monitor POC GLC every 15-20 min until > 70 mg/dL, then hourly
  — If seizing, and does not respond to dextrose, treat with anticonvulsant
  — Glucocorticoids are not beneficial for treatment of acute hypoglycemia and may delay identifying the inciting cause

❗ DKA: Be alert — a child with gastroenteritis, bronchiolitis, or pneumonia may also be in DKA (diagnosis often missed)

2 ▶ Adrenal Insufficiency

CONGENITAL ADRENAL HYPERPLASIA (CAH)

BACKGROUND
- Group of disorders characterized by enzyme deficiency → decreased cortisol synthesis → hypersecretion of adrenocorticotropic hormone (ACTH) → adrenal gland hyperplasia
- Varying degrees of mineralocorticoid and cortisol deficiency
  — Excess precursors can shunt to sex steroid pathway

Types
- Salt-losing
  — Severe, commonly infants 10-20 days of life
  — Nearly absent 21-hydroxylase activity
  — Decreased aldosterone synthesis, cortisol deficiency, life-threatening salt wasting, hyperkalemia, hyponatremia
- Classic non-salt losing
  — Less severe form in infants, little to no sodium-deficiency symptoms
- Nonclassic (late onset)
  — Late childhood or adolescence
  — Reduced but not absent 21-hydroxylase activity
  — Androgen excess / virilization

Newborn screen
- Developed to identify male infants with salt-wasting CAH
- High false-positive rate 98%, false negative rate up to 22.4%
- Even if initial labs normal can develop severe symptoms later during first month of life

EVALUATION
- **High Yield History**
  — Poor feeding, weight loss, failure to thrive, vomiting, dehydration
- **Exam**
  — Ambiguous genitalia in females due to shunting of steroid precursors to male sex hormones
    - Male genitalia usually normal or subtly virilized (enlarged phallus)
  — Hyperpigmentation due to increased ACTH secretion
    - α-melanocyte stimulating hormone is a breakdown product of ACTH
  — Adrenal crisis: hypotension and shock unresponsive to fluid boluses

- **Diagnostics**
  - Labs
    - Save 1 red-top tube of blood PRIOR to initiating treatment
    - BMP: hyponatremia, hyperkalemia, metabolic acidosis, hypoglycemia
    - Confirmatory tests: 17-hydroxyprogesterone (17-OHP), cortisol
  - EKG (electrolyte abnormalities)

LATE-ONSET PRESENTATION

BACKGROUND
- Non-salt-wasting forms: symptoms can be mild, easily missed
- Infection, trauma, other stressor can rarely cause acute decompensation

EVALUATION
- **High Yield History**
  - Severe acne, early puberty
  - Females (menstrual irregularity, hirsutism)
  - Syncope
- **Exam**
  - Acne, hirsutism, hyperpigmentation, cliteromegaly
  - Normal stature but usually shorter than both parents
- **Diagnostics**
  - POC GLC, BMP, 17-OHP, cortisol
  - EKG

MANAGEMENT
- Adrenal crisis
  - Hydrocortisone 25 mg IV infants, 50 mg IV children, 100 mg IV teens
  - Normal saline boluses 10-20 mL/kg IV, repeat PRN
  - Correct electrolyte imbalances, hypoglycemia
  - Endocrinology consult

DISPOSITION
- Salt-wasting / adrenal crisis: PICU
- Milder forms: discharge with endocrinology follow-up
  - Counsel on stress dose steroid indications

BEWARE

- ❗ Do not be reassured by a negative newborn screening
- ❗ May mimic pyloric stenosis with lethargy and vomiting, but pyloric stenosis patients typically have a hypokalemic alkalosis
- ❗ Need medical alert bracelet

3 ▶ Thyroid Disorders

HYPOTHYROIDISM

BACKGROUND

- Congenital hypothyroidism is usually diagnosed via newborn screening
- Acquired — increased risk: Down, Turner, Klinefelter, DiGeorge, William, Prader-Willi syndromes, Type 1 diabetes, celiac disease

EVALUATION

- **High Yield History**
  - Infants: developmental delay, poor growth and feeding, prolonged jaundice
  - Adolescents: fatigue, constipation, cold intolerance, delayed puberty, menstrual irregularities
- **Exam**
  - Congenital: may have umbilical hernia, enlarged tongue, coarse facies, poor muscle tone, hypothermia, large fontanelle, jaundice
  - Acquired: goiter, dry skin, xerostosis, coarse hair, bradycardia, non-pitting edema
- **Diagnostics**
  - Thyroid studies: TSH, free T4, T3, antithyroid peroxidase, antithyroglobulin antibodies

MANAGEMENT

- Levothyroxine (IV if myxedema coma, else oral)
- Consult pediatric endocrinology for levothyroxine dosing and further management

HYPERTHYROIDISM

BACKGROUND
- Uncommon in children, 90% caused by Graves' disease
- Other causes: toxic adenoma, multinodular goiter, McCune Albright
- Neonatal thyrotoxicosis: transplacental maternal thyroid-stimulating antibodies
- Thyroid storm or decompensated hyperthyroidism can be precipitated by infection/sepsis, surgery, trauma
- Excess thyroid hormone → increased cardiac output, decreased SVR, increased metabolism, increased sensitivity to catecholamines

EVALUATION
- **High Yield History**
  — Poor weight gain, frequent bowel movements, weight loss, nervousness, sleeplessness, hyperactivity, tremor
  — Vague ophthalmologic complaints with Graves' disease: foreign body sensation, pain, diplopia
  — Thyroid storm: fever, vomiting, diarrhea
- **Exam**
  — Increased HR and cardiac output, decreased SVR → "water hammer pulses"
  — Eyelid retraction from increased ocular muscle adrenergic tone, lid lag
  — Brisk reflexes, tremulousness, goiter, hyperthyroid-induced craniosynostosis
  — Thyroid storm: AMS, fever, arrhythmia, wide pulse pressure, hypotension, heart failure (gallop rhythm, hepatomegaly)
- **Diagnostics**
  — TSH, free T4, T3, TSH receptor antibody levels
  — EKG

MANAGEMENT
- Thyroid storm
  — Treat inciting/underlying cause (infection, trauma)
  — Aggressive cooling, acetaminophen, volume resuscitation (account for accelerated metabolic rate)
  — Consider broad spectrum antibiotics until culture negative
  — Antithyroid medication
    - Methimazole 0.5 mg/kg/day PO divided in three doses (max 30 mg/day)

- Iodide
    - Lugol's 5% solution (potassium iodide 10% and iodine 5%): 1 drop q8hrs (neonate), 4 drops q8hrs (children)
    - Give at least 1hr after the first dose of methimazole
- Beta-blocker
    - Propranolol
        - IV: 10 mcg/kg over 10-15 min or
        - PO: 0.5 mg/kg four times daily (neonate) or 10-40 mg four times daily in older children
    - Atenolol 1mg/kg/day PO if hx of bronchospasm
    - Esmolol infusion may be necessary
- Hydrocortisone 5 mg/kg (max 100 mg) or dexamethasone 0.2 mg/kg IV
- Stable hyperthyroidism: methimazole
- Consult pediatric endocrinology for dosing, further management

DISPOSITION

- Myxedema coma, thyroid storm: PICU admission
- Mildly symptomatic, stable: discharge with close endocrinology follow-up

BEWARE

- ❗ Maintain high index of suspicion for thyroid storm
    - Misdiagnosed as anxiety/panic attack, psychiatric disorders, sepsis, heat stroke
- ❗ Do NOT use propylthiouracil (PTU) in children — risk of hepatotoxicity

Section VIII
Environmental

1 ▶ Bites and Envenomations

MAMMALIAN

Mammals	Dog	Cat	Human
Bites	Young children: head & neck Older children: extremities	Puncture wounds	Occlusive Clenched fist ("fight bite") on knuckles
Organisms	*Streptococcus, Staphylococcus,* anaerobes, often polymicrobial		
	Pasteurella, Capnocytophaga canimorsus	*Pasteurella*	*Eikenella*
Infection rate	10-20%	30-50%	10% occlusive to > 25% fight bite

EVALUATION

- **High Yield History**: animal & its health status, time & circumstances of bite, anatomic location, # of bites, PMH (immunocompromised), vaccinations
- **Exam**: location, size, depth of wound(s), tendon injury, joint capsule, neurovascular status infection, foreign bodies
- **Diagnostics**: X-ray for fracture, joint pathology, foreign body

MANAGEMENT

- Exploration, irrigation, debridement
- Closure
  - Primary closure for cosmetically important areas (face)
  - Do not close hands, infected wounds, or high-risk (puncture, fight bite, > 12 hrs)
- Prophylactic antibiotics
  - Hands, punctures, late presentation, immunocompromised, human or cat, sutured bite
  - Amoxicillin-clavulanate 22.5 mg/kg (max 875 mg) PO two times daily for 5 days

- Clindamycin 10 mg/kg (max 600 mg) PO three times daily for five days **PLUS** TMP/SMX 5 mg/kg (max 160 mg) PO two times daily for 5 days
- Update tetanus
- Rabies prophylaxis for high-risk animals
- Consult surgical subspecialty for: deep infection, neurovascular compromise, serious cosmetic injury

DISPOSITION

- Discharge with wound check within 48 hrs if minor, no evidence of serious infection
- Admit if needs parenteral antibiotics, surgical repair

BEWARE

- ⚠ Fight bites (high risk for foreign body or joint involvement)
- ⚠ Foreign body (teeth)

MARINE ENVENOMATIONS

BACKGROUND

- Children → higher relative venom dose
- Severity varies greatly by local species
- Epidemiology
  - Jellyfish (true): mauve stinger (Atlantic, Pacific); lion's mane (Atlantic, Pacific); sea nettle (Chesapeake Bay); thimble, aka seabather's eruption (Caribbean, Florida)
    - Mild toxicity, systemic symptoms unlikely
  - Stingrays: southern (southeastern U.S. coasts) and round (California through Central America) stingrays
    - Injury when stepping on stingray
    - Retroserrated spine in tail bathed in venom
  - Sea snakes: tropical waters (Indo-Pacific), California coast
    - Relatively painless fang-sized bites
    - Symptoms within minutes or up to 8 hrs (delayed)
  - Sea urchins & sea stars: ubiquitous
    - Venomous spines
    - Injury to hand/foot from handling or stepping on creature

EVALUATION

- **High Yield History**: geographic location; symptoms: immediate vs. delayed, severity, local vs. systemic; prior envenomation/antivenom

- **Exam**
  - Typical findings
    - North American jellyfish: mild pain, irritant dermatitis
    - Stingrays: severe pain, gaping laceration +/– cyanotic edges; nausea/vomiting, cramps, arrhythmias when severe
    - Sea snakes: if envenomation → ptosis, dysphagia, hypersalivation, rapid myalgias weakness, blurry vision, ascending paralysis, rhabdomyolysis
      - Severe → renal failure, respiratory arrest
    - Sea urchin: multiple erratic punctures
    - Box jellyfish: excruciating pain, hypotension, paralysis, rapid blistering
  - Evaluate traumatic injuries, retained foreign body
  - Assess for systemic effects (hypotension, nausea/vomiting, dysrhythmias)
- **Diagnostics**
  - X-ray and US: foreign body (stingray, sea urchin)
  - CBC/CMP, UA if systemic symptoms; CK if sea snake

MANAGEMENT

- Treat allergy/anaphylaxis
- Remove tentacles/spines
- Hot water (up to 45°C/113°F) immersion or as tolerated for 60-90 min
- Supportive care, analgesia, wound care
- Prophylactic antibiotics ×3-5 days for stingrays, sea urchins, cone snail, deep puncture wounds
  - Cephalexin 25 mg/kg (max 500 mg) PO two times daily **PLUS**
  - Doxycycline 2.2 mg/kg (max 100 mg) PO two times daily for Vibrio coverage
    - Caution if < 8 yrs; consult with ID
- Update tetanus
- Antivenom for box jellyfish, stonefish, sea snakes if severe
  - Consult Toxicology

DISPOSITION

- Admit for abnormal vital signs, persistent systemic signs
  - Observation if sea snake (risk of delayed systemic symptoms)
- Discharge if symptoms resolved
  - Follow-up in 3-4 days if penetrating, 1 week if received antivenom
  - Sooner if severe

SNAKE BITES: PIT VIPERS & CORAL SNAKES

BACKGROUND
- 3000-6000 cases in U.S./year
- Children → higher relative venom dose
- Lower extremity most likely
- Main types
  - Crotalidae (pit viper): triangular head, elliptical pupils
    - Copperheads: NE to FL, west to Texas, southern Midwest
    - Cottonmouths: SE U.S. and along Gulf Coast
    - Rattlesnakes: more common at lower latitudes Atlantic to Pacific coasts
  - Elapidae (coral snakes): red, yellow, black banding (red adjacent yellow in U.S.)
    - Eastern coral snake: Southeast U.S.
    - Texas coral snake: west of Mississippi in LA, AR, TX

EVALUATION
- **High Yield History**: time/location of bite(s), comorbidities (anticoagulants), prehospital treatment, previous snakebite/antivenom, systemic symptoms
- **Exam**
  - Pit vipers: local (swelling, pain, ecchymosis, hemorrhagic bullae), systemic (nausea/vomiting, hypotension, paralysis, airway edema, rhabdomyolysis), hematologic (bleeding, thrombocytopenia)
  - Coral snakes: local (swelling, punctures), systemic (diplopia, ptosis, dysphagia, dysarthria, stridor, respiratory paralysis, muscle weakness)
- **Diagnostics**
  - CBC, PT/INR, PTT, fibrinogen
  - Systemic toxicity: CMP, CK, UA
  - EKG, CXR if cardiac or respiratory symptoms

MANAGEMENT
- Prehospital: remove constrictive jewelry/clothing, clean, immobilize & elevate limb, mark & time leading edge
  - Tourniquets NOT recommended
- ABCs
- Analgesia: opioids, avoid NSAIDs
- Contact medical toxicology or local Poison Control Center

- Pit viper
  - Monitor swelling, ecchymosis, pain
  - Antivenom
    - Indications: more than minimal/progressive swelling, abnormal labs, systemic symptoms
    - 2 commercially available FDA-approved antivenoms
      - Crotalidae Polyvalent Immune Fab Ovine (CroFab): initial dose 4-6 vials
      - Crotalidae Immune Fab Equine (Anavip): initial dose 10 vials
    - Consider maintenance dosing in conjunction with poison control center recommendations
    - If new or worsening symptoms, give more antivenom
- Coral snake
  - Monitor respiratory status, intubate for paralysis, or Negative Inspiratory Force (NIF) < 20 cm H2O
  - NACSA (North American Coral Snake Antivenom)
    - Indications: envenomation or systemic signs/progressive paralysis
    - 3-5 vials IV, repeat if progression
    - May develop anaphylaxis; treat as indicated
  - Hourly neurological assessments
- Update tetanus

DISPOSITION

- Pit Vipers
  - Observation if no antivenom or progression & normal labs
    - Dry bite - observe 8-12 hrs, normal repeat labs before discharge
  - Admission
    - No antivenom but symptom progression or abnormal labs: observe 12-24 hrs
      - Repeat labs at 4-6 hrs and before discharge
    - Antivenom used
      - Repeat coags at 2-4, 5-7 days for rattlesnake or abnormal heme labs
- Coral snakes
  - Admit all to ICU for 12-24 hrs observation

SPIDER BITES: BLACK WIDOW, BROWN RECLUSE, TARANTULA

BACKGROUND

- Black widow
  - Every state (rare in Alaska, Maine)
  - Alpha-latrotoxin → NE, GABA, ACh release → muscle cramps, autonomic symptoms
  - Black +/– ventral red hourglass
- Brown recluse
  - South-central U.S.
  - Fiddle-shaped marking on thorax
- Tarantula
  - Western U.S., pets

EVALUATION

- **High Yield History**: geography, bite location & timing, systemic symptoms, painful vs. painless
- **Exam**
  - Black widow: local (erythema with halo), systemic (myalgias, hypertension, tachycardia, nausea/vomiting, diaphoresis)
  - Recluse: local (erythema with blue/grey macule, necrotic ulceration), systemic (coagulopathies, hypotension, DIC, seizures, jaundice, renal failure, hemolytic anemia)
  - Tarantula: local (erythema, pruritus / urticaria for abdomen hair contact)
- **Diagnostics**
  - Black widow: CBC, BMP, CK, lactate, UA, EKG
  - Recluse: CBC, PT/INR, PTT, UA, Cr, LFTs if systemic symptoms

MANAGEMENT

- Wound care
- Black widow
  - Benzodiazepines for spasms, NSAIDs/opioids for pain
  - Consider antivenom if: seizures, hypertensive crisis, respiratory compromise, intractable pain, failing supportive care
    - Call medical toxicologist/poison control center (U.S.) 1-800-222-1222

- Recluse
  - Antihistamines, analgesics, cold compresses, elevation
  - Consider systemic corticosteroids or antihistamines
- Tarantula
  - Antihistamines, topical steroids, analgesics
  - Ocular exposure to hairs: Ophthalmology consult +/– topical steroids
- Update tetanus
- Antibiotics if infection

DISPOSITION

- Discharge if symptoms resolved
- Admission if persistent systemic symptoms

BEWARE

- Brown recluse: systemic reaction rarely correlates with lesion severity
- Black widow: antivenom NOT 1st line

2 ▶ Hyperthermia

BACKGROUND

- Core body temperature > 38°C/100.4°F due to failure of thermoregulation
- Risk factors: heat waves with high peak temperatures, extended exposure, low socioeconomic status, inability to escape hot environments (child locked in car), mental illness and other comorbidities, lack of air conditioning, physical activity in hot environments
- Classic heat stroke (vs. exertional) more common in young children due to immature thermoregulatory mechanisms
- DDx: infection, sepsis, toxin (sympathomimetic, anticholinergic), thyroid storm, neuroleptic malignant syndrome, malignant hyperthermia, serotonin syndrome

	Definition	Symptoms
Heat Exhaustion	<ul><li>Mild to moderately severe illness due to loss of salt and water during exposure to heat</li><li>Core temp may be low, normal, or high (but < 40°C/104°F)</li><li>NO severe CNS involvement</li></ul>	**Neuro**: dizziness, HA, fatigue, confusion that resolves with rest/cooling **CV/Pulm**: tachycardia w/o hypotension, tachypnea **GI**: nausea/vomiting/diarrhea **Skin**: warm, sweaty, flushed **MSK**: cramps

	Definition	Symptoms
Heat Stroke	• Core temperature ≥ 40°C/104°F with CNS dysfunction • Passive hyperthermia secondary to impaired mechanisms for heat dissipation or inability to escape a heated environment (generally develops over days) • Exertional hyperthermia secondary to exercise + heat exposure (develops rapidly)	**Neuro**: AMS, seizures, delirium, syncope, coma **CV/Pulm**: hypotension, arrhythmia, heart failure **GI**: hematemesis, hematochezia, liver failure **Renal**: renal failure **Skin**: sweaty or dry, purpura **MSK**: tetany

EVALUATION

- **High Yield History**
    - Duration and type of exposure
    - Drugs, medications, illicit drugs, PMH
    - Pre-hospital treatments
- **Exam**
    - Vital signs, core body temperature (rectal, esophageal, bladder)
    - Evaluate for mental status/encephalopathy, cardiovascular collapse/shock
- **Diagnostics**
    - Heat stroke associated with Multiple Organ Dysfunction Syndrome (severe inflammatory process that leads to multiorgan dysfunction)
    - Consider POC GLC, ABG, CBC, CMP, Phos, CK, PT/INR, PTT, troponin, lactate, UA, Utox, CXR, EKG

MANAGEMENT

- ABCs, 2 large-bore IVs
    - Rehydration with room temperature fluids
    - Initial fluid bolus 20 mL/kg NS
- Remove clothing
- Rapid cooling: cold water tubs or ice water immersion
    - Associated with shivering
        - Give benzodiazepines if severe (midazolam 0.05-0.1 mg/kg IV, max 2 mg)
    - *Caution*: cold water immersion may cause reflex bradycardia in infants & younger children, consider evaporative cooling in this age group
- Evaporative cooling: spray with tepid water or apply wet sheets and continuously fan patient, cooling blanket
    - Stop when core body temperature reaches 38°C

- Correct electrolyte derangements
- Benzodiazepines if seizures
- Monitor and treat complications (rhabdomyolysis, dehydration, acute renal injury, DIC, cardiogenic shock, liver failure)

DISPOSITION

- Discharge: mild illness, vital signs and symptoms normalized
- Admit to PICU: severe illness, significant lab abnormalities, end-organ damage, shock

BEWARE

⚠ Antipyretics should not be used since elevated temperature is not due to cytokines.

3 ▶ Hypothermia

BACKGROUND

- Definition: core temperature < 35.0°C
  — Mild: 32-35.0°C
  — Moderate: 28.0-32°C
  — Severe: < 28.0°C
- Deaths: infants 1 per million, children age 5-14 years 0.2 per million
- Younger children = higher risk
  — Higher surface area to body mass ratio
  — Infants < 6 mo cannot shiver
  — Limited glycogen stores for heat production
- Common causes: environmental exposure, endocrine dysfunction, burns, trauma, sepsis, toxins, abuse/punishment

EVALUATION

- **High Yield History**
  — Exposure duration, type
  — Ambient temperature
  — Submersion/wet skin
  — Medications, concurrent illness, abuse
- **Exam**
  — Core temperature: may need special low-reading temperature probe
  — Bradycardia, hypotension, delayed capillary refill
  — Shivering, severe → rigidity

- Mental status
- Severe → dilated, fixed pupils
- **Diagnostics**
  - POC GLC, CBC, CMP, lipase, type and screen, blood gas, PT/INR, PTT, UA to evaluate for end-organ damage
  - Imaging if concern for trauma, abuse, lung injury
  - EKG, cardiac monitoring given high risk for arrhythmias
    - J-wave (Osborn wave) not always present

MANAGEMENT

- Stabilize patient in horizontal supine position
- Avoid rough handling, may precipitate arrhythmia
- ABCs
  - If pulseless or in non-perfusing rhythm, start CPR, aggressively fluid resuscitate with 20 mL/kg warm NS
  - Defibrillate VFib/pulseless VT as per PALS guidelines
    - If initial shock unsuccessful, warm to 30°C then re-attempt
  - Consider epinephrine, antiarrhythmics if temperature < 30°C vs. wait until core temperature > 30°C
- Rewarming
  - Passive: remove wet clothing, apply dry blankets
  - Active external: forced-air warming blanket
    - Warm torso first to avoid "afterdrop" if severe
- Peripheral vasodilation → cold blood from extremities cools core
  - Active internal: warmed/humidified O2, warmed IV fluids (40-44°C)
  - Invasive for severe: thoracic, gastric, peritoneal, bladder lavage with warm fluid (40-44°C); ECMO or cardiopulmonary bypass provide fastest rewarming
- Resuscitate until core temperature 34-35°C
- Tetanus update if digits affected

Severity	Treatment
Mild	Passive and active external rewarming, supportive care
Moderate	Active external warming, warmed IVFs, correct lab abnormalities, if hemodynamically unstable, consider ECMO
Severe	Active internal rewarming, invasive, strongly consider ECMO

DISPOSITION

- Discharge: mild hypothermia
- Admit: moderate and severe hypothermia
  — If hemodynamically unstable → PICU with ECMO capability

BEWARE

- ⚠ IV access will be challenging; place IO line if there is a delay
- ⚠ Use femoral vein if central access needed (risk of ventricular fibrillation with irritable myocardium with IJ or subclavian)
- ⚠ Meaningful neurologic outcome is possible even with substantial downtime
- ⚠ Check pulses for up to 60 sec (patient may be severely bradycardic)

4 ▶ Submersion Injuries

BACKGROUND

- Drowning is a leading cause of death in children aged < 5 yrs
  — 10 die daily in U.S.; 2 are children < 14 yrs
- Pathophysiology
  — Submersion → voluntary breath holding → aspiration of water & laryngospasm → disruption of gas exchange → hypoxemia, hypercarbia, acidosis → cerebral hypoxia with AMS & cardiac dysfunction/dysrhythmias
- Clinical outcome depends on extent of hypoxic injury

EVALUATION

- **High Yield History**: circumstances, associated trauma, submersion time, resuscitation efforts (description, duration, rescuer training), PMH
  — Poor prognostic indicators
    - Prolonged immersion time > 5 min
    - CPR duration prior to ROSC > 25 min
    - GCS on ED arrival < 5
    - Persistent apnea/requiring CPR in ED
    - Chronic health conditions
    - Male sex
    - pH < 7.1 on arrival
- **Exam**
  — Vitals including rectal temp, continuous pulse oximetry
  — Alertness, cardiovascular dysrhythmias, pulmonary (tachypnea, wheezes, rhonchi), signs of trauma to head/neck/chest/abdomen

- **Diagnostics**
  - Labs
    - If alert, asymptomatic, normal pulse ox, do not need labs/imaging
    - ABG to guide respiratory management
    - POC GLC to assess for hypoglycemia
    - CBC, CMP, CK, PT/INR, PTT if critically ill
  - Imaging
    - CXR if symptomatic or respiratory abnormalities, abnormal pulse ox
      - Repeat prior to discharge
    - CT if signs or concerns for trauma
  - EKG on all symptomatic patients

MANAGEMENT

- ABCs
  - Reversal of hypoxemia is priority
    - High flow O2 for respiratory distress in patients who are protecting airway
    - Intubation if not oxygenating, ventilating, or protecting airway
      - May develop noncardiogenic pulmonary edema or ARDS and require high levels of PEEP
  - Consider NGT
  - IV fluids 20 mL/kg warmed NS boluses for shock
- Look for signs of trauma and treat as indicated
- Treat hypothermia
- Maintain normothermia, normoglycemia, and avoid hypotension to maximize good neurologic outcome

DISPOSITION

- Discharge: following 4-8hr ED observation if asymptomatic and no deterioration or mildly symptomatic and symptoms resolve, and if CXR at end of observation is clear
  - Close follow-up with PCP
- Admit
  - Asymptomatic/mildly symptomatic patients who deteriorate in ED
  - Moderate to severely symptomatic patients — PICU

BEWARE

- ❗ Consider NAT/abuse if delays in seeking care, inconsistent histories
- ❗ Consider underlying medical conditions & possible traumatic injuries
- ❗ Educate patients and families: 80% of drownings are preventable
- ❗ Aspiration → risk for pneumonia

Section IX
Gastroenterology

1 ▶ Acute Gastroenteritis

BACKGROUND

- Inflammation of stomach and intestines → vomiting and diarrhea
  - Vomiting only in viral gastritis, diarrhea may come later
- Causes
  - Viral (*rotavirus, norovirus*), most common accounting for up to 80%
  - Bacterial (*Salmonella, Shigella, Campylobacter, E. coli*) less common, often more severe
  - Parasites (*Giardia*) uncommon in developed countries
  - Preformed toxins (*S. aureus, B. cereus*)
- Usually mild and self-limited, may lead to severe dehydration requiring hospitalization

EVALUATION

- **High Yield History**
  - Time since onset, nausea, vomiting, emesis color (bilious, bloody), diarrhea (blood, mucous), fever, oral intake, urine output, sick contacts, recent travel, recent antibiotic
- Exam
  - Dehydration delayed capillary refill, decreased tears, dry mouth, sunken eyes, poor skin turgor
  - Abdomen: nontender or mild, diffuse tenderness
    - Focal tenderness suggests alternative diagnosis
- **Diagnostics**
  - Labs
    - Mild/moderate dehydration and diagnosis clear: no labs indicated
    - Severe dehydration, dehydrated neonate, AMS, failed oral hydration
      - POC GLC, BMP
      - If diagnosis unclear, consider: CBC, CMP, ESR, CRP, lipase, UA
      - Low bicarbonate = higher suspicion for severe dehydration

- Stool studies: not routinely necessary
  - Stool culture indications: fever, diarrhea > 3 days, bloody diarrhea, recent international travel, toxic appearing
- Imaging: only if diagnosis uncertain

MANAGEMENT

- Hydration
  - Mild-mod: oral rehydration with a formulated oral rehydration solution (ORS) or dilute apple juice at 50-100 mL/kg over 3-4 hrs
  - Severe or inability to tolerate ORS: IV or NGT fluid resuscitation
    - Initial IV bolus of 20 mL/kg crystalloid, repeat PRN
- Antiemetics
  - Ondansetron 0.15 mg/kg (max 4 mg) IV/PO given 15-30 min prior to attempting ORS
    - Avoid in children < 6 mos
- Antibiotics: consider for *Shigella, Campylobacter*
  - Azithromycin 10 mg/kg (max 500 mg) PO daily × 3-5 days
  - NO antibiotics for *E. coli* O157:H7 as toxin release→ hemolytic uremic syndrome
  - Caution antibiotics for *Salmonella* — increases carrier state
    - Treat neonates, immunocompromised, prolonged symptoms
- Antidiarrheals not recommended for children

DISPOSITION

- Non-toxic appearing and tolerating PO: home with follow up
- Severely dehydrated, or not tolerating PO: admit for IV rehydration
- Consider other diagnoses if toxic-appearing

BEWARE

- Hemolytic uremic syndrome triad: acute renal failure, thrombocytopenia, and microangiopathic hemolytic anemia as gastroenteritis improving
- Suspect inflammatory bowel disease if prolonged bloody diarrhea, abdominal pain, weight loss, unexplained anemia
- Appendicitis may present with vomiting and diarrhea, consider if RLQ abdominal tenderness

2 ▶ Appendicitis

BACKGROUND
- Nonspecific obstruction of appendiceal lumen
- Epidemiology
  — 1-8% of children presenting to ED with abdominal pain
  — Lifetime risk 8.6% for boys, 6.7% for girls
  — 5% of all cases occur < 5 yrs, higher perforation rate

EVALUATION
- **High Yield History**
  — Anorexia, periumbilical pain, migration of pain to RLQ, vomiting
  — Symptoms vary depending on age (from most to least frequent):
    - 0-30 days: distention, vomiting, decreased oral intake, lethargy/irritability
    - < 5 yrs: abdominal pain, fever, vomiting, anorexia, diarrhea
    - 5-12 yrs: anorexia, vomiting, fever, diarrhea, nausea, pain with movement
- **Exam**
  — Tenderness at McBurney's point (one-third distance along line from anterior superior iliac spine to umbilicus)
  — Pain with coughing or hopping (also bouncing in car ride to hospital)
  — Psoas, obturator, Rovsing signs not sensitive
  — Signs of peritonitis/perforation: rigidity, rebound tenderness
  — Analgesia does NOT obscure exam
- **Diagnostics**
  — Labs: CBC with differential, CMP, UA
    - Consider CRP, procalcitonin, lipase, T&S
  — Imaging
    - Ultrasound
      ◆ Preferred initial diagnostic study to prevent ionizing radiation
      ◆ Sensitivity 88%, specificity 94%, operator dependent
      ◆ Non compressible tubular structure, overall diameter > 6 mm
      ◆ Corroborative: wall diameter > 2 mm, appendicolith, RLQ free fluid, hyperemia
    - CT abdomen/pelvis with IV contrast
      ◆ Higher yield than US, but delivers radiation
      ◆ Sensitivity 94%, specificity 95%
      ◆ When US equivocal and suspicion still high

- ◆ Fluid-filled tubular structure > 6mm diameter, periappendiceal inflammation, +/– appendicolith
- ▪ MRI abdomen/pelvis
  - ◆ Avoids radiation, less available
  - ◆ Sensitivity 96%, specificity 96%
— Scoring Tools
  - ▪ Pediatric appendicitis score (PAS), Alvarado score, Pediatric Appendicitis Risk Calculator (pARC)

MANAGEMENT

- Pain control ((morphine 0.05-0.1 mg/kg, max 4 mg IV), NPO, IV hydration, antiemetics PRN
- Antibiotics
  — Ceftriaxone 50 mg/kg (max 2 g) IV once daily
  — Metronidazole 10 mg/kg (max 500 mg) every 8 hrs
- Beta-lactam allergic: gentamicin 2.5 mg/kg IV every 8 hrs + metronidazole
- Surgery consult
  — Operative management typically standard
  — Non-operative management: primarily adult data shows good outcomes in patients *without* appendicolith
    - ▪ ~ ⅓ ultimately require appendectomy

DISPOSITION

- Admit unless surgeon recommends medical management

BEWARE

- ❗ Appendix may not be visualized early in course by US
- ❗ Patients < 5 yrs have high occurrence of misdiagnosis and increased complications
- ❗ Appendicitis commonly misdiagnosed as or mimicked by acute gastroenteritis (yersinia), constipation, Crohn's disease, UTI, mesenteric adenitis, pelvic disease (ovarian torsion, ectopic pregnancy), strep throat

3 ▶ Biliary Pathology

BACKGROUND

- Biliary atresia: inflammation and fibrosis → blockage of biliary tree lumen
  — Incidence: 1/12,000
  — Two forms
    - ▪ Perinatal or postnatal (90%): likely virally mediated

- Fetal or embryonic (10%): often associated malformations (cardiac, GI)
- Choledochal cysts: cystic dilations of the extrahepatic (and rarely intrahepatic) biliary ducts, usually congenital
  — Incidence: 1/13,000-1/100,000
- Cholecystitis/cholelithiasis
  — Acalculous cholecystitis much more common in children than adults
  — Risk factors: sickle cell disease, Crohn's disease, obesity, cystic fibrosis, Wilson's disease, prolonged total parenteral nutrition
  — See EMRA's *EM Fundamentals* chapter for further information

EVALUATION

	Biliary Atresia	Choledochal Cysts
History	• Jaundice (esp. > 1 week old), acholic stools, dark urine • Late disease: weight loss, failure to thrive	• Classic triad: RUQ mass, abdominal pain, jaundice • Vomiting, fever, acholic stools • Associated with (recurrent) cholangitis, pancreatitis
Exam	• Hepatosplenomegaly • Jaundice • Late disease: stigmata of liver failure	• Hepatosplenomegaly • Jaundice
Labs	• Direct hyperbilirubinemia, transaminitis, ↑ alkaline phosphatase, ↑ GGT	
Diagnosis	• US: abnormal or absent gallbladder (normal does not rule out atresia) • Liver biopsy usually diagnostic • ERCP if biopsy ambiguous • Intraoperative cholangiography if all previous workup ambiguous	• US: cystic lesions with normal or distended gallbladder • MRCP confirmatory • Similar presentation to biliary atresia, imaging differentiates

- ED work-up
  — Labs: CBC with differential, BMP, direct and total bilirubin, LFTs, GGT, PT/INR, PTT
    ▪ Direct hyperbilirubinemia > 1.0 mg/dL or > 20% total bilirubin should prompt investigation into pathologic causes of jaundice
  — Imaging: hepatobiliary ultrasound

MANAGEMENT

- Biliary atresia
  — Consult GI, pediatric surgeon
  — Kasai procedure
    ▪ Jejunum attached to porta hepatis, allowing any residual bile flow from intrahepatic ducts to drain into jejunum

- Complications: cholangitis occurs in up to 50% of cases
— Early diagnosis is key!
  - Surgery at < 60 days of age: good bile flow in 80%
  - Surgery performed later: only 20-30% achieve good bile flow
— Liver transplant eventually required in up to 70-80% of patients who have a Kasai procedure
- Choledochal cyst
  — Consult Surgery for excision

DISPOSITION

- Admit: biliary atresia, choledochal cyst, suspected cholangitis
- Discharge with prompt Surgery follow-up: stable choledochal cyst

BEWARE

- Prolonged jaundice past first week of life, direct hyperbilirubinemia, malnutrition, poor weight gain, recurrent cholangitis, recurrent pancreatitis (↑ suspicion for biliary atresia/choledochal cysts)
- Maintain high index of suspicion for cholangitis in febrile patient who has had a Kasai procedure
  — Sepsis work-up, admit for empiric IV antibiotics

4 ▶ Bowel Obstruction

BACKGROUND

- Partial or complete interruption in forward flow of small or large bowel contents
- Intussusception (most common cause in < 2 yrs), malrotation with midgut volvulus, incarcerated inguinal hernias common causes of SBO in children vs. intestinal adhesions in adults

Neonatal	Childhood
• NICU/Nursery —Duodenal atresia —Omphaloceles/Gastroschisis • May present to ED —Malrotation of bowel with midgut volvulus (most common in first month of life) —Meconium ileus —Necrotizing enterocolitis	• Adhesions • Annular pancreas • Duodenal hematoma • Foreign body ingestion/bezoar • Hernias (inguinal, mesocolic) • Intussusception • Malrotation of bowel with midgut volvulus • Pyloric stenosis

EVALUATION

- **High Yield History**
  — Colicky, cramping abdominal pain with vomiting (often bilious), +/– distention, +/– obstipation of gas or stool, +/– blood per rectum
  — Neonate/Infant
    - Bilious vomiting concerning for malrotation
    - Irritable, inconsolable crying, poor feeding, flexed hips to decrease tension, possibly altered/lethargic/somnolent
  — Older children avoid motion due to pain
  — Bilious/bloody emesis, projectile vomiting, bloody stools
  — PMH: prior abdominal surgeries, hernia, IBD, lymphoma, immunocompromised state
- **Exam**
  — If obstruction high in intestinal tract, abdomen may not be distended
  — Lower intestinal obstruction → abdominal distention, tympany, diffuse tenderness, hyperactive/hypoactive/absent bowel sounds
  — Peritonitis if bowel perforation or vascular insufficiency
    - Signs of sepsis
  — Genitourinary: incarcerated hernia
    - Tender inguinal mass, reducibility
      - Don't attempt reduction if overlying skin discoloration
- **Diagnostics**
  — Labs: CBC, CMP, lactate
    - Hypochloremic hypokalemic metabolic alkalosis from recurrent vomiting
    - Metabolic acidosis and hyperkalemia in bowel strangulation
  — Imaging
    - KUB (include upright or left lateral decubitus for air-fluid levels, free air)
      - SBO: dilated small bowel loops with absence of air in lower abdomen
      - Double-bubble sign for duodenal atresia or malrotation with volvulus
    - POCUS: dilated bowel loops
    - Upper GI series with small bowel follow-through can help determine obstruction location
    - Need for CT depends on suspected diagnosis

MANAGEMENT

- ABCs
- Analgesia, consider morphine at 0.1 mg/kg (max 4 mg) IV if severe pain
- Evaluate for sepsis, give fluids, and correct electrolyte imbalances as needed

- Early bowel decompression with NGT
- Broad spectrum antibiotics when necrosis or perforation is suspected
  - Ceftriaxone 50 mg/kg (max 2 g) IV every 12 hrs + metronidazole 10 mg/kg (max 500 mg) IV every 8 hrs
  - Piperacillin/tazobactam 75 mg/kg (max 4 g) IV every 6 hrs
- Surgery consult
- Intussusception will need enema reduction

DISPOSITION
- Admit

BEWARE
- ❗ Ladd procedure (malrotation) predisposes children to postoperative intussusception, wound infection, feeding difficulties, ascites, pneumonitis, constipation
- ❗ Peristalsis-inducing medication (metoclopramide) contraindicated in complete mechanical bowel obstruction

5 ▶ Constipation

BACKGROUND
- Classification
  - Functional: painful defecation resulting in withholding behavior and eventual incontinence
  - Organic: bowel obstruction, cystic fibrosis, Hirschsprung's disease, diabetes insipidus, imperforate anus, spinal cord abnormalities, heavy-metal poisoning, medication side effects, metabolic (hypothyroidism, hypercalcemia, hypokalemia), neurologic disorders, infantile botulism
- Normal stooling patterns
  - Newborn: 3-4 stools/day in first week
    - Breastfed infants: 7 days between bowel movements can be normal if no excessive straining or pebble-like stools
  - Toddler: 2 stools/day
  - Preschool: 1 stool/day to every other day
- Hirschsprung's disease (aganglionosis of rectosigmoid colon)
  - Delayed meconium passage > 48 hrs, chronic constipation
  - Complications: toxic megacolon (distended abdomen, bilious vomiting), enterocolitis (diarrhea, rectal bleeding, distention, fever)

EVALUATION

- **High Yield History**
  - Age at onset
  - Meconium passage
  - Frequency, consistency, size of stools, bloody or painful, fecal incontinence
    - Withholding behavior suggests functional constipation
    - Straining, grunting, turning red in face can be normal in young children
      - Not constipation if stool frequency and consistency normal
  - Abdominal pain
  - Systemic symptoms
  - Diet, stressors, laxative use
  - Family history
  - Red Flags: onset < 1 mo old, delayed meconium passage, abdominal distension, intermittent/explosive diarrhea, empty rectum (Hirschsprung); failure to thrive; sacral dimple/ tuft (spinal dysraphism)
- **Exam**
  - Growth
  - Abdominal exam
    - Functional constipation normal exam or mild diffuse tenderness, palpable stool
  - Perineum/perianal exam for sensation, fissures, anal tone, reflexes (cremasteric, anal wink), consider digital rectal exam
  - Thyroid, spine anomalies
- **Diagnostics**
  - Functional constipation, no studies indicated
  - Labs depending on suspicion: TSH, BMP, lead and drug levels, tissue transglutaminase/ IgA for celiac, sweat test for cystic fibrosis
  - Imaging
    - KUB: NOT routinely recommended
    - Barium enema for suspected Hirschsprung's

MANAGEMENT

- No encopresis (stool leakage) or red flags
  - Diet: increase fiber, diluted prune juice, 1 oz per mo of life (max 4 oz/day)
  - Polyethylene glycol 3350 1 g/kg (max 17 g/dose) with 8 oz fluid daily, for > 6 mo old
    - Continue for 2 months or until no constipation ×1 month

- Encopresis without red flags
  - Disimpaction
    - Glycerine suppository (infants)
    - Enema: pediatric fleets 3-12 years, adult fleets > 12 years
    - Manually
  - Bowel regimen: dietary modification, behavior modification, polyethylene glycol
- Secondary constipation/red flags: GI consult, workup, treat underlying disease

DISPOSITION
- Discharge if functional or non-emergent organic cause

BEWARE
- Constipation increases risk for UTIs

6 ▶ Enteral Feeding Tube Complications

BACKGROUND
- Placed surgically, endoscopically, or radiographically for supplemental nutrition
- Types: Percutaneous Endoscopic Gastrostomy (PEG) tube, gastrostomy tube (G-Tube), jejunostomy tube (J-Tube), gastrojejunostomy Tube (GJ-Tube)
  - Most extend several inches outside the body and have 2-3 ports (feeding, medication, +/– balloon port)
  - Gastric or jejunal buttons have a lower profile and 2 ports (feeding/medication, +/– balloon port)
  - Secured by water-filled balloon or bumper
- Tube-related complications: dislodgement, clogging, leaking, reflux, gastric ulceration, gastric outlet obstruction due to malposition
- Stomal complications: hypergranulation, peristomal cellulitis/abscess, fungal infection

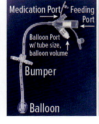
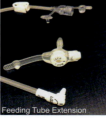
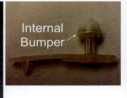

EVALUATION

- **High Yield History**
  - When was the tube placed?
  - What is the tube used for? Any oral intake?
    - Supplementation vs. all feeds
  - Type/size of tube?
  - How long has the tube been dislodged (if relevant)?
  - Pain, irritability, vomiting, hematemesis, hematochezia
- **Exam**
  - Rebound, guarding, abdominal distention may indicate peritonitis or obstruction
  - Leakage: check for gastric contents vs. pus vs. coffee ground drainage
  - Stoma site redness or purulent discharge may indicate infection
  - Check tube position: deeper than usual tube depth may indicate balloon migration into pylorus
- **Diagnostics:** assess location/confirm placement
  - Check pH of tube aspirate
  - Listen over stomach while insufflating air through tube
  - KUB with 10-20 mL water soluble contrast injected into tube
  - Bedside US

MANAGEMENT

- Dislodged PEG/G-Tube
  - Tract > 6-12 weeks old: may be mature, can replace tube in ED
    - Expeditious replacement or Foley placement reduces risk of stoma closure (< 3 hrs)
  - Tract < 6-12 weeks old: may be immature, consult specialist
  - If unable to pass same size tube, downsize or use Foley to dilate tract
  - If cannot easily withdraw gastric fluid after reinsertion, use contrast injection imaging to confirm placement in stomach
- Dislodged GJ-Tube/J-tube: consult specialist
- Clogged tube: instill warm water or carbonated beverage for 15-20 min, then flush
  - Consider alkalinized pancreatic enzymes if flushing unsuccessful
  - If cannot unclog, consider tube replacement (consult specialist if tract < 6-12 weeks old)
- Leaking gastric contents around tube: ensure balloon is inflated and abuts internal GI mucosa, ensure appropriate tube size

- Gastric ulceration if tip of G-tube or balloon over-dilation irritates stomach mucosa
  — Perform saline lavage, if nonbloody, can start H2-blocker antacid, sucralfate, schedule upper endoscopy
- Gastric outlet obstruction: tube tip accidentally migrates to pyloric channel or esophagus
  — Pull back until snug against abdominal wall; if unsuccessful, remove tube
- Hypergranulation around stoma: silver nitrate cauterization, topical steroids (triamcinolone cream 0.5% two times daily), barrier creams, polyurethane foam dressing
- Peristomal cellulitis: oral ABx covering skin flora

DISPOSITION

- Discharge most cases +/– specialist follow-up
- Admit: severe peristomal cellulitis/abscess, intra-abdominal infection, GI obstruction, unable to re-insert tube and needing hydration/nutrition

BEWARE

- Replacing tubes with tracts < 6-12 weeks old or using too much force risks creating a false tract
- If a tube with a plastic bumper cannot be rotated but flushes into the stomach, consider buried bumper syndrome (bumper eroded into abdominal wall) and consult specialist

7 ▶ Gastrointestinal Bleeding

BACKGROUND

- Upper GI bleed (UGIB): proximal to ligament of Treitz, hematemesis, melena or hematochezia
- Lower GI bleed (LGIB): distal to ligament of Treitz, melena or hematochezia
- Epidemiology
  — Most ED visits for pediatric GI bleeding in 15-19 yrs (40%) and 0-5 yrs (38%)
  — 80% do not need hospitalization or intervention
  — UGIB greater mortality than LGIB
- Non-GI DDx: bleeding diathesis, coagulopathy, swallowed maternal blood or epistaxis

DIFFERENTIAL BY AGE

Age	Upper GI Bleed	Lower GI Bleed
Neonate	<ul><li>Esophagitis, gastritis, stress ulcers</li><li>Gastrointestinal duplication</li><li>Hemorrhagic disease of the newborn</li><li>Malrotation/volvulus</li><li>Swallowed maternal blood</li><li>Vascular anomalies</li></ul>	<ul><li>Anal fissure</li><li>Hirschsprung-associated enterocolitis</li><li>Infectious colitis</li><li>Necrotizing enterocolitis</li><li>Malrotation/volvulus</li><li>Meckel's diverticulum</li><li>Milk protein intolerance</li></ul>
Infant (1 mo to 2 yrs)	<ul><li>Epistaxis</li><li>Esophagitis</li><li>Foreign body</li><li>Gastritis</li><li>Gastrointestinal duplication</li><li>Mallory-Weiss tear</li><li>Malrotation/volvulus</li><li>Peptic ulcer disease (PUD)</li><li>Pyloric stenosis (< 2 mo)</li></ul>	<ul><li>Anal fissure</li><li>Intussusception</li><li>Milk protein allergy</li><li>Polyps</li><li>PUD</li><li>Meckel diverticulum</li></ul>
Children & Adolescents (2+ yrs)	<ul><li>Epistaxis</li><li>Esophageal varices</li><li>Esophagitis (pill esophagitis)</li><li>Gastritis</li><li>Hemobilia (trauma)</li><li>Mallory-Weiss tear</li><li>PUD (*H. pylori*, stress)</li><li>Toxic ingestion (caustic substance)</li><li>Vascular malformation</li></ul>	<ul><li>Anal fissure</li><li>Colitis (ischemic, pseudomembranous)</li><li>Enteric infections (*Salmonella, Shigella, E. coli O157:H7, C. difficile*)</li><li>Hemolytic Uremic Syndrome</li><li>Hemorrhoids</li><li>Inflammatory bowel disease</li><li>Intussusception</li><li>Meckel's diverticulum</li><li>Polyps</li><li>PUD</li><li>Rectal prolapse</li><li>Vasculitis (Henoch-Schonlein Purpura)</li><li>Vascular malformation</li></ul>

EVALUATION

- **High Yield History**
  - Color, location, timing, volume of bleeding, food/foreign body ingestion
  - Associated symptoms: fever, dizziness, fatigue, palpitations, abdominal pain, diarrhea, weight loss
  - Birth history, PMH (hepatitis, heart failure, biliary atresia), prior UVC line placement (risk of portal vein thrombosis), medications, family history of IBD/colon cancer/coagulopathy
  - Consider biliary atresia in jaundiced > 2 wks old
  - UGIB: nausea, color and content of vomit (bilious or bloody), NSAID or SSRI use, recent trauma, recent illnesses
  - LGIB: travel history, stool pattern and consistency, pain with defecation, tenesmus, allergies
- **Exam**
  - Assess for signs of shock
  - Skin assessment: conjunctival pallor, scleral icterus, delayed capillary refill, petechiae, mucosal bleeding, spider telangiectasias
  - Abdominal exam: hepatosplenomegaly, ascites, epigastric or RUQ tenderness, rebound tenderness, surgical scars, mass
  - Stool occult blood, anal fissures, hemorrhoids
- **Diagnostics**
  - Labs: CBC, CMP, PT/INR, PTT, lipase, type and cross, ABG & lactate if in shock
    - ↑ BUN:creatinine ratio > 30 suggests UGIB over LGIB
      - Normal does not rule out GI bleed
    - Consider stool studies for LGIB with likely infectious cause
    - ESR, CRP, fecal calprotectin if concern for IBD
    - Apt-Downey test can differentiate neonatal from maternal blood
  - Imaging
    - US if suspect intussusception
    - KUB if suspect foreign body, NEC, obstruction, perforation
    - CT abdomen/pelvis w/ contrast if emergent concerns regarding inflammation, extraintestinal complications, surgical problems
    - Technetium-99 (Meckel) scan for painless rectal bleeding
  - Endoscopy or colonoscopy if indicated

MANAGEMENT

- UGIB — hemodynamically unstable
  - ABCs
  - Volume resuscitation
    - Crystalloids (LR, NS) at 20 mL/kg initially
    - PRBC at 10 mL/kg for Hgb < 7 g/dL or Hgb < 10 g/dL and unstable
    - Enough to maintain adequate perfusion, overexpansion can lead to rebleeding; goal post-transfusion Hgb 7-8 g/dL
  - Correct coagulopathies if actively bleeding: IV Vitamin K, FFP 10 mL/kg
  - Platelet transfusion 5-10 mL/kg if < 50,000
  - Consider NGT lavage with room temperature saline or water to evaluate for ongoing bleeding
  - Pantoprazole 1 mg/kg (max 80 mg) IV bolus + 0.1 mg/kg/hr (max 8 mg/hr)
  - Octreotide 1-2 mcg/kg bolus (max 50 mcg) with 1-2 mcg/kg/hr infusion (max 4 mcg/hr) for suspected variceal bleeding
  - Antibiotics: potential for sepsis, especially in bleeding varices
  - GI consult for emergent EGD for diagnosis and intervention
- LGIB
  - Rarely life-threatening
  - Supportive care: rehydrate, correct electrolyte imbalance/anemia, treat superinfection
  - Assess for potential complications needing surgical intervention
  - Colonoscopy for suspected colonic lesions, polyps, vascular malformations with active bleeding
- Peptic Ulcer Disease (stable)
  - Outpatient diagnostic testing
  - H2-receptor antagonists: famotidine 0.5 mg/kg (max 40 mg) PO daily at bedtime
  - Proton pump inhibitor: omeprazole 1 mg/kg (max 40 mg) PO daily
  - Sucralfate 10-20 mg/kg (max 1 g) PO four times daily, 1 hr before meals and at bedtime, not given with other medications

DISPOSITION

- Discharge: stable, reliable close follow-up in 48-72 hrs
- Admit
  - Large-volume blood loss
  - LGIB and abdominal pain, unless clear diagnosis and outpatient treatment plan

BEWARE

- ⓘ Is it blood? Rule out foods or medications that may mimic blood in stool or vomitus
  - Bright red blood: food coloring, juices, red candy, beets, tomato skins, cefdinir, rifampin
  - Melena: bismuth, iron preparations, spinach, blueberries, licorice, chocolate
- ⓘ Is it GI? Consider vaginal bleeding, hematuria

8 ▶ Inflammatory Bowel Disease (IBD)

BACKGROUND

- Crohn's Disease (CD): discontinuous transmural inflammation of GI tract, particularly terminal ileum and colon, discrete aphthous or linear ulceration
  - 20% with perianal involvement (skin tags, fissures, fistulas, abscesses)
- Ulcerative Colitis (UC): continuous mucosal inflammation confined to colon/rectum, possible terminal ileitis in pancolitis
- Epidemiology: 25% of IBD patients present < 20 yrs old, 18% < 10 yrs old, 4% < 5 yrs old

EVALUATION

- **High Yield History**
  - Abdominal pain, rectal bleeding, bloody diarrhea, stool characteristics, number of stools/day, nocturnal stools, limitation of physical activity
  - Extra intestinal manifestations (EIMs): erythema nodosum, pyoderma gangrenosum, arthritis, growth failure, osteopenia, osteoporosis, episcleritis, uveitis, iritis, nephrolithiasis, pancreatitis, anemia, venous thromboembolism
  - Associated conditions: ankylosing spondylosis, primary sclerosing cholangitis, autoimmune hepatitis
- **Exam**
  - Fever ≥ 38°C, tachycardia, dehydration, AMS, hypotension
  - Abdominal: tenderness, rebound tenderness, guarding
  - Mucosal ulcerations, anal fissures
  - Rash
- **Diagnostics**
  - Labs
    - CBC w/diff, CMP, ESR, CRP, albumin, lipase, +/− lactate
    - Stool studies, culture for *Salmonella, Shigella, Campylobacter, Yersinia, E. Coli O157, C. difficile* toxin, ova and parasites, occult blood
    - Fecal calprotectin, fecal lactoferrin

- Imaging
  - KUB to rule out toxic megacolon
    - Transverse colon diameter ≥ 56 mm for ≥ 10 yrs or > 40 mm in < 10 yrs
  - US: > 2 mm wall thickness small intestine, > 3-4 mm wall thickness large intestine
  - Consider abdominal CT or MRI if signs of peritonitis/unexplained deterioration but negative KUB
- Esophagogastroduodenoscopy (EGD), ileocolonoscopy with biopsy

MANAGEMENT

- IV hydration, correct electrolyte abnormalities
- Pain control: morphine 0.1 mg/kg IV (max 4 mg/dose); avoid NSAIDs
- Consult GI early (corticosteroids, immune modulators, ABx, etc.)
- Infectious colitis
  - Ciprofloxacin 10-15 mg/kg (max 500 mg) PO two times daily [not routinely used in young children] + metronidazole 7.5 mg/kg (max 500 mg) PO three times daily
  - Vancomycin 10 mg/kg (max 125 mg) PO four times daily until *C. difficile* status known
- Some experts avoid salicylates in acute flares (may worsen symptoms)
- Immunomodulators typically continued during flares; discuss with GI specialist

DISPOSITION

- Admit: significant flare requiring IV steroids or immunosuppressive agents
- Discharge with close outpatient GI follow-up: mild flare, no infectious source

BEWARE

- Suspect IBD: child falling off the growth curve, chronic diarrhea, unexplained anemia
- Suspect toxic megacolon → consult surgery
- Complications to watch out for: intestinal obstruction, fistulae / perforation

9 ▶ Intussusception

BACKGROUND

- Invagination or "telescoping" of one bowel segment into another (most common ileocolic)
  - Compression of vessels within segments can → bowel ischemia, necrosis, perforation
- Epidemiology: most cases 5-9 mo of age, ⅔ occur < 12 mo
  - Males 2:1 predominance

- Common causes: most idiopathic; ~5% pathologic lead points
- Predisposing conditions: Meckel's diverticulum, polyps, lymphoid hyperplasia, cystic fibrosis, Henoch-Schönlein Purpura

EVALUATION

- **High Yield History**: classic triad (colicky abdominal pain, vomiting, bloody stools) present in < 40%
  - Atypical presentations: AMS (irritability, lethargy), transient hypertension, sepsis, syncope
- **Exam**: often normal if not currently intussuscepting or ischemic bowel
  - May have palpable abdominal mass, often RLQ
  - Assess for peritonitis, shock
- **Diagnostics**
  - Labs: often normal
    - CBC, BMP for significant vomiting, pre-op
  - Imaging: US imaging of choice, nearly 100% sensitive/specific, may show target, bullseye, doughnut signs (transverse view) and pseudokidney or sandwich sign (longitudinal view)
    - KUB not sensitive/specific; can help evaluate perforation

MANAGEMENT

- Early Radiology consult with surgeon available for complications
- Fluid resuscitation (often dehydrated)
- NGT only if evidence of obstruction, persistent vomiting
- Enema reduction
  - Air enemas preferred; less caustic than barium in case of perforation
  - Perforation is the most common complication, < 1% occurrence
- Laparotomy reduction
  - Unsuccessful enema reduction, unstable, perforation/peritonitis, rectal bleeding > 48 hrs, known pathological lead point
  - Prophylactic IV ABx covering enteric flora
- 10% intussusceptions reduced non-operatively will recur
  - Manage with repeat enema if first was partially/completely successful

DISPOSITION

- Discharge: stable, benign abdomen, tolerating clear fluids within 2 hrs after enema reduction, reliable to return with precautions
- Risk of early (< 48 hr) recurrence < 4%
- Pediatrician vs. pediatric surgery clinic follow up within 1-2 days

BEWARE

- ⊙ Clinical suspicion is key: a child may appear well with no exam/US findings if bowel is not telescoped at presentation (intermittent intussusception)
  - Suspect in lethargic toddler even if no GI symptoms
- ⊙ Fever is common after reduction, attributed to inflammatory response

10 ▶ Pyloric Stenosis

BACKGROUND

- Epidemiology: 2- 3.5 per 1000 live births
- First-born, male, young mother, infant 2-6 weeks of age, rare after 12 weeks
- Risk factors: maternal smoking, bottle feeding, family history, macrolide use, prematurity

EVALUATION

- **High Yield History**: immediate postprandial non-bilious projectile vomiting, strong appetite, low urine output
- **Exam**: evaluate for dehydration, palpate for olive-like mass at the lateral edge of the rectus abdominis muscle in the right upper quadrant (pathognomonic)
  - Difficult to feel — lack of finding doesn't exclude
  - Tip: give sugar water to relax infant; examine immediately after an episode of emesis
- **Diagnostics**
  - Labs (abnormalities less common due to earlier presentation)
    - Hypochloremic, hypokalemic, metabolic alkalosis
    - BUN and creatinine to assess for dehydration and renal insufficiency
    - Unconjugated hyperbilirubinemia can be seen, and is associated with icteropyloric syndrome
  - Imaging
    - US preferred due to safety profile
      - Operator dependent, sensitivity and specificity > 95%
      - Evaluate for target sign on transverse view
      - Pyloric muscle thickness > 3 mm and pyloric muscle length > 10-14 mm
        - Tip: Pi = π = 3.14 (remember: π-loric stenosis)
    - Upper GI: second line option, due to radiation exposure
      - Evaluate for elongated pyloric canal (string aka apple core sign)

MANAGEMENT
- NPO
- IVF: correct electrolyte abnormalities, dehydration prior to surgical management
  — IV bolus 20 cc/kg NS if dehydrated
  — If euvolemic with normal electrolytes, start maintenance IV fluids
- Consult Surgery for pyloromyotomy

DISPOSITION
- Admit with surgical consultation for rehydration and surgical management

BEWARE
- Premature infants may not have the classic US measurements
- Due to earlier clinical presentations, patients may appear well without dehydration or electrolyte abnormalities, and may not have US findings

Section X
Genetics/Metabolism

1 ▶ Common Syndromes

Syndrome	Clinical Features	Comorbidities	ED Considerations

Turner Syndrome (45 ×0, may have mosaicism)	• Short stature (< 5%ile)
	• Lack of sexual development
	• Shield chest
	• Pectus excavatum
	• Webbed neck
	• Down-turned mouth, ptosis, low ears
		• 50% with cardiac anomaly:
		  — Aortic coarctation
		  — Bicuspid aortic valve
		  — QT prolongation
		• Hypertension (25%)
		• Renal anomalies (10% horseshoe kidney)
		  — Recurrent UTI
		• Learning difficulties
		• Chronic otitis media
		• Autoimmune disease
			• Difficult intubation: micrognathia, high-arched palate, short-neck
			• ↑ risk of aortic dissection
			• Prone to cardiac dysrhythmias
			• Increased risk of autoimmune: DM, Hashimoto's, celiac, IBD

Down Syndrome (Trisomy 21)	• Flattened facies with upslanting palpebral fissures • Macroglossia • Brushfield spots • Hallux valgus • Palmar simian crease • Developmental delay • Growth retardation	• CHD (50%) • Atlanto-axial instability • Increased risk of hematologic disorders / malignancy • GI malformations • Stroke • Early onset Alzheimer's • Endocrine abnormalities (thyroid)	• Difficult airway: Macroglossia, C-spine instability (requires neutral neck placement for intubation) • ↑ risk leukemia, DM, thyroid disorders

Syndrome	Clinical Features	Comorbidities	ED Considerations

Marfan Syndrome (Autosomal dominant connective tissue disorder)	• Long arms/legs with mobile joints
	• Pectus excavatum or carinatum
	• Scoliosis/kyphosis
	• Hindfoot valgus
	• Ectopia lentis (50-80%)
		• Cardiac (> 80%)
		  — Aortic dissection
		  — Thoracic aortic aneurysm
		  — Mitral valve prolapse
		• Upward lens dislocation
			• High risk for aortic dissection, retinal detachment, pneumothorax, joint dislocation

Muscular Dystrophy (X-linked recessive mutations in dystrophin gene)	• Onset of weakness between 2-4 years (Duchenne), 5+ years (Becker) • Winged scapulae • Pseudohypertrophy of calf muscles • Gowers' sign • Poor growth	• Dilated cardiomyopathy • Scoliosis • Elevated CK • Recurrent fractures • Recurrent pneumonia	• Avoid succinylcholine: higher risk for hyperkalemia, rhabdomyolysis • Patients often on long-term corticosteroids
Williams Syndrome (Autosomal dominant gene deletion in chromosome 7, most sporadic)	• Elfin facies • "Cocktail party" personality • Progressive hypertension • CHD 80-90%	• Supravalvular aortic stenosis • Cardiac hypertrophy and failure • Failure to thrive • Systemic arterial stenosis • Hypercalcemia • Recurrent UTIs	• Difficult airway: mandibular hypoplasia • Consider diagnosis if failure to thrive + murmur • Do not give multivitamins, Vit D → hypercalcemia
Pierre-Robin Sequence (Etiology unclear)	• Triad of micrognathia, retroglossoptosis, cleft palate • Conductive hearing loss • Failure to thrive	• Epilepsy • Undescended testes • Ocular anomalies • Cardiovascular anomalies • Recurrent otitis media • Obstructive sleep apnea	• Very difficult intubation; rapid facial growth 3-12 months lessens difficulty • Viral illnesses may worsen laryngomalacia

Syndrome	Clinical Features	Comorbidities	ED Considerations
Treacher Collins (Autosomal dominant gene mutation)	• Cleft palate • Malar hypoplasia • Micro/retrognathia • Normal intelligence • Absent eyelid lashes	• Choanal stenosis, atresia • Vision loss, cataracts • Conductive hearing loss • Feeding difficulties	• Very difficult intubation due to severe micrognathia
Prader-Willi Syndrome (absence of paternally derived gene on chromosome 15)	• Failure to thrive first months of life • Hyperphagia, food seeking, obesity • Developmental delay • Hypogonadism • Hypotonicity	• Diabetes • Fatty liver disease • Obstructive Sleep Apnea • Hypothyroidism • Osteoporosis • Frequent cellulitis due to skin picking	• Difficult airway: Obesity, difficult to ventilate w/ O2 saturation decreasing rapidly

EVALUATION

- **High Yield History**
  - Prior work-up and complications of their disorder
  - Advance directives, limitations of care, family goals
  - Ask family about pain, mental status, symptoms
  - Utilize family and PCP notes for background on baseline mental status, neuro exam
- **Exam**
  - Identify proper equipment sizes (airway equipment, G-tube, etc.)
    - Children with genetic syndromes often small for age
  - Look for signs of neglect, NAT, sexual abuse
  - Evaluate for skin breakdown/infection (sedentary, skin picking in Prader-Willi syndrome)
- **Diagnostics**
  - ↑ risk of electrolyte disturbances
  - ↑ DM, thyroid disorders

MANAGEMENT

- Airway management considerations
  - General
    - Avoid procedural sedation in ED

- If need to intubate, assume difficult airway
- Consult Anesthesia early
- Have surgical airway backup ready
- Consider laryngeal mask airway, video laryngoscopy, or fiberoptic intubation
— Pierre-Robin, Treacher Collins
  - Micrognathia and obstructing tongue make for difficult intubation
  - Tongue-jaw lift
  - Placement of OPA may help with bag ventilation
  - Consider LMA
— Prader-Willi
  - May be difficult to maintain airway, prepare to intubate early
  - Oxygen saturation may ↓ more quickly (obesity)
— Muscular Dystrophy
  - Do NOT use succinylcholine; higher risk for hyperkalemia and rhabdomyolysis
  - Poor reserve and ↑ risk for rapid hypoxia & hypercapnia
— Down Syndrome
  - Atlantoaxial instability: keep neck in neutral position
  - Macroglossia
- Other considerations
  — Maintain high index of suspicion for cardiac complications/associated CHD
  — Avoid multivitamins in Williams syndrome; Vitamin D may worsen hypercalcemia
  — Consider c-spine injury in children with Down Syndrome involved in acceleration/deceleration injuries
- Consult geneticist

2 ▶ Inborn Errors of Metabolism (IEM)

BACKGROUND

- Disorders affecting metabolism of fats, amino acids, organic acids, carbohydrates, commonly resulting in incomplete metabolism and/or production of toxic metabolites
- Most common types
  — Carbohydrate metabolism defects
  — Urea cycle defects
  — Select amino acid disorders
  — Organic acid disorders
  — Fatty acid oxidation defects

- More important to have suspicion for IEMs as a whole than to diagnose specific IEM in ED
- Neonatal screen identifies most IEMs early; pts will present with "Emergency Protocol" sheets
  - IEM test results often do not return until 2 weeks of life
  - False negative newborn screening can occur
  - Testing is per-state; caretakers can decline in some states
- Incidence as many as 1 in 2,500-5,000 live births
- Most autosomal recessive or X-linked inheritance
- May be immunocompromised with ↑ risk for sepsis during metabolic crises

EVALUATION

- **High Yield History**
  - Neonate
    - Vomiting, diarrhea, poor feeding, hemodynamic instability, jaundice, hepatomegaly, irritability, lethargy, coma, seizures, abnormal tone
    - Can present hours to days after birth if IEM defect severe
    - Recent change from breastfeeding to formula (due to protein content)
    - Commonly pyruvate carboxylase deficiency, urea cycle defects, organic acidemias
  - Infant/young child
    - Recurrent vomiting, lethargy out of proportion to vomiting, ataxia, seizures, coma, developmental delay, dysmorphism, failure to thrive, hypertrophic cardiomyopathy, hepatomegaly
    - Often presents when advance from formula/breastmilk to food
    - Commonly: glycogen and lipid storage diseases, fructose intolerance
  - Older child/teen
    - Subtle neurologic or psychiatric abnormalities, behavioral problems, profound developmental delay, anxiety, emotional lability, panic attacks, paranoia, seizures, peripheral neuropathy, exercise intolerance
    - Commonly: fatty-oxidation defects, partial urea cycle defects, glycogen storage diseases
  - Stressors that can induce catabolic state
    - Change in feeding intervals or change in content of diet (advancement of diet to include fruits, milk etc.)
    - Infection, sepsis
    - Puberty
    - Trauma/surgery

- When to suspect IEM
  - Multiple admissions for dehydration/lethargy that improves with fluids and glucose
  - Recurrent admissions for "infections" of unclear etiology
  - Unexplained severe acidosis/ketosis or metabolic derangements that are not correcting as expected after initial resuscitation
  - Continued vomiting despite multiple formula changes
  - DDx for any critically ill neonate
- **Exam**
  - General: AMS, lethargy, coma, abnormal odor, hypothermia
  - HEENT: cataracts, retinopathy, dysmorphic features
  - Cardiovascular: can have bradycardia or tachycardia
  - Pulmonary: tachypnea
  - Abdominal: hepatomegaly, splenomegaly
  - Neuro: developmental delay, weakness, ataxia, hypotonia
- **Diagnostics**
  - Labs (MUST collect before treating)
    - Include extra red top tubes and save urine for further studies
    - Classic findings in very ill
      - Hypoglycemia: Primary defect vs. consumptive process
      - Metabolic acidosis
      - Hyperammonemia

IEM	Blood Glucose	Ketones	Ammonia
Amino Acidopathies	↓	↑	←→
Organic Acidemias	↓	↑↑	↑
Urea Cycle Defects	←→	↑	↑↑
Fatty Acid Oxidation Defect	↓↓	↓↓	←→
Carbohydrate Disorders	↓↓	↑	←→

- Initial workup: CBC, CMP, blood gas, PT/INR, PTT, ammonia, LDH, CK, lactate, urinalysis (for reducing substrate and ketones)
  - Anion gap > 30-50 likely = organic acidemia
- Workup guided by metabolic specialist consult

MANAGEMENT

- ABCs
- Can initiate ED management without knowledge of exact diagnosis
  — Goals: stop catabolism, reduce toxic metabolite formation, correct electrolyte and acid-base abnormalities
- NPO (prevents further accumulation of toxic metabolites)
- Fluids: bolus 10-20 mL/kg NS
  — Avoid LR (worsening lactic acidosis in some IEMs)
- Hypoglycemia
  — Correct any hypoglycemia, even mild, with dextrose bolus: 0.25 to 1 g/kg D10 (neonate) or D25 (child)
    - Neonate: 2 mL/kg D10 = 0.2 g/kg
    - Child: 5 mL/kg D10 = 0.5 g/kg or 2mL/kg D25 = 0.5 g/kg
  — Follow with D10NS at maintenance to provide 8-12 mg/kg/min of glucose
    - To give 8 mg/kg/min of glucose: infusion rate in mL/hr = 8 mg/kg/min × weight(kg) × 60 / (dextrose concentration in gm/dL × 10)
      - Ex: 10 kg child, using D10: (8 × 10 × 60)/(10×10) = 48 mL/hr
    - Empirically, begin with 1-1.5x maintenance
  — Maintain serum glucose 120-170 mg/dL
- Metabolic acidosis
  — For severe acidosis, (pH < 7.0) treat with sodium bicarbonate 1 mEq/kg IV then 0.25-0.5 mEq/kg/hr
    - Treat acidosis of organic acidemia more aggressively at pH < 7.2 or bicarbonate 14-16 mmol/L
    - Caution, rapid correction may precipitate rapid fluid shifts, cerebral edema/hemorrhage, and decreased urine excretion of ammonia
    - Prevent hypernatremia with coadministration of potassium acetate 0.1-0.25 mEq/kg/hr
  — Hemodialysis is definitive treatment
- Hyperammonemia
  — Hemodialysis most rapid option when ammonia levels > 300-350 mcg/dL
  — Ammonia > 200 mcg/dL: give sodium phenylacetate and sodium benzoate for suspected urea cycle disorder
    - Eliminates nitrogen via alternative pathway
    - Dose 250 mg/kg = 2.5 mL/kg for patients ≤ 20 kg
    - 55 mL/m^2 = 5.5 g/m^2 IV for patients > 20 kg

- Dilute in 25 mL/kg of D10, give IV over 90-120 min
            - Replace potassium as needed with potassium acetate
        - Consider arginine HCl 10% IV 200-600 mg/kg over 2 hrs, then 600 mg/kg over 24 hr drip
        - Avoid steroids → induce protein catabolism → exacerbate hyperammonemia
- Evaluate and manage sepsis
    - High index of suspicion for concurrent sepsis in ill-appearing
    - BCx, empiric broad spectrum antibiotics as indicated
    - Galactosemia associated with *E. Coli* sepsis risk
- Carnitine important cofactor in many metabolic pathways and part of tx for organic acidurias and fatty acid oxidation disorders
    - Carnitine 50-200 mg/kg IV bolus safe for undifferentiated but highly suspected
- Coagulopathy may be amenable to treatment with Vitamin K 1-2 mg IM in infant, 5-10 mg IM in child
- Consult Metabolic Specialist early (empiric cofactors pyridoxine, folinic acid, biotin, riboflavin, cobalamin)

DISPOSITION

- Admit most; may take days to weeks to resolve and IVF/dextrose needed to prevent metabolic problems (hypoglycemia/ketosis)
- Do not discharge unless metabolic problem resolved and pt can maintain adequate oral caloric intake
- If child dies, important to obtain specimens for IEM diagnosis; counsel regarding risk to siblings, parents, or future children

BEWARE

❗ Be suspicious of the neonate that had normal good health ranging from hours to weeks of life and then deteriorates

❗ May present with intracranial bleeds or retinal hemorrhage due to coagulopathy; can be mistaken for NAT

Section XI
Genitourinary Complaints

1 ▶ Female-Specific Pathology

BACKGROUND
- GU diagnoses common in adolescent females with abdominal complaints

EVALUATION
- **High Yield History**
  - Age at menarche, LMP, cycle length, duration/amount of flow, intermenstrual/postcoital bleeding
  - Vaginal discharge, itching, use of bubble bath, douching
  - Sexual activity (type, dyspareunia, abuse/assault), contraception, prior STI/ vaginitis
  - Anemia, fatigue, fever
- **Exam**
  - Examine with chaperone
  - Note Tanner stage
  - Positioning: frog leg, knee chest
  - External: trauma (vulvar hematoma, labial tear, hymenal injury, laceration), lesions, masses, foreign bodies, congenital anomalies
  - Pelvic exam
    - Indications: pelvic trauma, foreign body, tumor, prolapsed organ causing acute urinary retention, unstable with vaginal bleeding
    - Potentially: pelvic pain/vaginal discharge/dysuria + sexually active
    - Consult Gyn if virginal
- **Diagnostics**
  - Labs
    - Urine pregnancy test for all post-menarcheal: quantitative beta-hCG PRN

- Vaginal bleeding (severe, pregnant): CBC, PT/INR, PTT, TxS, +/− von Willebrand (vWF) panel
- STI suspected
  - Urine or vaginal/cervical swab for chlamydia, gonorrhea
  - Wet mount for trichomonas, bacterial vaginosis (clue cells), *Candida*
  - HIV, RPR, hepatitis panel
— Imaging
  - POCUS for free fluid in Morrison's pouch if concerned for ectopic
  - Transabdominal US for pregnancy
    - Gestational and yolk sac at 5-6 wks
    - Fetal pole at 6-7 wks
    - Cardiac activity at 7-8 wks
  - Transvaginal US for adnexal torsion, abnormal uterine bleeding if associated pain, distension, or mass
    - CT not superior to US for identifying torsion

SPECIFIC CONDITIONS

Dysmenorrhea

- Cyclic menstrual cramps/pain with menstruation
- 50-70% of adolescents
- Cramping pain within pelvis, lower abdomen, back, anterior thighs
  — Typically begins with menses onset, lasts 8-72 hrs
- DDx: pregnancy, UTI, STI, ectopic pregnancy, endometriosis, PID, appendicitis, ovarian torsion, ruptured ovarian cyst, Mittelschmerz
- Management: NSAIDs, consider OCPs

Abnormal uterine bleeding

- Abnormal regularity, frequency, duration, or volume
  — 10% have regular cycles but heavy menses
- Etiology most often anovulatory noncyclic menstrual bleeding due to immature hypothalamic-pituitary-gonadal axis
  — PCOS common cause
  — ~20% have a coagulopathy
  — Vaginal bleeding in female neonates common as maternal hormonal levels wane
- Heavy: > 7 days, soaking 1 pad/tampon per 1-2 hrs, clots > 1 inch
- Labs: urine pregnancy or quantitative beta-hCG, CMP, CBC, PT/INR, PTT, TxC
  — +/− vWF, STI panel, thyroid panel

- Management
  - Iron supplementation
  - Hemodynamically stable, hemoglobin 10-12 g/dL
    - Monophasic estrogen-progestin oral contraceptives OR
    - Progestins: medroxyprogesterone acetate 10 mg/day or norethindrone acetate 5 mg/day for 10-12 days/month
  - Severe bleeding or hemodynamically unstable
    - Initial fluid resuscitation
    - Transfusion for hemorrhagic shock, Hgb < 7
    - Estrogen for adolescents: 25 mg IV q4-6hrs until bleeding stops
    - Non hormonal therapies
      - TXA, aminocaproic acid, desmopressin (vWF), clotting factors if known deficiency
      - Continued severe bleeding → D&C procedure

Imperforate hymen

- Remnant of the urogenital membrane
- Most frequent female GU obstructive anomaly
  - 1 per 100 - 200,000 population
- Adolescent with secondary sexual characteristics but no menarche
  - Chronic, vague abdominal pain, urinary symptoms
- Diagnosis
  - Exam: bulging membrane +/- blue color, covering introitus
    - Accumulated menstrual blood (hematocolpos)
  - Confirm with pelvic US if unsure
- Consult Gynecology for urgent hymenotomy in adolescents, elective in younger

Ovarian torsion

- 15% torsions in childhood due to hypermobile ovaries (peak 9-14 yrs)
- R > L, sigmoid colon protective on left; DDx ectopic, appendicitis
- Sudden sharp abdominal pain, may be intermittent/insidious, nausea/vomiting, +/- fever
- Diagnosis
  - US: enlarged ovary with ↓ blood flow
    - Absence of doppler flow specific, but normal flow does not rule out
    - Ovarian cyst > 4 cm risk factor for torsion
    - Pelvic free fluid if hemorrhage
  - Diagnostic laparoscopy if high clinical suspicion with indeterminate US and MRI unavailable

- Management: surgical emergency — Gynecology for detorsion
  - 40% salvage rate after 8 hrs, 33% after 24 hrs

Urethral prolapse
- 1 in 3,000; more common prepubertal (2-10 yrs), Black
- Painless spotting on underwear, +/− dysuria, urinary incontinence, retention
- Diagnosis clinical
  - Red-purple doughnut-shaped mass with central dimple
    - Venous congestion from distal urethra prolapsing beyond the meatus
  - Can pass a urinary catheter through central opening to confirm if unsure
- Management
  - Sitz baths, topical estrogen cream × 2wks
  - Treat constipation; straining exacerbates prolapse
  - Refractory/necrotic tissue → surgical management

Vaginitis
- Vulvovaginitis most common gynecologic disorder of childhood
- Causes: chemical irritants, infections, poor hygiene, tight underwear
  - Group A strep self-inoculation from nose/mouth
  - *Candida* less common as pre-pubertal vaginal pH alkaline
    - Consider DM or immunocompromised state
  - Pubertal: STI
  - Consider: atopic / contact dermatitis, lichen sclerosus, psoriasis
  - Consider sexual abuse
- Erythema, pain, itching, dysuria, bleeding
- Diagnosis
  - Exam usually sufficient
    - Rule out foreign body (toilet paper, retained tampon)
    - Characterize vaginal discharge
  - STI screening of high-risk patients (illicit drug use, sexually active, history of pregnancy)
- Management
  - Improved hygiene (wipe front-to-back); avoid irritants / tight clothing
  - Sexually active, as indicated:
    - Cover *gonorrhea* and *chlamydia*
      - Ceftriaxone 500 mg IM (1 g for patients > 150 kg) + doxycycline 100 mg PO two times daily for 7 days

- - - *Trichomonas*, bacterial vaginosis
    - ◆ Metronidazole 500 mg PO two times daily for 7 days
  - — Vaginal Candidiasis
    - Nystatin 100,000 U/gm topical two times daily for 14 days
    - Clotrimazole 1% cream two times daily for 14 days
    - Fluconazole 15 mg PO single dose — adolescents only

Labial adhesion

- Prepubertal labial adhesions caused by irritation (harsh soaps, tight clothes)
  - — 1.8 - 3.3% in 1-6yrs old
- Pubertal: rule out STI
- Often asymptomatic, occasional dysuria, difficult urethral catheterization
- Diagnosis: exam sufficient
  - — Raphe = thin, fused white line extending from posterior superiorly toward clitoris
- Management
  - — Often resolves spontaneously during puberty
  - — Do not manually separate: unnecessarily painful, will recur
  - — Estrogen cream two times daily for 2-4 wks to separate, then petroleum jelly for 2-3 wks to maintain separation
  - — Alternative to estrogen: betamethasone cream 0.05%

DISPOSITION

- Admit
  - — AUB if severe
  - — PID if ill-appearing, cannot tolerate PO, immunocompromised, tubo-ovarian abscess, pregnant
  - — Significant trauma/complication (expanding hematoma, deep laceration, active or rectal bleeding, inability to urinate)
    - Consult Gynecology, evaluate for sexual abuse/trafficking
- If discharged, follow-up with PCP or gynecologist or adolescent specialist

BEWARE

- ❗ Obtain history from adolescents one-on-one and emphasize confidentiality
- ❗ Pregnancy and sexual health treatable under mature minor clause (most states)
  - — Confidential between adolescent patients and treating physicians
- ❗ UTI and STI can occur concomitantly; both can cause dysuria
- ❗ Always consider sexual abuse or trafficking

2 ▶ Male-Specific Pathology

BACKGROUND
- Male GU complaints = ~ 0.5% - 2.5% of all ED visits
  — Testicular torsion 1 in 4000 annually
- Pathology varies by age

EVALUATION
- **High Yield History**
  — Circumcision: age performed, location (hospital, home, etc.)
  — Pain
    - Location: testicular, scrotal, penile
    - Onset, duration: acute vs. gradual
    - Worse with position, palpation, urination
  — Associated fever, nausea, vomiting, discharge
  — Sexual activity, sexual abuse
- **Exam**
  — Testicles/scrotum
    - Descended — may need to "milk" down the inguinal canal
    - Tenderness, swelling, erythema
      - Epididymis (overlies posterolateral testis)
      - "Bag of worms" for varicocele
    - Prehn's sign: elevate scrotum → alleviates epididymitis pain
      - Ddx from torsion pain
    - Lie: position of testicle within scrotum, normally vertical
      - May be altered in torsion
    - Blue dot sign: tender blue nodule on testis upper pole
      - Torsed testicular appendage
    - Cremasteric reflex: stroke skin of the inner thigh → cremaster muscle contracts, pulls ipsilateral testicle up toward inguinal canal
      - Absent in testicular torsion
    - Mass: malignancy
  — Penis and foreskin
    - Swelling, erythema
      - Balanitis (glans penis), posthitis (foreskin)

- ♦ Candidiasis: "balanitis thrush" = erythema of glans, irritation, swelling, pruritus, thick +/− lumpy discharge under foreskin, foul odor, phimosis, penile dyspareunia, dysuria
  - Penile discharge: color, character
  - Foreskin retractability (if uncircumcised)
- **Diagnostics**
  - Labs
    - Urinalysis
      - ♦ Pyuria (normal < 5 WBC/HPF)
      - ♦ Abnormal bag urines need cath specimen confirmation
    - STI
      - ♦ Urine gonorrhea, chlamydia NAAT
      - ♦ RPR, HIV, Hepatitis panel
      - ♦ If penile discharge, trichomonas
  - Imaging: scrotal US

SPECIFIC CONDITIONS AND MANAGEMENT

Acute scrotum

- Umbrella term, includes variety of pathologies
- **High Yield History**
  - Painful or painless
  - Onset: within minutes or up to 1 to 2 days
  - Associated nausea/vomiting
  - Scrotal swelling, erythema, discoloration
- **Diagnostics:** scrotal US with color Doppler
- DDx
  - **Testicular torsion**
    - Bimodal age distribution: first year of life & early adolescence
    - Abrupt onset pain, unilateral diffuse testicular tenderness, high-riding testicle with transverse/horizontal lie, absent cremasteric reflex, nausea/vomiting common
    - Pain may be preceded by trauma, physical activity, or have no inciting event (e.g. sleeping)
    - Typically afebrile, no dysuria, normal labs
    - Tx
      - ♦ Manual detorsion
        - ✦ Rotate the testicle medial-to-lateral, "opening a book"

- Emergent Urology consult for surgical exploration, detorsion, likely orchiopexy
- Testicle salvage rate: pain onset to surgery

< 6 hrs	6-12 hrs	12-48 hrs
~100%	80-88%	2.6%

- **Epididymitis/epididymo-orchitis**
  - Most common 10-14 yrs
  - Gradual onset posterior testicular pain, +/– urinary symptoms, may have fever
  - Swollen, tender epididymis and/or testicle, normal lie, +Prehn's sign
  - Etiologies: most common pediatric epididymitis viral
    - Sexually active: *Chlamydia, Gonorrhea*
    - Reflux of urine into ejaculatory ducts
    - Consider mumps if isolated orchitis
  - Labs: UA w/culture, STI testing
  - Tx
    - Analgesia, scrotal support
    - Antibiotics
      - Pre-pubertal: antibiotics for typical UTI pathogens if UA is positive
      - Sexually active: ceftriaxone 500 mg IM (1 g for patients > 150 kg) + doxycycline 100 mg PO two times daily for 7 days
- **Torsion of appendix testis**
  - Most common 7-12 yrs
  - Similar symptoms to testicular torsion but more insidious, less severe pain, no systemic or associated symptoms
  - "Blue dot" sign
  - Normal testicular flow on US
  - Analgesia, self-limited

Balanitis and balanoposthitis

- Risk factors
  - Chemical irritation, poor hygiene, contact dermatitis, local trauma, persistent manual manipulation
- Symptoms
  - Erythema and swelling, typically sparing penile shaft
  - Dysuria, penile discharge, bleeding, glans ulceration possible
  - Phimosis (uncommon)

- Management
  - Consider POC GLC if concern for DM
  - Hygiene: gentle foreskin cleaning
  - Sitz baths
  - Antifungal
    - Nystatin 100,000 U/gm topical two times daily for 14 days
    - Clotrimazole 1% cream two times daily for 14 days
    - Fluconazole 15 mg PO single dose — adolescents only; for severe, recurrent, DM
  - Antibiotics
    - Mupirocin 2% topical two times daily for 5-10 days
    - Oral: Cephalexin 25 mg/kg (max 500 mg) PO three times daily for 7 days in severe cases where suspect streptococcal etiology
  - Anti-inflammatory: hydrocortisone 1% cream two times daily for 7 days
  - Ensure able to urinate prior to discharge
  - Referral for circumcision if severe / recurrent

Paraphimosis

- Uncircumcised foreskin retracted behind glans → entrapped, unable to reduce
  - Venous congestion, possible ischemia
- Pain, swelling of glans, dysuria
  - May be so swollen that is difficult to see the paraphimotic foreskin
- Management
  - Evaluate for hair tourniquets, penile foreign body
  - Pain treatment
    - Penile block: 1% lidocaine w/o epinephrine injected around base of penis (ring block) or at 2:00 & 10:00 positions (dorsal penile block) OR
    - Analgesics or procedural sedation
    - Ice pack to reduce pain, swelling
  - Reduce edema
    - Manual compression, ace wrap, granulated sugar, D50W-soaked gauze
  - Manual reduction: place index fingers on leading edge of foreskin, thumbs on glans, direct pressure inward with thumbs to pull foreskin over glans
  - Urologist consultation
    - If reduction unsuccessful, emergent urologist consultation
    - Referral for circumcision

Phimosis
- Distal foreskin cannot be retracted back to completely visualize glans penis
- Physiologic vs. pathologic
  - Physiologic normal in infants, typically retractable in 90% by age of 6yrs
  - Pathologic: older age, symptomatic
- Symptoms: abnormal urine stream, urinary retention, ballooning with urination, UTIs
- Management
  - Hygiene instructions
  - Topical steroid betamethasone 0.05% daily × 4-6wks
  - Follow-up with PCP

Priapism
- Erection lasting ≥ 4 hrs, commonly patient with SCD
- Low-flow (ischemic) or high-flow, corpus cavernosum blood gas can DDx
- Analgesics, consult Urology

Zipper injury
- Mechanism: entrapment of glans, shaft, or foreskin in pants zipper
- Management
  - Analgesia, anxiolysis
  - Mineral oil and gentle release
  - Fastener release: cut zipper median bar

DISPOSITION
- PCP vs. Urology follow-up
  - Immediate Urology consult: testicular torsion, Fournier's disease, persistent priapism, non-reduced paraphimosis, significant trauma
  - Outpatient Urology follow-up: resolved priapism, reduced paraphimosis, minor trauma
  - PCP: all others
- Admit: unclear diagnosis with intractable pain/vomiting, unreliable follow-up

BEWARE
- Perform GU exam on any boy with abdominal pain; may not localize pain or be too embarrassed to discuss GU pain
- Persistent scrotal swelling and "bag-of-worms" appearance concerning for obstruction from tumor
- Be sure your definition of "sexually active," "circumcised" etc. matches the patient's

Section XII
Hematology/Oncology

1 ▶ Anemia

BACKGROUND
- Definition: Hgb < 1 g/dL + 0.1 × (age in yrs [pre-pubertal]) or < 2.5%ile for age/sex/race
- Sequelae: ↓O2 delivery, symptomatic anemia, high output heart failure, poor growth

EVALUATION
- **High Yield History**
  - Symptoms: fatigue, headache, dizziness, SOB, palpitations, weakness
  - Diet: exclusive breastfeeding, high cow's milk intake, "picky eater"
  - PMH: prior anemia, jaundice, chronic disease (malnutrition, rheumatologic, renal, cardiac, hepatic, bone marrow failure, malignancy)
  - Family history: anemia, jaundice, splenectomy, gallstones
- **Exam**
  - ↑HR, orthostatic hypotension, systolic murmur, cyanosis, respiratory distress, pallor (including conjunctiva and skin creases), jaundice
- **Diagnostics**
  - CBC w/peripheral smear, reticulocyte count, TxS
    - Consider iron studies, LDH/haptoglobin
  - Normocytic and ↑reticulocytes:
    - Antibody-mediated: isoimmune (ABO, Rh incompatibility), autoimmune (infectious, malignant, rheumatologic, medications)
    - Non-Antibody-mediated: hemorrhagic, microangiopathic hemolytic anemia (HUS, DIC), membrane (hereditary spherocytosis), enzyme deficiencies (G6PD, pyruvate kinase), hemoglobin (SCD, thalassemia)
  - Normocytic and ↓reticulocytes
    - Aplastic anemia, infiltrative malignancy, drugs/toxins, bacterial/viral suppression (parvovirus B19), pure RBC aplasia (Diamond-Blackfan, Transient Erythroblastopenia of Childhood)

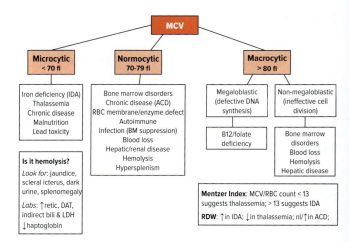

MANAGEMENT

- Asymptomatic, isolated anemia: start iron supplement
- Symptomatic anemia: PRBC transfusion (10 mL/kg or 250 mL unit if adolescent or older)
  - Expected Hgb rise
    - 2-3 g/dL per transfusion in children
    - 1 g/dL per unit in adolescent

DISPOSITION

- Consult Hematology for new/severe anemia, suspicion of malignancy, bone marrow disorder
- Admit: critically ill or ongoing bleed
- Discharge with PCP follow-up if asymptomatic, isolated

BEWARE

- ❗ Draw labs *BEFORE* transfusion of donor blood
- ❗ Match transfusion rate and volume to etiology: rapid transfusion for rapid blood loss vs. small aliquot transfusions (no > 2-3 mL/kg/hr) in chronic well-compensated anemia
- ❗ Raising Hgb too quickly in sickle cell patients can cause volume overload
- ❗ Remember to reassess during & after transfusions for adverse reactions

2 ▶ Bleeding Disorders

Coagulation Disorder	Deficiency	Presentation	Notes
Hemophilia		Hemarthrosis, intramuscular bleeds, bruising, ICH	M >> F Most are inherited (X-linked recessive), but can be spontaneous ~35% of males with hemophilia have severe disease
Hemophilia A (85%)	Factor VIII		Severity of disease determined by factor level: Mild: 6-50% — no tendency for spontaneous bleed, bleeding w/surgery or severe trauma Moderate: 1-5% — bleed w/ minor trauma Severe: < 1% — spontaneous bleeding
Hemophilia B (15%)	Factor IX		
Hemophilia C (< 1%)	Factor XI		M=F, more common in Ashkenazi Jews
Von Willebrand Disease Type 1: *deficiency* (75%) Type 2: *dysfunction* (22%) Type 3: *absence* (3%)	vWF — quantitative or qualitative defects	Epistaxis, bruising, menorrhagia, prolonged oozing from superficial cuts, bleeding after dental extraction	Most common hereditary bleeding disorder (1% population affected) Autosomal dominant with variable expression Can be acquired in autoimmune conditions Factor VIII may be decreased since vWF acts as its carrier
Vitamin K Deficiency (neonates & infants) aka hemorrhagic disease of the newborn	Vitamin K	Bleeding from umbilical stump, circumcision site, mucous membranes (nose, mouth), GI tract, ICH	Early (within 24 hr): maternal vitamin K antagonist use Classic (1st wk) and Late (1-6 mos): vitamin K refusal at birth, malabsorptive states, hepatic disease, dietary deficiency, antibiotic suppression of intestinal flora
Platelet disorder	Destruction, under-production, or adhesion defect	Petechiae, purpura bruising in the absence of trauma or in unusual places (palms, soles), mucosal bleeding, hematuria, hematochezia	Wide etiology range, including congenital, acquired, immunologic, nonimmunologic, sequestration

EVALUATION

- **High Yield History**
  - Neonate: scalp hematoma, ICH, bleeding with cord separation or circumcision
  - Toddler: mucocutaneous bleeding beyond expected, hemarthrosis, GI bleeding
  - Adolescent: heavy menses, bleeding with tooth extraction/minor surgery
  - Family history bleeding disorders
    - 30% hemophilia due to spontaneous mutations
  - If known hemophilia: ask if patient has known inhibitors, what dose/factor patient needs, if have home factor with them
- **Exam**
  - Mucocutaneous bleeding
  - Skin/HEENT: petechiae, purpura, gingival bleeding, epistaxis
  - Extremity: hemarthrosis, hip flexion contracture (iliopsoas bleed)
  - Abdomen/GU: hepatosplenomegaly, GU bleeding
    - Leg paresthesias can indicate retroperitoneal bleed
  - Neurologic: AMS in coagulopathic patient is ICH until proven otherwise
- **Diagnostics**
  - Labs: CBC w/peripheral smear, TxS, PT/INR, PTT, fibrinogen, CMP (renal, hepatic function), consider vWF testing, specific factor levels, mixing study if concern for inhibitors
    - PTT abnormality in hemophilia, should correct after factor replacement except if patient has inhibitors
  - Imaging as indicated

MANAGEMENT

- Treat first, diagnose second
  - Unknown diagnosis, give FFP (contains Factors VIII, IX, XI, vWF) 10 mL/kg IV
- Hemophilia
  - Indications for factor replacement
    - Mild/moderate bleed: replace factor level up to 50%
      - Epistaxis
      - Suspected bleeding into joint or muscle
    - Severe/life-threatening bleed: replace factor up to 100%
      - Head or neck trauma
      - New or concerning headache
      - Any bleeding around neck (airway compromise)
      - GI bleeding

- Retroperitoneal bleeding
- Deep hematoma
- Severe mechanism of injury even without evidence of bleeding — concern for delayed bleeding

Hemophilia A	1U/kg Factor VIII increases activity by 2%
Mild/Moderate	Dose Factor VIII = weight (kg) × desired level × 0.5
Severe	Dose Factor VIII = weight (kg) × desired level × 0.5
Hemophilia B	1U/kg Factor IX increases activity by 1%
Mild/Moderate	Dose Factor IX = weight (kg) × desired level
Severe	Dose Factor IX = weight (kg) v desired level
Desired level: use percentage as integer "50" for mild/moderate, "100" for severe	

- — If known inhibitors, higher risk of bleeding
  - Consult Hematology before treatment
- von Willebrand Disease
  - — Type I and 2A: DDAVP 0.3 mcg/kg (max 20 mcg) IV or 1 spray (150 mcg) for < 50 kg, 1 spray each nostril for ≥ 50 kg
  - — Types 2B, 2N, 2M, 3: factor VIII and vWF concentrate
- Vitamin K deficiency
  - — Phytonadione 1-2 mg SC/IV
  - — FFP 10 mL/kg IV, may repeat
- Hemarthrosis
  - — Ice, compression bandage, pain control; no arthrocentesis
- Adjunct therapies
  - — TXA topically or systemically for oral hemorrhage
  - — DDAVP increases factor VIII in mild hemophilia, may be useful in minor bleeds

DISPOSITION

- Admit: major or uncontrolled bleeding
- Discharge: stable vitals after serial exams; not requiring repeat dosing of blood product

BEWARE

- Development of inhibitors common in hemophilia → use recombinant factor VIIa
- Consult Hematology/Pharmacy early to prepare appropriate blood product
- Consider NAT with any unusual bruise or bleed

3 ▶ Immune Thrombocytopenia (ITP)

BACKGROUND

- Autoantibody-mediated platelet destruction within spleen
- Children < 10 yrs, peak 2-5 yrs, often viral or immunologic trigger
- DDx: hematologic malignancy, drug-induced thrombocytopenia, TTP, infection (HIV, hepatitis C, meningococcemia), hypersplenism, HUS, DIC
  — Henoch-Schonlein Purpura: normal platelets

EVALUATION

- **High Yield History**
  — Mucocutaneous bleed with minimal to no trauma; preceding URI/GI symptoms
  — Blood in vomit, stool, or urine
- **Exam**
  — Petechiae, purpura, ecchymosis, epistaxis, gingival bleed
  — Absent: significant splenomegaly, lymphadenopathy, congenital anomalies
- **Diagnostics**
  — Diagnosis of exclusion (isolated thrombocytopenia)
  — CBC with peripheral smear
    - Plts < 100,000, but usually much lower if bleeding/bruising
    - Rest of CBC normal
  — CT Head w/o contrast if concern for ICH (AMS +/− preceding trauma)

MANAGEMENT

- Most resolve spontaneously, serious bleeding is rare
  — 10-20% develop chronic ITP
- Observation; avoid contact sports and NSAIDs
  — Monitor menses, consider iron supplementation, hormonal therapy to lessen menorrhagia
- Indications for treatment
  — Plts < 20,000 + active bleeding
  — Plts < 10,000
  — Severe bleeding
- Treatment of severe bleeding (in consultation with hematologist)
  — IVIG: 1 g/kg with repeated dose 24 hrs later if plts < 40,000
  — Platelet transfusion 10 mL/kg, repeat as needed
  — Methylprednisolone 30 mg/kg (max 1 g) IV

- Anti-D immune globulin 75 mcg/kg IV
    - For Rh(D)-positive patient and direct antiglobulin negative
    - Utility in splenectomized patients unclear
- Consider plasmapheresis

DISPOSITION
- Admit and consult Hematology: plts severely low and/or active hemorrhage

BEWARE
- ❗ Consider malignancy, bone marrow failure, infection, prior to diagnosing ITP
- ❗ AMS in setting of thrombocytopenia is ICH until proven otherwise

4 ▶ Oncologic Emergencies

- Cancer ↑ risk of emergencies due to complications of malignant process or therapeutics
- Oncologic emergencies may be metabolic, infectious, hematologic, or due to tumor burden

NEUTROPENIC FEVER
- Single oral temp 38.3°C or ≥ 38°C for 1 hr with ANC < 500 cells/mcL, or ANC < 1000 cells/mcL and predicted ↓ (recent chemotherapy)

EVALUATION
- **High Yield History**
    - Chills/rigors usually treated as fever even if temp normal
    - PMH: malignancy, recent chemotherapy, known neutropenia
- **Diagnostics**
    - Labs
        - CBC w/ differential, CMP, inflammatory markers, DIC panel if ill-appearing
        - Cultures: blood cultures (peripheral & indwelling catheters), UA (no I&O cath), urine culture, stool culture if diarrhea, respiratory PCR nasopharyngeal swab
    - Imaging: CXR if respiratory symptoms, other as indicated

MANAGEMENT
- IV bolus 20 mL/kg NS if dehydrated/shock; repeat if septic (caution: avoid pulmonary edema)
- Shock: early consideration of vasopressors, IV hydrocortisone

- Empiric antibiotics as soon as possible (within 1 hr of presentation)
  — Cefepime 50 mg/kg (max 2 g) IV or meropenem 20-40 mg/kg (max 1-2 g) IV if concern for multidrug resistant organisms (higher dose for CNS infections) OR piperacillin-tazobactam 80 mg/kg IV for < 9 mo, 100 mg/kg (max 3 g) IV otherwise
  — Add vancomycin 15 mg/kg (max 1 g) IV if concern for indwelling catheter infection, prior MRSA, signs of shock, DIC, and/or respiratory distress
  — Add metronidazole 10 mg/kg (max 500 mg) IV if GI tract infection or *C.diff* suspected

DISPOSITION

- Admit and consult Oncology; PICU if hemodynamically unstable
- Consult ID for antimicrobial guidance (may need antifungals)

BEWARE

! Avoid rectal temperature, I&O cath in neutropenic patient

NEUTROPENIC COLITIS

- Invasive infection from mucosal breakdown, usually in cecum (typhlitis) but may involve entire intestines, rapidly progresses to perforation, peritonitis, and/or shock

EVALUATION

- **High Yield History**: abdominal pain, fever, vomiting, diarrhea, hematochezia, difficulty ambulating (may mimic appendicitis)
- **Exam**: abdominal tenderness (often RLQ) in setting of neutropenia
- **Diagnostics**
  — Labs: CBC w/ differential, CMP, blood cultures, DIC panel
  — Imaging
    - CT abdomen/pelvis with IV contrast: bowel wall thickening (> 3mm), pneumatosis intestinalis, soft tissue edema
    - US: bowel wall thickening, free fluid if ruptured

MANAGEMENT

- Antibiotics (doses as above for neutropenic fever) covering E. coli, gram-negative enteric organisms, anaerobes, pseudomonas
  — Cefepime 50 mg/kg (max 2 g) IV every 8 hrs PLUS metronidazole 10 mg/kg (max 500 mg) IV every 8 hrs metronidazole **OR**
  — Piperacillin-tazobactam 75 mg/kg (max 4 g) IV every 6 hrs **OR**
  — Meropenem 20 mg/kg (max 1 g) IV every 8 hrs or imipenem 20 mg/kg (max 1 g) IV every 6 hrs if resistance or severe allergy to above
- Bowel rest, NG suction, parenteral nutrition, blood transfusion as needed

DISPOSITION
- Admit to PICU; consult Oncology, ID, Surgery if perforation, uncontrolled sepsis, or GI bleeding

TUMOR LYSIS SYNDROME
- Metabolic emergency caused by tumor cell death, rapid release of intracellular contents

EVALUATION
- **High Yield History**: high tumor burden, rapid cell proliferation (leukemia, lymphoma), chemotherapy initiation → greatest risk
- **Diagnostics**
  — Labs: CMP, uric acid, LDH, Mg, PO4
  — Cairo-Bishop criteria: ≥ 2 or more of hyperkalemia, hyperphosphatemia, hyperuricemia, hypocalcemia
  — If end-organ damage, serum creatinine and/or LDH may be elevated
  — EKG: arrhythmia if severe derangements

MANAGEMENT
- IV fluids (no K+) 2x maintenance rate to improve renal perfusion and excretion
  — Goal urine output 2 mL/kg/hr (4-6 mL/kg/hr for ≤ 10 kg)
- Hyperuricemia: allopurinol and/or rasburicase (dose per Oncology)
- Hyperkalemia: refer to "Fluids and Electrolytes" chapter
- Consider dialysis if critically ill and/or severe refractory electrolyte derangements

DISPOSITION
Admit to PICU, consult Oncology, repeat labs frequently

HYPERLEUKOCYTOSIS
- Markedly elevated blasts in microcirculation promotes sludging, local ischemia, thrombosis secondary hemorrhage
- Possible cerebrovascular, cardiac, pulmonary, renal involvement

EVALUATION
- **High Yield History**: headache, lethargy, blurry vision, chest pain, diaphoresis, SOB, decreased urine output
- **Exam**: fever, AMS, stupor, coma, papilledema, retinal hemorrhage, petechiae, purpura, poor perfusion, tachypnea, hypoxemia, oliguria

- **Diagnostics**
  - Labs: CBC w/ differential (elevated WBC > 100,000)
  - Imaging
    - CT head without contrast (ICH, mass effect)
    - CXR for pulmonary infiltrate
    - US: echocardiogram, renal with doppler (renal venous thrombosis)

MANAGEMENT
- IV fluids 2x maintenance rate (no K+)
- Platelet transfusion (10 mL/kg) to maintain platelets > 20-30,000
- May require STAT induction chemotherapy, plasmapheresis

DISPOSITION
- Admit PICU, consult Oncology

BEWARE
- Patients at high risk for tumor lysis syndrome

SUPERIOR VENA CAVA (SVC) SYNDROME
- Mechanical obstruction of SVC by mediastinal mass
- Possible airway compromise commonly from lymphoma

EVALUATION
- **High Yield History**: cough, orthopnea, dyspnea, hoarseness, wheeze, stridor
- **Exam**: engorged collateral veins in chest/abdomen, swelling/plethora of face, possible distal cyanosis and AMS if poor gas exchange
- **Diagnostics**
  - Labs: CBC w/ differential, tumor lysis labs as above
  - Imaging: CXR may detect mediastinal mass, CT chest with IV contrast to define tracheal compression, vascular involvement

MANAGEMENT
- Avoid sedation and recumbency given mass effect on adjacent vital structures
- Urgent echocardiogram to define degree of cardiovascular compromise

DISPOSITION
- Admit PICU, team-based management with Anesthesia, Pediatric Surgery, Oncology, Radiology, Critical Care

SPINAL CORD COMPRESSION

- Mechanical compression of spinal cord due to primary or metastatic disease
- Most commonly sarcomas but also lymphoma, leukemia, neuroblastoma, germ cell tumors, and "drop" CNS metastases

EVALUATION

- **High Yield History:** localized back pain, progressive symmetric weakness, difficulty ambulating, bowe/bladder dysfunction
- **Exam:** neurologic deficits (motor, sensory level, patellar reflexes, gait disturbance), saddle anesthesia
- **Diagnostics:** MRI entire spine w/ IV contrast

MANAGEMENT

- IV Dexamethasone to decrease local edema, dosing per Neurosurgery

DISPOSITION

- Admit for chemoradiation and/or surgical decompression; consult Oncology, Neurosurgery

5 ▶ Sickle Cell Disease

BACKGROUND

- Autosomal recessive hemoglobinopathy (HbS)
- May be combined with other hemoglobin (Hgb) mutations (thalassemia, HbC) → various degrees of disease state, HbSS is most severe
- Chronic hemolysis, endothelial dysfunction, progressive end-organ damage

EVALUATION

Complication	Etiology	Presentation	Management
Acute Chest Syndrome (ACS)	Pneumonia (viral, bacterial), infarction, emboli, overhydration, hypoventilation	**New pulmonary infiltrate** on CXR + symptoms: pleuritic chest pain, cough, fever, hypoxia, dyspnea, wheeze	Empiric antibiotics; supplemental O2; cautious IV fluids and analgesia; bronchodilator; consider PRBC transfusion with Hematology consult
Aplastic crisis	Parvovirus infection, bacteremia or other viremia	Pallor, weakness, lethargy, splenomegaly. **Precipitous drop in Hgb and retic**	Supportive blood transfusions. Recovery within weeks

Complication	Etiology	Presentation	Management
Cholelithiasis	Hemolysis → high bilirubin → stone formation	RUQ abdominal pain, anorexia, emesis, jaundice, fever, Murphy sign	Elevated bilirubin, liver enzymes; WBC (cholecystitis); lipase (gallstone pancreatitis); RUQ US; GI, Surgery
Priapism	¼ of males. Ischemia in corpus cavernosum	Painful, rigid penis. Difficulty with urination	Hydration, pain control; Exchange transfusion if persists; Urology
Sepsis	Functional asplenia → encapsulated organisms (*S. pneumoniae*, *H. influenzae*), salmonella	**Fever ≥ 38.5°C** may be the sole presenting symptom; poor perfusion, AMS	CBC, reticulocytes, blood culture Urine, CSF studies, CXR depending on symptoms Empiric antibiotics (within 60min of triage)
Splenic Sequestration	Intrasplenic pooling of cells. Majority 5-24 months old (HbSS)	Rapid onset pallor, fatigue, LUQ pain, possible shock. **Splenomegaly + Hgb drop**	Transfuse small aliquot PRBC in consultation with Hematologist (avoid autotransfusing trapped cells)
Stroke	Hemorrhagic or ischemic - stenosed/occluded vessels from chronic endothelial injury	Focal motor weakness, hemiparesis, speech deficit, headache, seizure, AMS	Head CT w/o contrast; blood or exchange transfusion, goal HbS < 30%; MRI/MRA when stable; All patients with stroke require chronic transfusions
Traumatic hyphema complications	Sickle cell disease *or trait* increases risk of complications in hyphema	Blood in anterior chamber	Consult ophthalmology for any size hyphema Rigid eye shield, bedrest, anti-emetics as needed
Vaso-occlusive crisis (VOC)	Local ischemia, infarct, inflammation in and around bone. Triggers: cold, illness, hypoxia, dehydration, altitude	Sudden or gradual pain in extremities, chest, abdomen, back. Dactylitis in 6-18 mo old (swollen digits, refusal to walk)	Clinical diagnosis, **trust patient's assessment of pain;** Consider septic arthritis if joint immobility, osteomyelitis if pinpoint tenderness, cholecystitis/pancreatitis if abdominal pain

MANAGEMENT

- Fluids
  - Maintenance or slightly above maintenance IV fluids typically used in VOC while more cautious fluid use in ACS
- Supplemental oxygen if SpO2 < 95%
- Pain management
  - NSAIDs
    - Ibuprofen PO 10 mg/kg (max 600 mg)
    - Ketorolac IV 0.5 mg/kg (max 15-30 mg), limit ×5 days (renal injury)
  - Oral opioids
    - Morphine 0.2-0.5 mg/kg (max 15-20 mg) every 2-4 hrs PRN
    - Hydrocodone 0.1-0.2 mg/kg (max 5-10 mg) every 4 hrs PRN
    - Oxycodone 0.1-0.2 mg/kg (max 5-10 mg) every 4 hrs PRN
  - IV opioids
    - Morphine 0.1 mg/kg (max 4-10 mg) every 2-4 hrs (depending on whether opioid naive)
    - Hydromorphone < 50 kg 0.01-0.015 mg/kg every 2-4 hrs, > 50 kg 0.2-0.6 mg every 2-4 hrs
- Antibiotics (ACS, fever/bacteremia, cholecystitis)
  - Cultures + empiric ABx for all febrile patients with sickle cell disease
  - Cover *S. pneumoniae*, *H. influenzae*, Salmonella; atypical bacteria in ACS
    - Ceftriaxone 50 mg/kg (max 2 g) IV daily **OR** clindamycin 10 mg/kg (max 600 mg) IV every 8 hrs if allergic
    - Azithromycin 10 mg/kg (max 500 mg) IV daily for ACS
    - Add vancomycin 15 mg/kg (max 1 g) IV every 8 hrs if critically ill
- Consider transfusion: stroke, aplastic crisis, splenic sequestration, severe ACS
  - Consult Hematology

DISPOSITION

- Admission criteria vary by institution; generally, admit if ill-appearing, significantly abnormal findings, uncertain follow-up
- VOC with pain controlled may be discharged

BEWARE

- Avoid sedation when giving analgesics → risk of inducing ACS (hypoventilation)
- Blood transfusions may lead to hyperviscosity

Section XIII
Infectious Diseases

1 ▶ Fever of Unknown Origin

BACKGROUND

- *Fever of unknown origin (FUO):* daily fever ≥ 100.4 for ≥ 8 days
- *Fever without a source (FWS):* daily fever ≥ 100.4 for ≤ 7 days
- DDx: infectious, autoimmune, oncologic, neurologic, genetic, factitious, iatrogenic
- Infectious: accounts for most pediatric FUO
  — Indolent infections
    - Generalized: cat scratch (bartonella), malaria, brucellosis, TB, salmonellosis, toxoplasmosis, viral infections
    - Localized: aseptic meningitis, osteomyelitis, endocarditis, intra-abdominal or parapneumonic abscess, septic joint, sinusitis, mastoiditis, UTI
  — Common infectious agents
    - Bacteria: S. pneumoniae, H. influenzae, N. meningitidis, Staphylococcus, Salmonella, Bartonella
    - Viruses: CMV, EBV, adenovirus, enterovirus, arboviruses, human metapneumovirus, HSV, HIV, COVID-19
    - Consider fungemia in immunocompromised host
- Noninfectious
  — Autoimmune
    - Juvenile idiopathic arthritis, Henoch-Schonlein Purpura, SLE, Kawasaki disease, dermatomyositis, inflammatory bowel disease, Behcet's disease, MIS-C (recent COVID-19 infection)
  — Malignancy
    - Leukemia, lymphoma
    - Less common: neuroblastoma, hepatoma, sarcoma, atrial myxoma
- Periodic fever syndromes
  — Familial Mediterranean fever, hyperimmunoglobulin D syndrome

EVALUATION
- **High Yield History**
  - Fever (pattern, measurement techniques)
  - Associated symptoms of Kawasaki, URI, gastroenteritis, UTI, arthritis, osteomyelitis
    - B symptoms: weight loss, night sweats
  - Exposures
    - Sick contacts
    - Animal contacts
    - Travel history
    - Medications
  - Ethnic background
    - Familial Mediterranean fever: non-Ashkenazi Jews, Turks, Armenians, Arabs, Greeks, Italians
- **Exam**
  - Vital signs, fever
  - Thorough initial physical exam
    - Conjunctivitis, dental, pharyngitis, otitis, sinusitis, lymphadenopathy, lung sounds, hepatosplenomegaly, limbs/joints, rash
- **Diagnostics**
  - Labs
    - CBC w/ differential, CMP, ESR, CRP, +/− procalcitonin (utility unclear)
    - Aerobic & anaerobic blood cultures
    - UA, urine culture
    - Consider CSF studies
    - Consider LDH, uric acid, ferritin
    - Infectious disease titers as indicated
  - Imaging
    - CXR
    - Echocardiogram if suspect endocarditis
    - MRI if suspect osteomyelitis

MANAGEMENT
- Empiric ABx: age-dependent decision, give if suspect life-threatening infection
  - Always start antibiotics in neonates: cefotaxime / ceftriaxone (if > 4 weeks old) or ampicillin + gentamicin (see Febrile Neonate & Infant chapter)
  - Older children: empiric antibiotics may delay diagnosis

- Antipyretics
  — Avoid aspirin (risk of Reye's syndrome)
  — Acetaminophen 15 mg/kg (max 650 mg -1 g) PO every 4 hrs (do not exceed 75 mg/kg/day) ibuprofen 10 mg/kg (max 400 mg) PO every 6 hrs
- Trial of discontinuing medications potentially causing drug-induced fever
- Ill-appearing: consult ID, Rheumatology, Heme-Onc

DISPOSITION

- Admit ill-appearing, risk factors for severe illness (malignancy, immunodeficiency, neonate ≤ 28 days old)
- Stable: may work up as outpatient

BEWARE

⚠ Consider factitious fever (Munchausen by proxy): very high fever reported, but exam non-localizing and patient does not develop a witnessed fever

2 ▶ Infectious Mononucleosis

BACKGROUND

- Infectious mononucleosis = most common presentation of primary symptomatic Epstein-Barr virus (EBV) infection
- Transmission requires close personal contact, typically through saliva
- Viral replication starts in oropharynx → spreads to bloodstream, forms reactive CD8+ T-lymphocytes
- Incubation period 30-50 days

EVALUATION

- **High Yield History**: fever, fatigue, sore throat, lymphadenopathy
  — Close contacts with similar symptoms
- **Exam**
  — Exudative pharyngitis, tonsillar enlargement, lymphadenopathy (classically posterior cervical chain but can be generalized)
  — Hepatosplenomegaly
    - Rare splenic rupture, can be atraumatic!
  — Generalized rash, especially with beta-lactam antibiotic
- **Diagnostics**
  — CBC w/ differential
    - Lymphocytosis with > 10-20% atypical lymphocytes

- Some patients develop an autoimmune hemolytic anemia due to IgM cold-agglutinins cross-reactivity to RBCs
- Consider splenic rupture if low hematocrit, especially in patients with abdominal pain
- Mild transaminitis common
- Monospot test: detects serum heterophile antibodies (IgM antibodies that agglutinate sheep or horse RBCs)
  - Not reliable in children < 4yrs
  - May produce false negatives during the first week of clinical illness
- EBV titers

MANAGEMENT

- Classic: symptomatic treatment only
- Marked tonsillar swelling / pain: consider prednisone 1-2 mg/kg (max 60 mg) daily PO × 3-7 days
- Splenic rupture: non-operative management preferred to preserve splenic function
  - If patient unstable → splenectomy
- Airway management may be necessary if develop recumbent dyspnea secondary to tonsillar edema
- Consult infectious disease specialist if patient immunocompromised

DISPOSITION

- Most discharged with supportive care: adequate hydration, acetaminophen or ibuprofen for fever, myalgias, sore throat
- Avoid contact sports for 4 weeks to ↓ risk of splenic rupture

BEWARE

- Airway obstruction due to oropharyngeal inflammation = rare but serious complication
- AVOID treatment with penicillin (risk of rash)
- Children should also be assessed for strep throat and tested/treated as appropriate
- May be a cause of FUO

3 ▶ Influenza-Like Illness

BACKGROUND
- Fever (temp ≥ 37.8 °C) and a cough and/or sore throat without a known cause
- Infections to consider:
  — Influenza, COVID-19, RSV (most common cause of lower respiratory tract infections in children < 1 yr)
  — Other viruses: adenovirus, parainfluenza, human metapneumovirus
  — Bacterial infections: pneumonia, tonsillopharyngitis, rhinosinusitis

EVALUATION
- **High Yield History**
  — Fever, acute onset, cough (often nonproductive), rhinorrhea, sore throat, malaise, myalgias
  — Headache = most prevalent non-respiratory influenza symptom (26%)
  — Vaccination status, ill contacts
- **Exam**
  — Rhinorrhea, pharyngeal erythema
  — Associated otitis media common
  — Lung auscultation non-localizing
    - Can have diffuse rhonchi and/or scattered wheezes
- **Diagnostics**
  — Labs
    - Influenza A/B antigen test if would treat with oseltamivir (see below) or positive test will change management (simplify fever work-up)
    - Consider COVID-19 testing, especially if known contact
    - CK if suspect viral myositis → significant muscle pain (usually legs, back) or unable to walk
      ◆ Influenza most common cause
    - Consider RSV testing if neonate (high risk for apnea) or if positive test will change management
    - Ill-appearing: CBC, BMP, BCx, +/– UA, UCx
  — Imaging
    - CXR (r/o bacterial lobar pneumonia) if significant hypoxia, respiratory distress, focal lung findings

MANAGEMENT

- Supportive care
  - Acetaminophen 15 mg/kg (max 650 mg - 1 g) PO every 4 hrs (do not exceed 75 mg/kg/day)
  - Ibuprofen 10 mg/kg (max 400 mg) PO every 6 hrs if ≥ 6 mos
  - Oral rehydration, encourage fluids, rest
- Antivirals for confirmed infection
  - Oseltamivir can shorten duration if administered within first 48 hrs after symptom onset
    - Adverse effects (nausea, vomiting, headache, rare neuropsychiatric in children)
    - CDC recommends treatment if < 48 hrs of symptoms AND high risk: age < 2 yrs, neurologic disorder, asthma, chronic disease, < 19 yrs and taking salicylate/aspirin, BMI ≥ 40, pregnant, being hospitalized (even if > 48 hrs of symptoms)

Age / Weight	Dose (two times daily for 5 days)
< 1 year old	3 mg/kg/dose
≤ 15 kg	30 mg
15-23kg	45 mg
23-40 kg	60 mg
> 40 kg	75 mg

- Education: hand hygiene, isolation from high-risk contacts, stay home until 24 hrs after fever resolves

DISPOSITION

- Admit: unable to tolerate PO, significantly ↑ WOB, ↑ CK concerning for rhabdomyolysis, significant comorbidities, bacterial superinfection (pneumonia) as indicated

BEWARE

- Avoid aspirin — risk of Reye's syndrome
- RSV symptoms tend to peak near day 4 of illness
- Do not test to identify specific viruses if results will not change management

4 ▶ Meningitis and Encephalitis

BACKGROUND

- Meningitis = meningeal inflammation
  - May be rapidly progressive over hours to several days
- Encephalitis = brain parenchyma inflammation

- High mortality with bacterial meningitis/viral encephalitis
  — High risk for long-term morbidity
- Common organisms
  — Bacterial meningitis

Age	Causative Organisms
0-28 days	Group B Strep
	E. coli
	Listeria monocytogenes
1-2 months	Neonatal pathogens
	S. pneumoniae
	N. meningitidis
	H. influenzae
> 2 months	S. pneumoniae
	N. meningitidis
	H. influenzae

  - Staphylococcus aureus uncommon
  — Aseptic meningitis:
    - Viral (most common): coxsackievirus, enterovirus, HSV2
    - Bacterial: Lyme, TB
    - Medications: NSAIDs, TMP/SMX, IVIG
    - Autoimmune: Sarcoid, Behçet's, SLE
    - Other: neoplasm, fungal and amoebic infections
  — Viral encephalitis: herpesviruses (HSV, CMV, EBV, HHV6, VZV), influenza, rabies, measles, enterovirus, West Nile, Eastern/Western equine & St. Louis encephalitis viruses

EVALUATION

- **High Yield History**
  — Meningitis:
    - Neonates/infants
      - Fever, seizure, lethargy, vomiting, poor feeding, poor tone
      - History of maternal HSV, GBS infection
    - Older children
      - Fever, photophobia, headache, neck pain/stiffness, vomiting, irritability, confusion, somnolence
  — Encephalitis: fever, seizure, AMS, behavior changes, delirium

- Risk factors: recent illness, neurosurgery, VP shunt, basilar skull fracture, extension from otitis media/sinusitis, cochlear implant, NICU admission, unimmunized, immunosuppressed, community residence (dorms, military barracks)
- Travel history

- **Exam**
  - Infants
    - Temperature instability: febrile, normothermic, or hypothermic (indicates severe sepsis)
    - Poor capillary refill, respiratory difficulty (grunting, tachypnea, nasal flaring) common
    - Inconsolable irritability or paradoxical irritability (infant cries more with attempts to console by rocking, indicates meningeal irritation)
    - Bulging fontanelle = late finding indicating elevated ICP
    - Nuchal rigidity often absent in neonates
  - Older children
    - AMS, nuchal rigidity ~30% of patients
    - Kernig (inability to straighten knee when hip/knee flexed at 90 degrees) and Brudzinski signs (flexion of lower extremities when neck flexed) specific but < 5% sensitive
    - Cushing's triad (hypertension, bradycardia, respiratory depression) late finding of increased ICP
  - Thorough skin exam to look for petechiae/purpura fulminans, vesicles

- **Diagnostics**
  - Labs: CBC, CMP, POC GLC, lactate, blood culture, CSF studies
    - Normal peripheral WBC does not rule out bacterial meningitis
  - Traumatic LP: correct WBC for RBC count (1 WBC per 1000 RBCs)
  - CSF pathogens PCR if available
  - Head CT prior to LP only if focal neurologic deficit, papilledema, immune deficiency, known CNS condition
    - HSV encephalitis: frontotemporal edema/hemorrhage

CSF Findings	Bacterial Meningitis	Aseptic Meningitis	Viral Meningitis
WBC	↑↑↑, neutrophils	↑↑ lymphocytes	↑ lymphocytes
Protein	↑	↑	Normal or ↑
Glucose	↓	Normal	Normal
Gram stain	Positive in 80%	Negative	Negative
RBC	if traumatic LP	if traumatic LP	HSV may be bloody

- Bacterial Meningitis Score: consider bacterial meningitis if CSF pleocytosis (CSF WBC > 10) and ANY of:
  — Positive CSF gram stain
  — CSF absolute neutrophil count (ANC) ≥ 1000
  — CSF protein > 80 mg/dL
  — Peripheral ANC ≥ 10,000
  — History of seizure

MANAGEMENT

- Bacterial meningitis
  — ABCs: assess/treat shock, ventilatory support as needed
  — Antibiotics: higher doses needed to cross blood-brain barrier
    - 0-28 days:
      - Ampicillin (covers *Listeria*) 100 mg/kg IV every 6 hrs PLUS
        - Gentamicin 2.5 mg/kg IV every 8 hrs PLUS
        - Cefotaxime 75-100 mg/kg (max 2 g) IV every 6-8 hrs OR ceftazidime or cefepime 50 mg/kg (max 2 g) IV every 8 hrs
        - Ceftriaxone contraindicated—risk of hyperbilirubinemia
      - Add vancomycin 15 mg/kg IV every 6 hrs (max 1 g) if history of NICU admission or recent operation
    - > 28 days:
      - Ceftriaxone and vancomycin (for possible resistant streptococcus)
  — Steroid use controversial
    - May reduce neurologic sequelae (especially hearing loss) in children with *H. influenzae* meningitis
      - Benefit for other pathogens unproven
    - If given, must be with first antibiotic dose, else no benefit
    - Not for infants < 2 mo
    - Dexamethasone 0.15 mg/kg IV every 6 hrs
- Aseptic meningitis
  — Supportive care
  — Consider IV antibiotics pending CSF culture
    - Viral meningitis may be indistinguishable from early bacterial meningitis
    - Add acyclovir 20 mg/kg neonates, 10-15 mg/kg child, 10 mg/kg ≥ 12 yrs IV every 8 hrs if concern for HSV
- Viral encephalitis
  — Acyclovir as above if HSV encephalitis suspected/confirmed, decreases mortality

DISPOSITION

- Admit bacterial meningitis/encephalitis to PICU
- Consider discharge with close follow up for aseptic meningitis
  - Often admitted for empiric IV antibiotics/monitoring pending CSF culture
  - Admit if neonate/infant, immunocompromised, ill-appearing
    - Neonates/infants at risk for dehydration

BEWARE

- ⚠ Complications: apnea, shock, hypoglycemia, hypothermia, hyponatremia, seizures
- ⚠ Consider bacterial meningitis if presentation consistent even if alternate infection identified (AOM, pneumonia, UTI) as young children may not contain infection

5 ▶ Meningococcemia

BACKGROUND

- Severe illness caused by *Neisseria meningitidis*
  - ~15% mortality; 20% of survivors have long-term disability (deafness, amputations, neurocognitive deficits)
- Rare in USA: 330 cases in 2018
  - Declining with vaccination
  - Highest in children < 1 yr, adolescents 16-23 yrs
  - Outbreaks: colleges, military
  - Epidemics in "meningitis belt" in sub-Saharan Africa
- Infects via nasopharyngeal route and evades immune response → peripheral vasodilation, capillary leak, disseminated infection
- 70% present with meningitis, 30% with bacteremia only

EVALUATION

- **High Yield History**
  - Initially nonspecific symptoms: fever, myalgias, pharyngitis
  - Rapid progression to critical illness over hours
  - CNS involvement: headache, neck stiffness, photophobia, lethargy, irritability
- **Exam**
  - Shock (tachycardia, tachypnea, mottling, delayed capillary refill, hypotension)
  - Rash: begins as macules, papules, or urticaria → petechial within hours
    - Pressure regions (belt, socks)
    - Seen at presentation in ~50%

- Purpura fulminans: complication of DIC, vascular thrombosis → subcutaneous hemorrhage/skin necrosis → limb/digital ischemia
- May have myocardial dysfunction; assess for CHF
- **Diagnostics**
  - Labs: CBC, BMP, VBG, blood culture, lactate, LP if concern for meningitis
    - Can present in DIC—↑ PT/PTT, ↓ fibrinogen, ↑ D-dimer
    - LP contraindicated in DIC

MANAGEMENT

- ABCs: rapidly identify/correct shock, may need mechanical ventilation
  - Fluids: NS 20 mL/kg IV, often need repeat boluses
    - May clinically worsen if myocardial dysfunction present
  - Vasopressors: epinephrine 0.1 mcg/kg/min, norepinephrine 0.1 mcg/kg/min, titrate up to effect
  - Can present with Waterhouse-Friderichsen Syndrome (adrenal hemorrhage)
    - Steroids controversial, no benefit identified in *N. meningitidis*
  - Management of DIC: cryoprecipitate 10 mL/kg, FFP 10 mL/kg
    - Goal fibrinogen > 100 mg/dL, platelets > 50,000
- Antibiotics: ceftriaxone 100 mg/kg (max 2 g) first dose, then 50 mg/kg (max 2 g) IV every 12 hrs, or cefotaxime 75-100 mg/kg (max 2 g) IV every 6-8 hrs
- Droplet precautions
- Surgical consultation for debridement/amputation if limb ischemia
- Prophylaxis indicated for close household contacts, healthcare providers involved in intubation/suctioning/ETT management
  - Rifampin 5 mg/kg infants < 1 mo, 15-20 mg/kg (max 600 mg) older every 12 hrs for 2 days **OR**
  - Ceftriaxone 125 (< 15yr) – 250 mg IM once **OR**
  - Ciprofloxacin 20 mg/kg (max 500 mg) PO once

DISPOSITION

- Admit to ICU

BEWARE

- May be misdiagnosed early as viral syndrome or strep pharyngitis given nonspecific initial symptoms
- Suspect in febrile children with petechiae

6 ▶ COVID-19 and MIS-C

BACKGROUND
- SARS Coronavirus 2 (aka COVID-19) novel pandemic virus arose in 2019
  - Incubation period up to 14 days, most common 4-5 days
  - Asymptomatic infections common
  - Vast majority of children mild infections
    - Higher risk: infants, underlying chronic disease, Trisomy 21, pregnant
- Multisystem Inflammatory Syndrome in Children (MIS-C)
  - Rare complication of COVID-19 infection
  - Definition (all must be present):
    - Fever, laboratory evidence of inflammation, and *clinically severe illness requiring hospitalization (per CDC)* with > 2 organ involvement
    - No alternative diagnoses
    - Current or recent COVID diagnosed via RT-PCR, serology, antigen test or exposure within 4 weeks prior
- Epidemiology
  - Most commonly 1-14 years old, average 8 years
  - > 70% cases Hispanic/Latino or Non-Hispanic Black in U.S.
- Pathophysiology not well understood
- Similar to Kawasaki Disease presentation

EVALUATION

COVID-19
- **High Yield History**
  - Fever, cough, sore throat, vomiting, diarrhea, headache, myalgias
    - Loss of sense of smell or taste
  - Ill contacts
- **Exam**
  - Most similar to mild viral URI
  - Pulse oximetry, respiratory exam, hydration
- **Diagnostics**
  - RT-PCR or antigen testing
  - CXR rarely indicated
    - Bilateral consolidations, ground-glass opacities

MIS-C
- **High Yield History**
  - Persistent daily fevers, usually for 4-6 days at presentation
  - Most 2-4 weeks after COVID-19 infection
  - Abdominal pain, vomiting, diarrhea; cough uncommon
  - Tachypnea/labored breathing likely → shock
- **Exam**
  - *Ill-appearing!*
  - Nonspecific rash, conjunctivitis, mucous membrane involvement
  - Less common: swollen hands/feet, lymphadenopathy
- **Diagnostics**
  - Labs
    - CBC: lymphocytopenia, neutrophilia, mild anemia, thrombocytopenia (< 150,000)
    - Elevated CRP, ESR, D-Dimer, fibrinogen, ferritin, procalcitonin, IL-6 (inflammatory markers)
    - BMP, LFT, UA to assess kidney, liver function, electrolytes
    - PT/INR, PTT (hypercoagulability)
    - Cardiac enzymes/troponin, BNP (cardiac involvement)
  - Imaging
    - Most have normal CXR and CT chest
    - Echocardiogram
  - EKG (usually nonspecific)

MANAGEMENT

COVID-19
- Supportive care: antipyretics, hydration
- Education: natural history, isolation especially from high-risk contacts, return precautions

MIS-C
- ABCs, ventilatory support as needed
- Treat shock with fluid and vasoactive infusions (epinephrine, norepinephrine)
- If features of KD or incomplete KD:
  - IVIG (2 g/kg over 10-12 hrs) and low dose aspirin (3-5 mg/kg, max 81 mg/day) PO
- Consider methylprednisolone 1 mg/kg (max 30 mg) IV every 12 hrs
- Consider empiric broad-spectrum antibiotics given similarities with toxic shock
- Consider thrombotic prophylaxis given hypercoagulability

- Consider ID, rheumatology, cardiology, hematology consultations
  - IL-1 and IL-6 inhibitors may be recommended

DISPOSITION
- COVID-19: discharge most; admit hypoxia, respiratory distress, dehydration, complication
- MIS-C: admit to PICU/monitored bed

BEWARE
⚠ Many children present with GI rather than respiratory symptoms

Section XIV
Neonatal

1 ▶ Abdominal Pathology

ABDOMINAL WALL DEFECTS

- Gastroschisis
  - Full-thickness abdominal wall defect
  - Typically isolated gastrointestinal pathology
    - Up to 10% have intestinal atresia; all are malrotated
    - Can have necrosis, perforation, intestinal stenosis
- Omphalocele
  - Central abdominal wall defect at base of umbilical cord
  - Up to 80% have other congenital anomalies
    - Fetal aneuploidy, CHD, Beckwith-Wiedemann syndrome
- Risk factors: antidepressants, vasoconstrictors, young maternal age, substance use, cigarette smoking

EVALUATION

- **Exam**
  - Gastroschisis: located to the right of umbilical cord with evisceration of variable amount of intestines and organs exposed directly to the environment
  - Omphalocele: midline with herniation of intestines and organs outside of the abdominal cavity into a membrane covered by protective sac of peritoneum, Wharton's jelly and amnion
    - Normal cord inserts into sac
- **Diagnostics**
  - Prenatal US diagnosis and elevated alpha-fetoprotein

MANAGEMENT

- ABCs, mechanical ventilation as needed
  - Respiratory insufficiency may occur due to pulmonary hypoplasia
- Thermoregulation
  - High risk of hypothermia, place in warmer immediately
- Inspect and protect bowel
  - Emergent surgical consultation for ischemic bowel
  - Wrap bowel in warm sterile saline dressings with plastic bag overlying to prevent evaporative heat and fluid loss
  - Alternatively, can place baby's abdomen and legs in a plastic bag
- Lay newborn on either flank to minimize occlusion to narrow mesentery
- NPO, OGT for decompression
- Vascular access and maintenance fluids
  - Exposed bowel → ↑ insensible losses
- Prophylactic ABx (ampicillin 50 mg/kg IV every 6 hrs and gentamicin 2.5 mg/kg IV every 8 hrs)
  - Gastroschisis & ruptured omphaloceles
- Omphalocele
  - Unless ruptured, most do not need immediate surgical intervention
  - Prioritize cardiopulmonary stabilization
  - Judicious fluid management if suspect CHD

DISPOSITION

- NICU with pediatric surgeon

DIAPHRAGMATIC HERNIA

- Herniation of abdominal contents into thorax → pulmonary hypoplasia, pulmonary hypertension
- Associated anomalies: CHD, CNS lesions, esophageal atresia, adrenal insufficiency
- Female predominance, left side more common

EVALUATION

- **Exam**
  - Variable respiratory distress, absent breath sounds on ipsilateral side, barrel chest, scaphoid abdomen
- **Diagnostics**
  - Prenatal US: polyhydramnios, chest mass, mediastinal shift
  - Postnatal CXR: feeding tube and/or bowel visualized in thorax

MANAGEMENT

- Airway/Breathing
  - Prompt intubation to avoid BMV/HFO2 which causes gastric distension and lung compression
  - Lung protective settings: low peak inspiratory pressure
  - NPO, OGT for decompression permits lung re-expansion
- Circulation
  - Vascular access: umbilical arterial and venous lines
  - Maintenance fluids, inotropic agents PRN
- Pulmonary hypertension
  - Inhaled NO: selective pulmonary vasodilator improves oxygenation
    - Contraindicated with concomitant CHD dependent on right-to-left shunt, may → hypoperfusion and decompensation
  - Vasodilatory agents (PGE1, sildenafil): for persistent/severe cases
  - Surfactant not indicated - associated with poor outcome

DISPOSITION

- NICU with ECMO capabilities for refractory cases

HERNIAS

- Inguinal
  - Persistence of processus vaginalis allows communication between abdominal cavity and inguinal canal → indirect hernias (organs including bowel or ovary) or hydrocele (fluid only)
  - Associated with male sex, prematurity
- Umbilical
  - From incomplete closure of umbilical ring
  - ↑ low birthweight/premature and Black infants

EVALUATION

- **High Yield History**: mass (reducibility), vomiting, apparent pain, fever
- **Exam**
  - Inguinal
    - Exam may be normal given intermittent extrusion with increased intraabdominal pressure
    - Incarceration (inability to reduce hernia): irritability, vomiting, abdominal distension, firm palpable inguinal mass

- Strangulation: vascular compromise → bowel necrosis and perforation
  - Umbilical
    - Soft mass protrudes during crying, coughing, straining
- **Diagnostics**
  - US helps differentiate inguinal hernia from other groin masses
  - Umbilical hernia is clinical diagnosis

MANAGEMENT

- Inguinal
  - Reduction for incarceration without peritoneal signs: analgesic, Trendelenburg/frog leg position, apply steady pressure and traction distally while guiding bowel segments into the abdomen proximally
  - Definitive surgical repair required
- Umbilical
  - Caretaker reassurance: most spontaneously resolve
  - Surgical referral: symptomatic, persists beyond age 5yrs

DISPOSITION

- Emergent surgery consult for incarcerated or strangulated hernia
- Outpatient surgery for asymptomatic inguinal hernia
- Umbilical hernia → surveillance

NECROTIZING ENTEROCOLITIS (NEC)

- Intestinal ischemia/necrosis resulting from poor intestinal perfusion, abnormal bacterial colonization, diminished gut barrier function
- May occur in term infants (~10% of NEC cases) with associated risk factors (CHD, hypoxemic perinatal events, sepsis)

EVALUATION

- **High Yield History**: birth weight/gestational age, feeding intolerance/vomiting, abdominal distension, hematochezia
- **Exam**: abdominal tenderness and/or distension, abdominal wall erythema/crepitus, high gastric residuals, unstable vitals, lethargy
- **Diagnostics**
  - Labs: CBC w/ differential, CMP, CRP, PT/INR, PTT, blood cultures
  - KUB (pneumatosis intestinalis, pneumoperitoneum, portal vein gas)

MANAGEMENT

- ABCs
- NPO, OGT decompression
- IV fluids:
  — IV bolus NS 10 mL/kg as needed
  — IV maintenance fluids of D10W 80-100 mL/kg/day
    - May require more due to third spacing
  — Maintain urine output at 1-3 mL/kg/hr
- Antibiotics: broad spectrum per antibiogram
  — Ampicillin 50 mg/kg IV every 6 hrs + gentamicin 2.5 mg/kg IV every 12 hrs if ≤ 7 days old, every 8 hrs otherwise
    - And either clindamycin 10 mg/kg IV every 6-8 hrs or metronidazole 10 mg/kg IV every 8 hrs
  — Central line: add vancomycin 15 mg/kg IV every 6 hrs
- Emergent surgical consultation

DISPOSITION

- NICU with pediatric surgeon

PRUNE BELLY SYNDROME/EAGLE BARRETT SYNDROME

- Triad: abdominal muscle deficiency (wrinkly appearance of abdomen), urinary tract abnormalities, cryptorchidism
- Complications: renal disease (dysplastic changes), UTI/pyelonephritis (vesicoureteral reflux), pulmonary hypoplasia (oligohydramnios)
- Males > 95%

EVALUATION

- **High Yield History:** frequent UTIs, fever
- **Diagnostics**
  — UA, urine culture
  — Renal US, IV pyelogram

MANAGEMENT

- Antibiotic prophylaxis and UTI treatment PRN

DISPOSITION

- NICU with pediatric surgeon

2 ▶ Brief Resolved Unexplained Event (BRUE)

BACKGROUND

- **BRUE**: Event in an infant < 1yr old: observer reports sudden, **brief, unexplained** (not attributable to a clear cause), and now **resolved episode** of 1 or more of:
  - Cyanosis or pallor
  - Absent, decreased, or irregular breathing
  - ↑ or ↓ tone
  - Altered level of consciousness/altered mental status
- Replaces prior term (ALTE): Apparent Life-Threatening Event

AAP Guidelines Low Risk Definition
Age > 60 days
Gestational age ≥ 32 weeks and post conception age ≥ 45 weeks
First BRUE
Duration < 1 min
No CPR required by a trained provider
No alarming H&P findings

- High risk: any patient who does not meet all low-risk criteria above
- DDx: periodic breathing, breath holding spells, infection, apnea, UTI, metabolic disorders, seizure, reflux, choking, arrhythmia, child abuse

EVALUATION

- **High Yield History**
  - Description of event
    - Context: activities prior to event (sleeping, eating, vomiting)
    - Change in color, tone, breathing; seizure-like movements
    - Duration — have caretaker estimate using stopwatch
  - Have caretaker describe their response, including any CPR
  - Feeding: what, how much, how often, when was last feed prior
  - Birth history: prematurity, prenatal history, newborn screening abnormalities
  - Family history: seizures, arrhythmias, sudden unexplained death
- **Exam**: to rule out other cause
  - General: vital signs, craniofacial abnormalities, evidence of NAT
  - Cardiac: murmurs, arrhythmias, perfusion
  - Respiratory: hypoxia, tachypnea, rales/wheezing
  - Abdomen: organomegaly, masses, tenderness
  - Neurologic: tone, responsiveness, reflexes

- **Diagnostics**
  - Low risk: not required, can consider:
    - Pertussis, EKG
  - High risk: no official AAP recommendations, but strongly consider:
    - CBC, BMP, Ca, Mg, PO4, POC GLC, inborn error labs
    - UA, Utox
    - Respiratory pathogens panel including RSV, COVID, pertussis
    - EKG (look for long QT, dysrhythmia, evidence of CHD)
    - Imaging: CXR, consider head MRI/CT, skeletal survey

MANAGEMENT
- Consider observing on pulse oximetry (1-4 hrs) for low risk
- If underlying cause found, not a BRUE, specific management

DISPOSITION
- Admit high risk: continuous pulse oximetry monitoring, observation for repeat events, feeding evaluation, investigate suspected underlying cause
- Discharge low risk: PCP follow-up within 48 hrs
  - Caregiver education: CPR training, cocooning (caretaker pertussis immunization)

BEWARE
- ALWAYS consider NAT
- Neonatal seizures may be subtle (lip smacking, blinking, cycling of extremities)

3 ▶ Crying Infant

BACKGROUND
- Common ED complaint within first 3 months of life, with no accepted definition of "excessive crying"
- Most cases benign etiology, but must consider a wide differential
  - Common benign causes include "colic," otitis media, constipation
  - Most common serious cause is UTI
- Colic is a diagnosis of exclusion
  - No universally accepted definition
    - Can use the "Rule of 3s:" > 3 hrs of crying/day, > 3 days/week, for > 3 weeks, or Modified Wessel criteria (same as rule of 3s, but for 1 week)
    - Typically begins ~3 weeks old
  - Prevalence 1.5% to 11.9%

EVALUATION

- **High Yield History**
  - Duration, frequency, triggers, relationship to feeds
  - Consolable, soothing techniques
  - Eating: what, how much, how often
  - Urine output and stooling habits
  - Sleeping habits, some quiet alert time
  - Head to toe ROS: fever, URI symptoms, vomiting, diarrhea, bloody stools/urine, rash
  - Trauma
  - Birth history, neonatal complications, prenatal maternal drug use
  - Immunizations (including timing)
  - Caretaker support, who watches the baby, who is in the house?
- **Exam**
  - General: vital signs, weight gain, consolability, toxic-appearing, tone
  - Skin: rash, jaundice
  - HEENT: corneal abrasion, ears, blisters, thrush, fontanelles, meningismus
  - CV/Pulm: lung sounds, murmurs, pulses
  - Abdomen: masses, distension, tenderness, hepatomegaly
  - Genital exam: hernia, torsion, anal fissure
  - Extremities: hair tourniquet, fracture, abscess
  - NAT: frenulum exam (lips and tongue), bruising, retinal hemorrhage
- **Diagnostics**
  - H&P most important for diagnosis; add testing based on suspicion
  - Fluorescein exam controversial; consider if signs of corneal abrasion and no other obvious etiology
    - If abrasion, trial of anesthetic drop
  - Stool guaiac if concern for intussusception
  - Labs
    - UA, UCx, especially if < 1 mo
    - Sepsis work-up if febrile, hypothermic, toxic appearing
    - Utox if concern for neonatal or home drug exposure
    - LP: use similar decision-making as for febrile infant
  - Imaging
    - Not routine unless a specific etiology suspected based on H&P
    - CT head, skeletal survey if considering NAT
    - US if suspect intussusception, pyloric stenosis, appendicitis
  - EKG if suspect CHD, dysrhythmia

MANAGEMENT
- If no serious etiology:
    - Reassurance and caretaker education
        - Colic typically peaks ~6 weeks and is much better by ~12 weeks
    - "5 Ss:" Swaddling, Side/Stomach positioning (but not for sleeping), Shushing sounds, Swinging, Sucking (breast/pacifier)
    - Caretaker coping and assistance

DISPOSITION
- Admit: identified serious etiologies, toxic appearing, true persistent inconsolable crying in the ED

BEWARE
- Avoid extensive unnecessary workups; let H&P be your guide
- UA may not be positive in young infants despite positive cultures
- Maintain suspicion for NAT

4 ▶ Febrile Infant and Neonate

BACKGROUND
- Body temp ≥ 38.0°C
- Infant temperature should be taken rectally unless contraindicated
    - Axillary, oral, tympanic thermometers less reliable in this age group
- Neonatal sepsis is leading cause of infant mortality worldwide
- ≤ 28 days old, risk of serious bacterial illness (SBI) as high as 12% if febrile

EVALUATION
- **High Yield History**
    - Symptoms
        - Irritability, lethargy, home behavior, feeding
        - Vomiting, diarrhea, cough, congestion, rash
    - Birth History
        - Higher risk for SBI in preterm
        - Prenatal care: group B strep more prevalent if untreated
        - Maternal infections (HSV)
        - NICU/Nursery stay/course

- Sick contacts
- Vaccination history: which vaccines were given and when

- **Exam**
  - Vital signs
    - Fever may be only presenting sign of SBI
  - Signs and symptoms can be nonspecific
    - Fever, hypothermia (rectal temperature < 36.0°C), respiratory distress, cyanosis, apnea, irritability, hypotonia, seizures, bulging fontanelle, poor perfusion, bleeding problems, abdominal distension, hepatomegaly, hematochezia, jaundice, and "just not looking right"

- **Diagnostics**
  - Labs
    - CBC w/ differential
      - Poor sensitivity/high specificity
      - Preterm infants ↑ leukopenia
      - Full term ↑ leukocytosis
    - CRP
      - Poor sensitivity/high specificity
    - Procalcitonin
      - High sensitivity and specificity
      - Levels rise faster than CRP and stay elevated for longer
      - Newer, needs more research on diagnostic accuracy
    - BCx
    - UA, UCx via catheterized specimen
    - Respiratory pathogen panel
    - LP
      - All febrile infants ≤ 28 days old
      - \> 28 days if ill appearing; if well-appearing, use risk stratifying tool to determine
  - CXR
    - Hypoxia, respiratory distress/symptoms (grunting, nasal flaring, retractions)
  - Decision tools
    - Used for well-appearing, full-term infants to determine who needs admission and further workup
    - UA is considered positive if nitrite positive

	Philadelphia	Rochester	Boston	Step by Step	PECARN
Age	29-60 days	0-60 days	28-89 days	22-90 days	0-60 days
Temperature	≥ 38.2°C	≥ 38°C	≥ 38°C	≥ 38°C	≥ 38°C
Laboratory Values Low Risk * Stool only if indicated	CBC WBC < 15,000, Band:neutrophil ratio < 0.2 UA WBC < 10 CXR normal CSF WBC < 8 *Stool Neg	CBC WBC > 5000 and < 15,000 Bands < 1500 UA WBC ≤ 10 *Stool WBC ≤ 5	CBC WBC < 20,000 UA WBC < 10 CXR normal if obtained CSF WBC < 10	UA WBC none CRP ≤ 20 mg/L Procalcitonin < 0.5 ng/mL ANC ≤ 10,000	CBC ANC ≤ 4000 UA WBC ≤ 5 and LE/nitr neg Procalcitonin ≤ 1.7 ng/mL

MANAGEMENT

- Well appearing and ≥ 29 days → choose an algorithm to use and follow
  — High risk: pan-culture (blood, urine, CSF), admit, empiric IV antibiotics
  — Low risk: may be observed in the ED or hospital without empiric antibiotics or considered for discharge home with prompt follow-up
- Ill appearing — pan culture, empiric IV antibiotics
  — 0-28 days
    - Ampicillin 50-100 mg/kg IV every 6 hrs AND EITHER gentamicin 2.5 mg/kg IV every 12 hrs if ≤ 7 days old, every 8 hrs otherwise OR cefotaxime 50-100 mg/kg IV
    - Higher dose until meningitis ruled out
    - Cephalosporin preferred if suspect meningitis
      - Ceftazidime or cefepime 50 mg/kg IV every 8 hrs if cefotaxime unavailable
      - Ceftriaxone should be AVOIDED in this age group: bilirubin displacement → ↑ kernicterus
    - Gentamicin preferred if high likelihood Group B Strep
  — 29-90 days
    - Cefotaxime (or ceftriaxone 50-100 mg/kg IV daily if no hyperbilirubinemia, higher dose until meningitis ruled out) AND
    - Ampicillin if ≤ 60 days
    - Consider vancomycin 15 mg/kg IV every 8 hrs if MRSA suspected
  — Empiric acyclovir 20 mg/kg IV every 8 hrs if risk factors for HSV

DISPOSITION

- Admit neonate ≤ 28 days old with fever ≥ 38°C
- \> 28 days old: admit ill-appearing, risk factors, cannot risk stratify into low-risk group
  — Use decision tool + shared decision making to make the best disposition

BEWARE

- Heart rate increases by 9.6 (~10) BPM for every 1°C rise of fever
- Fever responsive to antipyretics (if given before ED evaluation) has no correlation to SBI risk

5 ▶ Jaundiced Neonate

BACKGROUND

- Epidemiology
  — 60% of full-term and 80% of preterm newborns in 1st week of life
  — Major reason for readmission to the hospital in first 2 weeks of life
- Definition
  — Total serum bilirubin (TSB) > 5 mg/dL
  — Conjugated (direct) bilirubin > 1 mg/dL or 20% of TSB is always pathologic
- Pathophysiology: bilirubin is a product of heme metabolism
  — Conjugated in the liver, excreted via bile
  — Enterohepatic circulation leads to increased levels
- Kernicterus: rare catastrophic sequela of hyperbilirubinemia
  — AKA Bilirubin Induced Neurologic Dysfunction (BIND)
  — Risk factors: higher bilirubin level, prematurity

DIFFERENTIAL DIAGNOSIS

Benign Causes	
Physiologic jaundice	Immature neonatal liver function results in physiologic increase after birth, peaks day 3-5 of life at up to 8-9 mg/dL, then declines
Breastfeeding jaundice	Exaggerated physiologic jaundice in exclusively breastfed infants due to limited maternal milk production leading to decreased intake & dehydration. Occurs in first week of life
Breast milk jaundice	Unclear pathophysiology. Later peak at 10-21 days of age, may persist several weeks

Pathologic Causes	
Unconjugated	Hemolysis (ABO incompatibility, hematoma, hemorrhage, G6PD deficiency, sickle cell, thalassemia, pyruvate kinase deficiency, spherocytosis), UTI, sepsis, obstructive GI disease (meconium ileus, duodenal atresia, Hirschsprung's, pyloric stenosis), genetic (Gilbert's, Crigler-Najjar, galactosemia, hypothyroidism)
Conjugated	Never benign. Infection (TORCH, sepsis, hepatitis), biliary obstruction (atresia, choledochal cyst, stricture, Alagille syndrome), drugs and toxins, inborn errors of metabolism

EVALUATION

- **High Yield History (high risk factors)**
  - Birth history
    - **Prematurity**
    - Jaundice **in first 24 hrs of life** / icterus, bilirubin levels, phototherapy
    - **ABO incompatibility**, known blood type of mom, baby
    - Hours since birth - important to know to assess risk
    - **Cephalhematoma, bruising**
  - **Hemolytic disease**
  - Dietary
    - Breast vs. bottle vs. both: frequency, quantity
    - Urine and stool output and color (dark urine, acholic stools)
  - Additional symptoms
    - Fever, vomiting, pallor
    - BIND (Kernicterus) symptoms: poor suck, irritability, shrill cry, change in tone, poor feeding; late findings: altered mental status, seizures
  - Family history
    - **East Asian race**
    - **Sibling that required phototherapy**
- **Exam**
  - Jaundice
    - Blanching skin with pressure may help to appreciate yellow color
    - Cephalocaudal progression with higher levels when lower half of body jaundiced (but physical exam is poor predictor of TSB level)
    - Scleral icterus often visible at TSB levels of 6-8 mg/dL
  - Vital signs, weight gain / growth chart, hydration
  - Cephalohematoma, bruising, petechiae, pallor

- Hepatosplenomegaly
- Neurologic exam: behavior, tone, abnormal movements (bicycling, choreoathetoid), retrocollis, opisthotonus
- **Diagnostics**
  - Transcutaneous bilirubin TcB ("bilimeter") screening in low-risk infants
    - Obtain serum levels if TcB > 70% of the concerning serum level for age OR > 13 mg/dL
    - Do not use in babies who previously received phototherapy
  - Labs for all with potentially significant hyperbilirubinemia
    - Total + direct serum bilirubin and hemoglobin level
    - If low risk level of unconjugated bilirubin and normal hemoglobin, no further labs needed
  - Labs for all with intermediate to high-risk bilirubin levels
    - CBC with smear to assess for anemia, hemolysis
    - Blood type and Coombs to assess for blood group incompatibility
      - Type and cross for possible exchange transfusion
    - Reticulocyte count
    - UA to rule out UTI as association exists
  - Labs if conjugated hyperbilirubinemia
    - BMP, LFTs including GGT, albumin level, total protein
    - Viral hepatitis panel
    - TORCH titers
    - Consider thyroid function tests (hypothyroidism), G6PD
    - Sepsis work-up as indicated
  - Imaging
    - RUQ ultrasound for conjugated hyperbilirubinemia

MANAGEMENT

- AAP has established thresholds for initiation of phototherapy and exchange transfusion based on age and risk factors
  - Can be accessed at bilitool.org
- Fluids and nutrition
  - Treat dehydration with oral and IV fluids as needed
  - Encourage frequent feeds to aid clearance
  - AAP recommends against discontinuation of breastfeeding
    - If needed, mothers may briefly pump and save breastmilk while feeding formula

- Phototherapy — converts bilirubin into water-soluble non-toxic excretable forms
  - Efficacy is proportional to the amount of skin exposed
    - Blankets and pads may be used under the infant
    - Triple or 360° phototherapy may be used with emergently high bilirubin levels
  - Eye protection and avoiding dehydration are important
  - Home phototherapy is sometimes available for select term low-risk infants
- Exchange transfusion rarely required, used for severely elevated / high risk for BIND
  - Performed by neonatal intensivist

DISPOSITION

- Admit if meets criteria for phototherapy or exchange transfusion, has conjugated hyperbilirubinemia, ill-appearing
- Discharge: well-appearing, adequate PO, not meeting criteria for phototherapy
  - Although sunlight exposure may reduce bilirubin, not recommended due to risk of sunburn
  - Discuss importance of maintaining good hydration, encourage breastfeeding

BEWARE

- Conjugated hyperbilirubinemia is always pathologic
- Cutoff levels for intervention are lower in infants born premature
- Maintain a high index of suspicion for sepsis

6 ▶ Neonatal Emergencies (THE MISFITS)

THE MISFITS Differential Diagnosis	
Trauma	Non-accidental trauma
Heart	CHD
	SVT (Consider if HR > 220)
Endocrine	Hypoglycemia
	Hypothyroidism, thyrotoxicosis
	Congenital adrenal hyperplasia (CAH)
Metabolic	Electrolyte, glucose abnormalities
Inborn error	Inborn error of metabolism
Seizure/CNS	Intracranial hemorrhage or infection
	Cerebral AVM, stroke

THE MISFITS Differential Diagnosis *(continued)*	
Feeding/Formula	Incorrect formula mixing
	Food protein-induced enterocolitis syndrome (FPIES)
Intestinal	Intussusception
	Malrotation ± midgut volvulus
	Necrotizing enterocolitis (NEC)
	Omphalitis
	Duodenal atresia
	Pyloric stenosis
	Hirschsprung → toxic megacolon
Toxicologic	Lidocaine (recent procedure or circumcision)
	Diphenhydramine (for fussiness)
	Dermal exposures (rubbing alcohol, maternal breast)
	Homeopathic remedies (gripe water)
Sepsis	GBS, Listeria, GNRs (incl *E coli*), staph, HSV, enterovirus, RSV, COVID-19

EVALUATION

- **High Yield History**
  — Symptoms
    - Fever
    - Vomiting, bilious/non-bilious
    - Irritability, lethargy
    - Respiratory difficulty, tachypnea
    - Seizure-like movements
      - Seizures can be subtle in neonates (staring, blinking, lip smacking, bicycling); most are subclinical
    - Feeding
      - Water to formula mixing ratio, any additives used, non-human milk, herbals/homeopathic remedies
    - Bloody stools (may indicate GI necrosis)
  — Birth History: gestational age at delivery, birth weight, complications, instrumentation and/or resuscitation at birth, NICU stay, newborn screening results
  — Maternal History: HIV, syphilis, hepatitis B, rubella, GBS, blood type
    - Maternal medications if breastfeeding
  — Family history of metabolic disorders, sibling deaths at young age

- **Exam**
  - Vital signs, signs of shock
  - Respiratory distress, work of breathing, unequal breath sounds
  - Perfusion: capillary refill, pulses (brachial AND femoral), cyanosis, mottling, warm/cool extremities, mental status
  - Cardiovascular (see CHD chapter)
    - Obtain BP & pulse oximetry in all 4 extremities
    - Murmur, gallop, hepatomegaly
    - Hyperoxia test with 100% oxygen: compare pre-ductal (right upper extremity) and post-ductal (lower extremity) SpO2 or PaO2
      - No improvement suggests extrapulmonary R→L shunting
  - Neurologic
    - Lethargy, irritability, muscular tone
    - Auscultate fontanelle: cranial bruit may indicate brain AVM
    - Reflexes: root, suck, gag, Moro
  - Skin
    - Rash: especially vesicles, petechiae
    - Hyperpigmentation (CAH)
    - Bruising
    - Jaundice
  - Abdomen / umbilicus: distension, discoloration, tenderness, hepatosplenomegaly
  - GU: strangulated/incarcerated hernia, testicular torsion
    - Hyperpigmented scrotum or ambiguous genitalia (CAH)
  - Head to toe exam for trauma
- **Diagnostics** (consider based on suspected etiology)
  - Labs
    - POC GLC
    - CBC with differential, blood cultures
    - CMP, Mg, PO4
    - Blood gas
    - UA, UCx, Utox
    - BNP if suspect CHD
    - Ammonia, lactate, pyruvate, urine organic acids
    - Respiratory pathogen panel
    - CSF studies if concern for CNS pathology

- Imaging
  - CXR
  - Acute abdominal series
  - Upper GI series with oral contrast if suspect malrotation
  - Head CT
- EKG

MANAGEMENT

- ABCs
- Vascular access (IV, IO)
  - Umbilical venous line if stump still present (up to age 10 days)
- Shock
  - 10-20 mL/kg NS bolus IV/IO
    - 5-10 mL/kg with frequent reassessment if concern for CHF
  - Epinephrine 0.1 mcg/kg/min IV if fluid-refractory
  - Consider hydrocortisone 25 mg IV/IO for shock refractory to vasopressors (CAH)
- Correct or prevent hypo/hyperthermia
  - Avoid rapid correction of hypothermia (use warmer's servo-control option set to 36.5°C skin temp)
- Hypoglycemia correction: D10W 2 mL/kg IV
- Electrolyte correction
  - Maintenance fluids D5W without electrolytes used day 1 of life
  - Hyponatremic seizure: 3% saline 5 mL/kg IV
  - Hyperkalemia with EKG changes: calcium gluconate 10% 60 mg/kg IV over 3-5 min, sodium bicarbonate 1-2 mEq/kg IV over 5-10 min, insulin 0.1 u/kg/hr IV ± D10W
  - Symptomatic hypocalcemia: calcium gluconate 10% 100-200 mg/kg IV
- Empiric antimicrobials (higher doses if meningitis)
  - Ampicillin 50-100 mg/kg IV/IM
  - Gentamicin 2.5 mg/kg IV/IM
  - Acyclovir 20 mg/kg IV
  - Cefotaxime 50-100 mg/kg IV
- Phenobarbital 20 mg/kg IV if still seizing after electrolyte correction
- Adenosine 0.1 mg/kg IV for SVT
- PGE1 0.05 mcg/kg/min titrated to effect (max 0.1 mcg/kg/min) with cardiology consult if suspect ductal-dependent lesion (failed hyperoxy test)
- Salt-losing CAH suspected: hydrocortisone 25 mg IV
- Inborn Error: NPO, maintenance IVF with dextrose, genetics consult
  - Nitrogen binding agent, dialysis if ammonia > 200-500µmmol/L

- Thyrotoxicosis: methimazole 0.25 mg/kg and propranolol 1 mg/kg PO
- Surgical consult if distended or acute abdomen

DISPOSITION
- Admit to PICU or NICU

BEWARE
- ⚠ Overall appearance is often the most important part of exam to identify the severely ill infant as may only have non-specific signs/symptoms
- ⚠ Tachycardia is usually the first sign of shock in children; hypotension is a late finding

7 ▶ Normal Feeding, Elimination, and Growth

BACKGROUND
- Expected feeding in first 0-6 months
  - Breastfeeding
    - Weeks 1-3: 10-20 min across both breasts, 8-12 feedings/day
    - Should be fed "on-demand" looking for signs of hunger: licking lips, rooting, hand to mouth repeatedly, fussiness, crying (late)
    - Should not sleep longer than 4hrs between feeds during first month
    - May take a few days for mother's milk to come in or for baby to learn to latch; refer to pediatrician or lactation specialist
    - After 2 mos may stretch feeds out to every 3-4 hrs, longer stretch at night
  - Bottle Feeding
    - Formulas: Cow's milk protein-based, Soy-based, Protein hydrolysate (hypoallergenic)
    - Standard 20 kcal/oz
      - Week 1: 1.5-2 oz/feed × 8-12 feedings/day
      - Weeks 2-4: 2-3 oz/feed
      - Month 2: 4-5 oz/feed × 6-8/day
      - Feeds increasing by 1 oz/mo until leveling off at 8 oz/feed
      - Concern for overfeeding with bottle feeding, should not exceed 32 oz/day
  - Introduction of solid foods
    - 6-8 mos: rice cereal, purees (thin first, then thick)
    - 8-10 mos: finger foods (finely chopped, soft foods)
    - Avoid choking hazards (hot dogs, nuts, grapes, raw carrots)
    - May safely introduce highly allergenic foods as tolerated

- No evidence that delayed introduction prevents atopic disease
- Growing evidence early introduction reduces allergies
- No honey for < 1 yr, risk of infant botulism
- Expected elimination in the first 0-6 mos
  — Wet diapers per 24 hrs: 1 on day 1 of life, 6-8 by day 6 onwards
  — Stools: thick, dark meconium on day 1
    - Expect change in stool frequency/character with changes in feeds
    - Breastfed: pale yellow/seedy by day 5, generally more frequent
    - Formula fed: firmer, yellow/brown stool, generally less frequent
- Expected weight gain in the first 0-12 mos
  — Normal for newborns to lose 7% of birthweight (BW) in first few days
    - Concern if ≥ 10% loss or if has not regained BW by 10-14 days
  — Infants gain ~30 g/day from 0-3 mos, 20 g/day from 3-6 mos, 10 g/day from 6-12 mos
    - Should double BW by 5 months, triple BW by 1 year
- Expected length and head circumference
  — < 2 yrs old, use WHO standard growth charts
  — ≥ 2yrs, use the CDC reference growth charts
  — Birth height doubles by age 3-4 yrs

EVALUATION

- **High Yield History**
  — Feeding frequency, quantity, duration, formula vs. breastfeeding, how mixing formula
  — Elimination (wet diapers, stool) frequency and character
  — Caretaker expectations and concerns
  — Birth history: birthweight, prematurity, complications
  — Family history: inborn errors of metabolism, genetic diseases
- **Exam**
  — Weight, length, head circumference (correct for prematurity to age 2yrs)

MANAGEMENT

- Observation of feeding
- Caretaker education

DISPOSITION

- Admit if failure to thrive: work-up, calorie evaluation, supplementation as needed
- Discharge with follow-up if growth, feeding, elimination within expected parameters
  — Lactation support PRN

8 ▶ Post-NICU Premature Baby

Birth weight	Gestational Age
Low birth weight (LBW): < 2500 g	Preterm: < 37 wks
Very low birth weight (VLBW): < 1500 g	Very preterm: ≤ 32 wks
Extremely low birth weight (ELBW): < 1000 g	Extremely preterm: < 28 wks

- — Corrected age = current age (weeks since birth) - number of weeks born preterm
- Weight gain in the first 1-12 months
  - — Infants should gain 26-40 g/day from 1-3 months, 12-25 g/day from 4-11 months, 9-12 g/day by 12 months
  - — Recommend 24 kcal/oz formula or breast milk fortified with iron and vitamin D
- Complications of prematurity (may have lasting sequelae)

Condition	Etiology	Notes
Retinopathy of prematurity (ROP) Failure of retinal vessels to develop normally, leading to visual impairment	Injury to developing retinal blood vessels from hypoxia, hypotension, or hyperoxia (free radical formation)	Schedule ophthalmology exam at age 1 mo for infants born ≤ 30 wks GA or ≤ 1500 g
Anemia of prematurity	Inefficient response to erythropoietin; worsened by low iron stores, phlebotomy	Hemoglobin nadir 7-10 g/dL at 4-8 weeks of life
Necrotizing enterocolitis (NEC) See: Neonatal — Abdominal Pathology chapter	Poor intestinal perfusion and abnormal bacterial colonization leading to intestinal ischemia and necrosis	• Symptoms: abdominal distension, erythema, crepitus, high gastric residuals • KUB: pneumatosis intestinalis, portal venous gas, pneumoperitoneum
Bronchopulmonary dysplasia (chronic lung disease, CLD)	Lung immaturity, oxygen toxicity, barotrauma, pulmonary edema (volume overload, PDA), inflammation leading to airway hyperplasia, interstitial fibrosis	• Symptoms: — Chronic wheeze or cough — Higher rates of respiratory infections • ↑ mortality from cor pulmonale, lower respiratory tract infection, sudden death

Condition	Etiology	Notes
Apnea of prematurity Prolonged respiratory pause of ≥ 20 sec, or association with bradycardia, color change, or desaturation	Central (immature respiratory control), obstructive (upper airway obstruction, chest wall/diaphragm collapsibility)	• Diagnosis of exclusion • Rule-out infection, seizure, electrolyte abnormality, hypoglycemia, anemia, CHD, GER, toxicological, medication effect, periodic breathing (respiratory pauses of ≤ 10 sec, benign in infants) • Typically resolves by 37 wks post-conceptual age

Intraventricular hemorrhage (IVH)
• Most common type of neonatal intracranial hemorrhage (mainly ≤ 32 wks GA or VLBW)
• 90% occur in first 3 days of life
	Preceding hypoxic ischemic injury that destroys highly vascular germinal matrix, infarcts periventricular white matter, impairs CSF absorption from post-hemorrhagic hydrocephalus	• Symptoms:
		  — Bulging fontanel
		  — AMS, posturing
		  — BP or Hct drop
		  — 20-25% asymptomatic
		• Screening cranial US by day of life 7 for ≤ 32 wks GA infants

Gastroesophageal reflux (GER) • Retrograde movement of gastric contents into esophagus and above • 50% of infants 0-3mo regurgitate ≥ 1x/day	Relaxation of lower esophageal sphincter	• Risk of aspiration, cyanosis, and vomiting in relation to GER • pH probe study (gold standard test for GER) often underestimates occurrence

EVALUATION

- **High Yield History**
  - Birth history
    - Gestational age, NICU course, complications, procedures
  - Current symptoms and concerns
    - Feeding routine and tolerance, supplementation, weight gain
    - Medications, apnea monitor, home oxygen, pulse oximetry
    - Palivizumab during RSV season
- **Exam**
  - Developmental milestones (based on corrected age)
  - AMS, bulging fontanel, posturing (IVH)
  - Chronic wheeze, cough (CLD)
  - Abdominal distension, crepitus (NEC)
  - Pallor (anemia)

- **Diagnostics**
  - Labs
    - Higher risk for hypoglycemia, anemia
    - Respiratory pathogen panel (higher risk for associated apnea)
  - Imaging
    - CXR with CLD (chronic changes, compare to previous)
    - Evaluation of VP shunt function: shunt series, CT

MANAGEMENT

Condition	Management
Anemia of prematurity	• Limit blood draws • Transfuse for severe anemia • Recombinant erythropoietin, iron supplementation
NEC	• Bowel rest, IVF, OGT decompression • Broad spectrum IV antibiotics, admit to NICU • Surgical consultation
CLD	• Maintain SpO2 between 90-95% (SpO2 > 95% increases risk for ROP). After 36wks GA, maintain SpO2 > 95% to prevent pulmonary hypertension and cor pulmonale (lower risk of ROP) • Diuretics, bronchodilators • Steroids increase risk of adverse neurologic outcome without lasting benefit. Exceptions: asthma-like exacerbations, ventilator-dependence, high O2 requirement
Apnea of prematurity	• Home monitoring not indicated if asymptomatic • Caffeine 10-20 mg/kg PO loading dose • Nasal oxygen or nasal CPAP PRN
IVH	• Correct coagulopathies • Decrease PaCO2 (to maintain cerebral perfusion, lower ICP) • LP (up to 10 mL CSF removal), furosemide or acetazolamide for post-hemorrhagic hydrocephalus • VP shunt if persistent, progressive hydrocephalus
GER	• Frequent small volume feeds • Upright position 20-30 min after feeds • Trial cow's milk protein-free formula or thickened feeds • Head of bed elevation has no effect

DISPOSITION

- Admit if high suspicion for dehydration, respiratory complications, need neurologic or cardiac monitoring
- If discharge: close follow up, return precautions

BEWARE

① Vulnerable child phenomenon → increased risk for NAT

9 ▶ Skin Findings

CONGENITAL DERMAL MELANOSIS (MONGOLIAN SPOT)

- Most common pigmented lesion
- Black-gray-blue patches over lower back, buttocks, legs
- Fades after first few years
- Consider GM1 gangliosidosis if diffuse

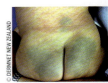

Congenital Dermal Melanosis

CUTIS MARMORATA

- Purple, reticular, blanching rash in areas exposed to cold
- Improves with warmth, usually resolves after first few months

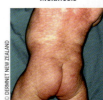

Cutis Marmorata

ERYTHEMA TOXICUM

- Most common newborn rash, especially in term infants
- Diffuse, papular-to-pustular rash with erythematous base, sparing palms and soles
- Occurs after first day of life, resolves spontaneously after 2 weeks

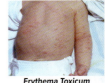

Erythema Toxicum

HARLEQUIN COLOR CHANGE

- Red in dependent regions and pale in non-dependent regions
- Secondary to immature autonomic system
- Occurs most commonly day of life 2-5, resolves after days-to-weeks

MILIA AND MILIARIA

- Milia: white, millimeter sized papules on scalp/face caused by keratin inclusion cysts
- Miliaria
  - Crystallina: small, clear vesicles on head, upper chest/back
  - Rubra "heat rash": small, erythematous papules on head, upper chest/back
  - Sweat gland obstruction from blankets, tight clothing, warm environments
- Resolve spontaneously

NEONATAL ACNE

- Comedones over face and chest
- Onset first month of life
- Spontaneously resolves by 4 months in most, avoid thick lotions

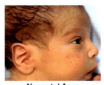
Neonatal Acne

NEONATAL HERPES

- +/– vesicular eruption
- First week to month of life
- Localized cutaneous infection, CNS infection, or disseminated infection
- Sepsis work-up with LP, admit, treat with IV acyclovir

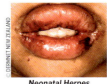
Neonatal Herpes

SEBORRHEIC DERMATITIS

- Yellow greasy scales, hair loss, and erythematous plaques over scalp, face, and skin creases, "cradle cap"
- First month of life
- Resolves spontaneously by 6 mos
- Treat with gentle scrubbing after softening with petrolatum/oil
- Mild topical steroids (1% hydrocortisone) and anti-fungal shampoos (2% ketoconazole or dilute selenium sulfide shampoo 2x/wk) for persistent rash

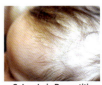
Seborrheic Dermatitis

Skin Findings

TRANSIENT NEONATAL PUSTULAR MELANOSIS

- Pustules pop → erythematous macules with fine collarette of scale
- Spontaneous resolution over 3-4 weeks

BEWARE

Skin Finding	Association
Nevus flammeus (port-wine stain)	Sturge-Weber (unilateral facial/trigeminal)
	Klippel-Trenaunay-Weber (lower extremity)
Fast-growing hemangiomas	Kasabach-Merritt
Hemangiomas near sensitive organs	May require intervention (vision obstruction)
Mandibular hemangiomas	Airway hemangiomas
Cafe-au-lait spots, neurofibromas	Neurofibromatosis
Pigmented macules with wheal when scraped	Urticaria pigmentosa
Linear erythematous blisters, wart-like growths, hyper/hypopigmentation, hair loss	Incontinentia pigmenti
Vesicles with erythematous base	Varicella

10 ▶ Umbilical Cord Issues

BACKGROUND

- Umbilical cord: two umbilical arteries, one umbilical vein, Wharton's jelly (supportive gelatinous substance)
- Cord typically dries and separates within 1-2 weeks
  - Delayed separation (> 3 weeks) associated with immunodeficiency (leukocyte adhesion deficiency), infection, urachal anomalies, antiseptic agents
- Omphalitis: polymicrobial soft tissue infection of periumbilical region, can present as cellulitis or more severe forms such as bacteremia, necrotizing fasciitis, peritonitis
  - Incidence < 1% in developed countries
  - Risk factors: non-sterile cord clamping, poor cord care, prematurity
- Umbilical granuloma: persistence of normal granulation tissue at base of the umbilicus after cord separation
- Umbilical polyp: epithelial remnant of either omphalomesenteric duct (intestinal mucosa) or urachus (uroepithelium)

EVALUATION

- **High Yield History** gestation/birth weight, birth history, cord care, umbilical discharge (color, odor, viscosity), systemic symptoms (fever, lethargy)
- **Exam**
  - Vital signs, general appearance, signs of shock
  - Periumbilical skin findings: erythema (local vs. circumferential), induration, warmth
    - Localized erythema from diaper irritation — leave diaper off for several minutes and observe for improvement
  - Discharge
    - Clear drainage: patent urachus
    - Mucopurulent/malodorous: infection
    - Serosanguinous/mucoid: umbilical granuloma
    - Bleeding: suggestive of omphalitis as infection delays thrombosis of umbilical vessels
    - Mild discharge may be normal without other signs of infection
  - Mass
    - Umbilical granuloma: red/pink friable lesion, 3-10 mm
    - Umbilical polyp: appears similar to granuloma but larger
- **Diagnostics**
  - Labs if suspect omphalitis: CBC with differential, CMP, wound culture/gram stain, blood cultures
  - UA, UCx if suspect patent urachus
  - Imaging: US, CT as indicated

MANAGEMENT

- Cord care: topical antiseptics are not superior to dry cord care in low-risk neonates
- Umbilical granuloma: silver nitrate
- Omphalitis
  - NS bolus 20 mL/kg
  - IV antibiotics: dosages depend on postnatal age, weight, trough levels
    - Antistaphylococcal penicillin or vancomycin if high suspicion for MRSA
    - Aminoglycoside
    - +/– Anaerobic coverage
  - Emergent surgical consultation for necrotizing fasciitis or abscess formation
- Umbilical polyp/patent urachus: surgical consultation

DISPOSITION
- Admission for suspected omphalitis
- Discharge with close follow-up for remaining conditions

BEWARE
- ❗ Omphalitis may cause inflammation and thrombosis of the portal vein → portal hypertension
- ❗ Umbilical mass unresponsive to silver nitrate is suggestive of a polyp

Section XV
Neurology

1 ▶ Ataxia and Paralysis

BACKGROUND

- Ataxia: acute onset, episodic or chronic gait instability, decreased coordination, usually due to cerebellar dysfunction
  — Consider in children presenting with partial or full paralysis, poor tone, refusal to ambulate
- Infectious/postinfectious and ingestions make up the vast majority of cases
  — Other causes: trauma, neurologic
- DDx: acute post infectious cerebellar ataxia (APCA) accounts for 30-75% of cases, toxic ingestion, Guillain-Barre syndrome (GBS), tick paralysis, infantile botulism, acute postinfectious demyelinating encephalomyelitis (ADEM), neoplasm, ICH, meningitis/encephalitis, vestibular migraine, benign paroxysmal vertigo (BPV)
- Previously healthy children typically have benign, self-limited etiologies

EVALUATION

- **High Yield History**
  — Access to medications, drugs, toxins (especially anticonvulsants)
  — Recent infection or vaccine administration
  — Trauma, stroke risk factors
  — Migraines, vomiting, visual changes
    - Family history of migraines → migraine, BPV
  — Chronicity
    - Acute: infectious/postinfectious, toxin, trauma
    - Subacute: GBS, metabolic
    - Insidious: tumor, other space occupying lesion
- **Exam**
  — Vital signs: Cushing reflex = ↑ICP, fever
  — HEENT: visual acuity, papilledema, nystagmus, otitis media, meningismus
  — Thorough neurologic exam

- Motor: weakness vs. ataxia
- Truncal vs. extremity ataxia, cerebellar signs
- Cranial nerve abnormalities suggestive of mass effect
- Opsoclonus myoclonus syndrome: ataxia, dancing eye movements, jerking (suggestive of neuroblastoma)
  - Skin exam for ticks, bites, rashes
  - GBS: extremity ataxia, ascending paralysis, decreased reflexes
  - Infantile botulism: hypotonia, hyporeflexia, weak cry, poor gag reflex
  - APCA: truncal ataxia, gait instability without mental status changes
  - ADEM: ataxia + other neurologic deficits AND altered mental status
- **Diagnostics**
  - Labs
    - Start with ingestions as identification can prevent further workups: Utox, blood alcohol level, drug levels if known ingestions, POC GLC
    - LP if suspect meningitis, encephalitis
  - Imaging
    - CT head if concern for trauma, ICH, mass, stroke
    - MRI when considering ADEM or posterior CVA
  - EEG if history suggests seizure

MANAGEMENT

- Supportive care often
- Antibiotics early in infection, antidotes PRN, IVIG for GBS
- Neurology vs. neurosurgery consult

DISPOSITION

- Typically admit for thorough workup and supportive care
- If mildly symptomatic with history suggestive of APCA, may consider discharge

BEWARE

! Conversion disorder is a diagnosis of exclusion (not made in the ED)

2 ▶ Headache

BACKGROUND

- Up to 90% of children have headaches; majority benign
- Primary vs. secondary (symptom of underlying condition)
- DDx: migraine, tension, cluster, medication overuse headache, space occupying lesion, hypertension, URI, strep throat, sinusitis, cerebral venous thrombosis, idiopathic intracranial hypertension (IIH), infection, bleed, substance use, intoxicants (CO, lead)

Etiology	Characteristics
Migraine	Onset hours-to-days
	May have an aura
	Usually unilateral (may be bilateral in younger children), throbbing/pulsating
	Associations: nausea, vomiting, photophobia, phonophobia
	May have positive family history
Tension	Onset minutes-to-days
	Band-like, bilateral
	Rare associations: nausea, photophobia, phonophobia
Cluster	Onset minutes-to-hours
	Usually unilateral frontal/periorbital
	Associations: lacrimation, conjunctival injection, rhinorrhea or congestion

EVALUATION

- **High Yield History**
  - Acute vs. chronic, progressive vs. stable
  - Precipitating/palliating factors, quality, location, severity, associated symptoms (aura, nausea, vomiting, photophobia, phonophobia, vision changes)
  - Current medications
  - Red flags: morning/supine headaches, migraine without family history, change in character/frequency, onset within 6 months, AMS, primarily occipital, focal neurologic findings, fever, pregnancy/OCP use
- **Exam**
  - Vitals including temperature
  - HEENT: extraocular movements, fundoscopy, visual acuity & fields, pupils, intraocular pressure, sinuses, ears, oral cavity, tonsils
  - Neck: bruits, rigidity, meningismus
  - Skin: purpura or petechiae + fever → concern for meningococcemia
    - Cafe-au-lait spots, neurofibromas, ash-leaf spots may → neurocutaneous disorder
  - Neurologic exam: strength, sensation, reflexes, coordination, cranial nerves

- **Diagnostics**
  - Urine pregnancy test
  - Consider UA - UTI may present as headache without dysuria
  - Labs otherwise rarely needed; consider CBC, blood cultures, LP with opening pressure PRN
  - Imaging rarely needed; consider CT head if red flags, mass, or clot suspected

MANAGEMENT

- Analgesia
  - Acetaminophen 15 mg/kg (max 1 g) PO every 4-6 hrs (do not exceed 75 mg/kg/day)
  - Ibuprofen 10 mg/kg (max 400 mg) PO every 6 hrs
- Acute migraine
  - IVF 20 mL/kg NS IV
  - Ketorolac 0.5 mg/kg (max 30 mg) IV
  - Prochlorperazine 0.15 mg/kg (max 10 mg) IV
    - Often with diphenhydramine 1 mg/kg (max 50 mg) IV
  - Sumatriptan 10-20 mg IN or 3-6 mg SQ
- Oxygen for cluster headaches
- Headache hygiene
  - Headache diary to identify triggers
  - Avoid common triggers
    - Lack of sleep, excessive screen time, skipping meals
    - Tyramine, sodium nitrite, MSG, caffeine withdrawal
  - Stress management, daily exercise
- Consult Neurology if red flags, abnormal neurologic exam, high frequency, poor response to analgesics
  - IIH: serial LPs, acetazolamide, furosemide

DISPOSITION

- Admit if secondary headache or red flags or unremitting pain requiring further workup/management

BEWARE

! Migraine symptoms in young children may be atypical: bilateral, shorter duration

3 ▶ Seizures

BACKGROUND

- Febrile seizures
  - Seizures associated with a fever of at least 38°C (100.4°F) but without evidence of intracranial infection, hypoglycemia, trauma, and with normal development
  - Usually 6 mos – 5yrs of age, affects 2-4% children
  - Complex: > 15 min, focal, ≥ 2 in 24 hrs
    - Simple: none of these
  - Risk of epilepsy following a simple febrile seizure slightly > general population
    - Increased risk if complex febrile seizure, seizure family history, abnormal development
- DDx afebrile seizures: metabolic derangements/electrolyte abnormalities, toxins, trauma (including NAT), ICH, space-occupying lesion, vasculitis
- Status epilepticus: duration > 5min OR consecutive seizures with no return to baseline in between
- Seizure mimics: breath holding spells, vasovagal syncope, pseudoseizures

EVALUATION

- **High Yield History**
  - Ingestions, head trauma, context prior to seizure episode
  - Elements suggestive of true seizures: AMS, lateral tongue biting, lip smacking, post-ictal phase
- **Exam**
  - Meningeal irritation, signs of trauma (including NAT), signs of increased ICP (bulging fontanelle, papilledema)
  - Signs of infection: full HEENT, skin, lung exam
  - Thorough neurologic exam
- **Diagnostics**
  - Simple febrile seizures with return to baseline status: work up the fever itself (labs/diagnostics as indicated for the febrile episode)
  - Labs rarely indicated but consider for patients with afebrile seizures:
    - Electrolytes: hyponatremia, hypoglycemia, hypocalcemia
    - Anti-epileptic drugs (AEDs) level as indicated
    - UA, UCx, Utox
    - LP if febrile status epilepticus or concern for meningitis, encephalitis

- Imaging: consider head CT in trauma, prolonged post-ictal phase, status epilepticus
  - Otherwise, outpatient MRI typically done
- Consider EKG to rule out long QT, Brugada
- EEG not typically done in ED

MANAGEMENT

- Currently seizing
  - ABCs: maintain airway, give O2 as indicated, establish IV
  - POC GLC always; treat hypoglycemia
  - Consider POC chemistry; treat abnormalities
- Medications in a stepwise fashion

1st line: Benzodiazepines	Dose
Lorazepam IV, IO, IM	0.05-0.1 mg/kg (max 4 mg)
Midazolam IM, IN, IV, IO, Buccal	IV, IO 0.1 mg/kg (max 5 mg) IN, IM, buccal 0.2 mg/kg (max 10 mg)
Diazepam PR	0.5 mg/kg for 2-5 yr 0.3 mg/kg for 6-11 yr 0.2 mg/kg ≥ 12 yr (max 20 mg)

- Benzodiazepine choice & route of administration less important than **time to administration ASAP**
  - **DO NOT** wait for an IV; consider other routes
  - Repeat 1-2 times; if no change, then move on to 2nd line therapies

2nd line: Anti-Epileptics	Dose
Fosphenytoin IV, IM	20 mg PE/kg (max 1500 mg PE)
Phenytoin IV	20 mg/kg (max 1 g)
Levetiracetam IV	60 mg/kg (max 4.5 g)
Valproic acid IV	20-40 mg/kg (max 3 g)

- If ongoing seizures despite 1st and 2nd line interventions:
  - Patient likely to require intubation
  - Pyridoxine 100 mg IV empiric in < 2 yrs for pyridoxine-sensitive epilepsy (rare)
    - Consider for reversal of Vitamin B6 deficiency, possible isoniazid overdose
  - Neurology consultation

3rd line: Anti-Epileptics	Dose
Phenobarbital IV (esp. infants)	20 mg/kg (max 1 g)
Midazolam infusion	0.2 mg/kg (max 10 mg) then 0.1 mg/kg/hr IV
Pentobarbital infusion	5 mg/kg then 0.5 mg/kg/hr IV
Ketamine infusion	1.5 mg/kg then 1 mg/kg/hr IV
Propofol infusion	2 mg/kg then 1 mg/kg/hr IV (caution children)
General anesthesia	Consult Anesthesia

DISPOSITION

- Admit: status epilepticus, prolonged postictal period and not back to baseline
- Discharge: work up negative, patient back to baseline
  — Febrile seizure: with antipyretics, return precautions, education (do not leave unattended in water), follow-up PCP 1-2 days
    - Antiepileptics do not reduce risk of epilepsy, not typically recommended
  — Afebrile seizure: follow-up PCP or Neurology with outpatient EEG, MRI

4 ▶ Stroke

BACKGROUND

- Incidence ranges from 1-5 per 100,000 per year, higher in neonates
- High morbidity and mortality
- 55% ischemic, 45% hemorrhagic
  — Ischemic strokes subdivided into arterial ischemic strokes (AIS, 75%), cerebral venous sinus thrombosis (CVST, 25%)
  — Hemorrhagic strokes mainly intracerebral and subarachnoid hemorrhages
- Risk factors associated with 90% of AIS: CHD, prothrombotic states, arteriopathy, vasculitis, head and neck infection/trauma, metabolic syndromes, Moyamoya syndrome, sickle cell disease, iron deficiency, cancer
- Risk factors for hemorrhagic stroke: AV malformation, aneurysm, thrombocytopenia, hemophilia, coagulopathy, sickle cell disease

EVALUATION

- **High Yield History**
  — Young children present more with nonspecific symptoms (AMS, seizures)
  — Older children: face, arm, or leg weakness, speech difficulty
  — Vomiting, headache neck pain, AMS
  — Recent head/neck infection or trauma

- **Exam**
  - Vital signs: fever, Cushing reflex → increased ICP
  - Auscultate head, eyes, carotids for bruits
  - Eyes: movement, pupil response, visual field deficits
  - Cardiac: murmurs, clicks, irregular rhythms
  - Complete neurological exam: weakness, cranial nerves, reflexes/clonus, neurologic deficit (laterality if any)
  - Infants with CVST: dilated scalp veins, periorbital swelling, bulging anterior fontanelle
- **Diagnostics**
  - Labs
    - CBC with differential, PT/INR, PTT, D-Dimer, fibrinogen
      - If fever: blood & urine cultures, CSF studies
    - Urine pregnancy test PRN
    - Consider electrolytes, BUN, creatinine, POC GLC, ESR, CRP, UA
    - When considering anticoagulation therapy, evaluate for hypercoagulable, prothrombotic states
  - Imaging
    - Head CT without contrast gold standard to detect ICH
      - May be normal 12-24 hrs following ischemic stroke and in up to 40% of CSVT
    - MRI most sensitive, can detect ischemic changes within hours of onset
    - MRA and MRV should be performed at the time of MRI to visualize cerebral artery flow, diagnose CVST
      - CTA if MRI unavailable
  - EKG: if suspicion for underlying cardiac disease

MANAGEMENT

- Keep head of bed flat to maximize cerebral perfusion
- Supplemental O2 to maintain SpO2 ≥ 95%
- Treat any hyperthermia
- Treat seizures with standard anticonvulsants
- Treat hypotension with crystalloid resuscitation / inotropic support to maintain cerebral perfusion (permissive hypertension up to 20% above 95th percentile for age)
- Closely monitor blood glucose q2hrs as hypoglycemia worsens neurologic outcome and hyperglycemia can worsen cerebral ischemia
- Consult Neurology as soon as stroke suspected or diagnosed

- Anticoagulation therapy considered once hemorrhagic stroke is excluded and no contraindications
  - Consult with pediatric neurologist, hematologist
  - Aspirin 3-5 mg/kg PO q24hrs
  - Unfractionated heparin 30 mcg/kg IV over 10 min (max 5000 units)
- Tissue plasminogen activator (tPA) for AIS presenting within 4.5 hrs of symptom onset
  - Children rarely present early enough to consider therapy
  - Administer in consult with Neurology
- Neurosurgery consult if hemorrhagic stroke
- Sickle cell patients
  - Exchange transfusion with goal ↓ hemoglobin S to < 30%
- Additional therapies individualized to the etiology

DISPOSITION
- Admit PICU

BEWARE
⚠ Consider stroke mimics: complex migraines, structural brain lesions, CNS infections, Todd paralysis, psychogenic causes

5 ▶ Ventriculoperitoneal Shunt Complications

BACKGROUND
- Catheter surgically inserted into brain or spinal cord to divert excess CSF away from brain
  - Drains into peritoneum → reabsorbed
- Indications: hydrocephalus (congenital stenosis, post-meningitis, etc.)
- Complications
  - Mechanical malfunction (most common)
    - Most common in first year after placement
    - Catheter obstruction from debris → decreased fluid drainage → CSF re-accumulation, recurrent hydrocephalus
  - Infection (8-15% overall)
    - Most in first month after placement
    - Common organisms: *Staphylococcus epidermidis*, *Staphylococcus aureus*, GNR
  - Overdrainage: can cause traction on vessels → subdural hematomas
  - Abdominal complications: pseudocysts, bowel perforation

- Ventriculopleural shunt: alternative option to VP shunt
  — Drains CSF from the cerebral ventricles into pleural space

EVALUATION

- **High Yield History**
  — Fever, headache, irritability, difficulty feeding, nausea/vomiting, drowsiness/somnolence, malaise, seizures
- **Exam**: bulging fontanelle, papilledema, meningismus, increased head circumference, lethargy, tense or full reservoir on palpation
- **Diagnostics**
  — CSF: tap shunt or perform LP to evaluate for infection or ↑ pressure
    - LP can miss shunt infections
  — CT head: evaluate for hydrocephalus from obstruction or overdrainage causing slit ventricle syndrome
  — XR shunt series: evaluate for discontinuity in the tubing
  — Abdominal CT/US to evaluate for pseudocyst formation or perforation PRN

MANAGEMENT

- Consult Neurosurgery
- Check VP shunt and reservoir (**Always in consult with Neurosurgery**)
  — Compress chamber and assess for rapidity at which it refills
    - Difficulty / slow can = obstruction
  — Shunt tap: performed under sterile technique with 25 gauge needle
    - CSF drained slowly until the pressure is < 15 cm H2O
- VP shunt infection
  — Suspect if fever without other likely source, recent shunt placement, headache, meningismus, peripheral leukocytosis, confirm with LP/shunt tap
  — Shunt removal or externalization + antibiotics
  — Vancomycin mg/kg (max 1 g) IV every 6 hrs + ceftriaxone 50 mg/kg (max 2 g) IV every 12 hrs

DISPOSITION

- Admit if shunt malfunction or infection

BEWARE

⚠ Evaluate for shunt malfunction if caretaker reports child behavior or activity level abnormal, even if you do not appreciate the finding

Section XVI
Ophthalmology

1 ▶ Preseptal and Orbital Cellulitis

BACKGROUND

- Epidemiology
  - Preseptal (periorbital) cellulitis
    - ↑ in children < 10 yrs
    - Usually an extension of an adjacent infection (hordeolum, dacryocystitis), trauma (insect bite, laceration/penetrating wound)
    - Occasionally preceded by URI
  - Orbital (postseptal) cellulitis
    - Major cause is extension from sinus infection, especially in older children
    - Linked to recent orbital trauma, orbital or nasal surgery, hematologic spread, local spread from preseptal or facial cellulitis
- Common organisms
  - Preseptal cellulitis
    - *S. aureus*, *Streptococcus spp.* most common
    - *M. catarrhalis*, *H. influenzae* less common but ↑risk in unvaccinated
  - Orbital cellulitis
    - Same as for preseptal cellulitis above
    - Mixed aerobes and anaerobes if dental source
    - Immunocompromised patients at risk of fungal infection
- Complications
  - Preseptal cellulitis can spread to postseptal tissues
  - Orbital cellulitis
    - Subperiosteal abscess, orbital abscess
    - Cavernous sinus thrombosis
      - ◆ Symptoms: headache, fever, CN III, IV, or VI deficits
    - Vision loss
    - Meningitis, epidural abscess, subdural empyema
    - Frontal bone osteomyelitis

EVALUATION

- **High Yield History**
  - Preseptal cellulitis
    - Fever, eyelid pain/erythema/warmth/swelling, preceding URI, purulent nasal discharge, preceding trauma or insect bite, vaccination status
  - Orbital cellulitis
    - Fever, sinus infection, bacteremia/severe infection, trauma or recent surgery, dental infection, immunosuppression/diabetes, AMS, diplopia, stiff neck, vaccination status
- **Exam**
  - Preseptal cellulitis
    - Eyelid erythema, warmth, tenderness, edema
    - May have minimal conjunctival injection and/or fever
    - Evaluate sensation in CN V1 and V2 distributions, examine periorbital area, palpate head and neck lymph nodes
    - NONE of the differentiating signs of orbital cellulitis below
  - Orbital cellulitis
    - Eyelid erythema, warmth, tenderness, edema
    - Differentiating signs from preseptal cellulitis: visual changes, greater than minimal conjunctival injection, chemosis, proptosis, restricted EOM, painful EOM, afferent pupillary defect in severe cases, increased intraocular pressure
    - Evaluate for AMS, meningeal signs, dental abscess, mouth/nose fungal infection in immunocompromised patients, sinus infection
- **Diagnostics**
  - Preseptal cellulitis is a clinical diagnosis
  - If diagnosis uncertain, concern for complicated/severe preseptal cellulitis, or concern for orbital cellulitis consider:
    - CBC, blood cultures, culture of drainage
    - CT orbit +/– brain, sinuses w/ contrast
      - Evaluate for orbital cellulitis, ocular/subperiosteal or epidural abscess/subdural empyema, foreign body

MANAGEMENT

- Preseptal cellulitis
  - Oral antibiotics × 10-14 days if mild case to be treated as outpatient
    - Potential sinus source
      - Amoxicillin/clavulanate 22.5 mg/kg two times daily for mild infections, 45 mg/kg two times daily (use 600 mg/5 mL formulation) for moderate-

- severe or if possible *S. pneumoniae* resistance (max 875 mg) PO two times daily
    - ◆ Cefdinir 7 mg/kg (max 300 mg) PO two times daily OR
    - ◆ Cefpodoxime 5 mg/kg (max 200 mg) PO two times daily
  - Potential skin source (including MRSA)
    - ◆ Cephalexin 25 mg/kg (max 500 mg) PO three times daily PLUS
    - ◆ TMP/SMX 5 mg/kg (max 160 mg) PO two times daily OR
    - ◆ Clindamycin 10 mg/kg (max 600 mg) PO three times daily
  - IV antibiotics (failed oral or severe infection) as below for orbital cellulitis
- Orbital cellulitis
  - IV antibiotics
    - Vancomycin 15 mg/kg (max 1 g) every 6 hrs PLUS
    - Ampicillin/sulbactam 50 mg/kg (max 2 g) every 6 hrs OR
    - Ceftriaxone 50 mg/kg (max 1 g) every 12 hrs OR
    - Piperacillin-tazobactam 75 mg/kg (max 4 g) every 6 hrs
- Consultations
  - Preseptal cellulitis
    - None in ED if mild, uncomplicated case to be managed as outpatient
    - Ophthalmology if severe or if unclear diagnosis
  - Orbital cellulitis
    - Ophthalmology
    - Consider ENT consult if concern for sinus source or abscess
    - Consider oral maxillofacial surgery consult for odontogenic source
    - Consider ID consult for severe or atypical presentations

DISPOSITION

- Preseptal cellulitis
  - Consider outpatient management: well-appearing, afebrile patients with mild infections
  - Requires next day follow-up, admission if progression to severe preseptal or orbital cellulitis, not improving in 1-2 days
- Admit orbital cellulitis

BEWARE

- ! Do not miss oro/nasopharyngeal fungal infections in immunocompromised patients as source
- ! Do not miss signs of CNS infection in altered patients, particularly in younger/less verbal children

2 ▶ Red Eye

Common Causes of Red Eye			
Accessory Structures	**Problem/Cause**	**History/Exam**	**Management**
Blepharitis	• Inflammation at eyelid margin • Meibomian gland dysfunction, *Staph*	• Tearing • Photophobia • Crusting at lashes • Pruritus	• Warm compresses • Gentle cleanse w/dilute baby shampoo • Artificial tears
Dacryocystitis	• Nasolacrimal duct infection • *Staph, Strep*	• Medial canthus erythema • Purulent discharge • Usually unilateral	• Admit, IV antibiotics • Ophthalmology consult
Entropion Ectropion Trichiasis	• Misdirection of eyelid/lashes causes eye irritation or dryness	• Pain • Photophobia • Tearing • Lashes inward (entropion)	• Artificial tears • Ophtho referral if persistent
Conjunctiva/Sclera	**Problem/Cause**	**History/Exam**	**Management**
Ophthalmicus Neonatorum	Conjunctivitis first 30 days of life	• Maternal infection • Age at onset	
Chemical	Postnatal erythromycin prophylaxis	• Inflamed lids • Watery discharge	Self-resolves in 2 days
Gonococcal	• *N. gonorrhoeae* • Day 2-7 of life	• Severe bilateral lid edema • Copious purulent discharge	• Admit, IV antibiotics (below) • Emergent Ophtho consult
Chlamydial	• *C. trachomatis* • Day 7-14 of life	• Uni- or bilateral • Watery to mucoid discharge	Oral erythromycin or azithromycin (below)
Herpetic	• HSV • Within first 6 weeks of life	• Lid edema • Dendrites on fluorescein exam • +/− skin, mucous membrane lesions	• Perform LP • Admit, IV acyclovir (below) • Emergent Ophtho consult
Other bacterial	• Rare • 2 weeks of life or later • *Staph*, rare *Pseudomonas*	• Usually unilateral • Purulent discharge	• Admit, IV antibiotics for *Staph, Pseudomonas*

Conjunctivitis, non-neonatal	• Bacterial • Viral • Allergic • Vasculitic	• Onset, ill contacts, associated symptoms • Contact lens use • Pain, pruritus • Perilimbic sparing = conjunctivitis (vs. iritis)	
Bacterial	• *S. Aureus* • *H. influenzae* • *S. pneumoniae* • Less common: gonorrhea, chlamydia • *Pseudomonas* w/ contact lens	• Normal vision • Eye discomfort but no pain • Mucopurulent discharge • "Glue eye" — stuck shut in AM • Usually unilateral	• Ophthalmic antibiotics (below) — Erythromycin ointment — Trimethoprim-Polymyxin B drops — Fluoroquinolone drops (esp if contact lens)
Viral	• Adenovirus • HSV, VZV	• Uni- or bilateral • Watery, mucoid discharge • Dendrites on fluorescein exam for HSV, VZV	• Cool compresses • Artificial tears • Admit, IV acyclovir (below), ophthalmology consult for HSV, VZV
Allergic	• Airborne allergens • Pet dander	• Pruritus, edema • Allergic "shiners" • Atopic history • Cobblestoning of tarsal conjunctiva	• Topical ophthalmic options • Naphazoline • Ketotifen • Olopatadine
Vasculitic	• Kawasaki disease • Other vasculitides	• Bilateral • Nonpurulent	• Disease-specific
SJS/TEN	Commonly a medication hypersensitivity reaction	• Bilateral • Purulent • Associated skin findings	• Stop offending medication • Treat SJS/TEN
Episcleritis	Episclera (between conjunctiva & sclera) inflamed	• Dull ache • Mild tenderness • Normal vision • Nodule w/radially oriented vessels	• Self-limited • Artificial tears • Oral NSAIDs
Scleritis	• Vasculitides • Connective tissue diseases	• Pain • +/− vision impaired • Focal or diffuse erythema • Violaceous or pink sclera	• Evaluate for and treat underlying systemic disease

Conjunctiva/Sclera	Problem/Cause	History/Exam	Management
Pterygium	• Chronic UV exposure • Sun reflection off water/snow (surfers, skiers)	• Yellow, fleshy mass with red vessels • Can grow over cornea	• Artificial tears • Prevention: sunglasses • Large: refer to ophthalmology
Subconjunctival hemorrhage	• Minor trauma • Valsalva (e.g. lift weights, cough)	• Bleeding disorder • Flat, demarcated, bright red region	Self-resolves over 2-3 weeks

Cornea	Problem/Cause	History/Exam	Management
Corneal abrasion, ulcer, erosion	• Minor trauma • Foreign body	• Contact lens ↑ risk • Pain, photophobia • FB sensation • Fluorescein uptake	• Remove FB • Topical anesthetic • Prophylactic topical antibiotic
Superficial Keratitis	• Contact lens use • UV exposure • Dry eyes	• Cornea inflamed • FB sensation • Photophobia • Fluorescein exam punctate lesions	• Topical antibiotic • Topical cycloplegic • Analgesics • Recheck in 24 hrs

Other	Problem/Cause	History/Exam	Management
Acute angle-closure glaucoma	• Trisomy 21, congenital rubella, neurofibromatosis • Rare in children	• Enlarged cornea • Haziness, edema • Globe may appear large • Increased IOP • Sluggish mid-size pupil	• Emergent ophthalmology consult
Iritis (aka anterior uveitis)	• Iris and ciliary body inflammation • Trauma • Systemic diseases	• Perilimbal injection (vs. conjunctivitis) • Pain • Consensual photophobia • Slit lamp: anterior chamber cell & flare	• Consult ophthalmology • Topical cycloplegics
Globe rupture	• Trauma	• Decreased vision • Teardrop pupil • Prolapsed uvea • Vitreous discharge • Seidel sign	• Emergent ophthalmology consult • Hard eye shield • Bedrest • Antiemetics PRN

EVALUATION

- **High Yield History**
  — Contact lens use, visual acuity change, pain, pruritus, FB sensation, discharge, symptom onset/duration, trauma (including use of any tool or construction where debris could hit eye), recent new or change in medications, systemic symptoms
- **Exam**
  — Eye "vital signs": visual acuity, IOP, visual fields, pupillary reaction, EOM
  — Examine surrounding structures: lids, lashes, glands, nasolacrimal duct, general appearance
  — Flip lid to evaluate for foreign body
  — Fluorescein exam if any concern for corneal pathology
  — Slit lamp exam
- **Diagnostics**
  — Typically not required
    - Culture eye discharge in infants and complicated cases

MANAGEMENT/DISPOSITION

- Depends on specific etiology
- Antibiotics for bacterial infections
  — Gonococcal conjunctivitis: emergent Ophtho consult; admit for IV antibiotics, frequent irrigation (avoid patching eye in effort to contain copious discharge; can ↑ bacteria concentration)
    - Cefotaxime or ceftazidime or ceftriaxone (if > 28 days old and no hyperbilirubinemia) 50 mg/kg/dose IV every 12 hrs
  — Suspected herpetic or varicella infection: emergent Ophtho consult, probable admission, acyclovir 20 mg/kg (max 800 mg) IV every 8 hrs or valacyclovir PO
  — Suspected neonatal chlamydial conjunctivitis: requires oral erythromycin 12.5 mg/kg PO every 6 hrs for 14 days OR azithromycin 20 mg/kg PO daily for 3 days
  — Routine bacterial conjunctivitis (treat 7-10 days)
    - Ophthalmic polymyxin-trimethoprim or fluoroquinolone, 1-2 drops every 2-3 hrs while awake
    - Erythromycin ophthalmic ointment ¼ inch ribbon four times daily alternative for infants
    - Avoid aminoglycosides and sulfonamides as can cause irritation
    - Return precautions if worsening / not improving after 5 days of therapy
  — Patients with contact lenses + infection: Ophthalmology consult, more frequent antibiotics, pseudomonas coverage

BEWARE

- ❗ Maintain high index of suspicion for associated systemic conditions such as Kawasaki disease, uveitis, disseminated gonorrhea
- ❗ Chlamydia or gonorrhea conjunctivitis after neonatal period: evaluate for NAT, child sexual abuse
- ❗ Do not confuse gonococcal ophthalmicus neonatorum with less-concerning childhood infectious conjunctivitis presentations

Section XVII
Orthopedics

1 ▶ Back Pain and Discitis

BACKGROUND
- Typically benign, but warrants evaluation & follow-up
  — Nonspecific musculoskeletal pain ≥ 50% of cases
- DDx
  — Congenital
  — Infectious: discitis, spinal epidural abscess, osteomyelitis
  — Inflammatory: reactive arthritis, sacroiliitis
  — Neoplastic
  — Nonspinal: cholecystitis, nephrolithiasis, pancreatitis, pneumonia, pyelonephritis, PID, sickle cell vaso-occlusive crisis
  — Overuse/trauma: disc herniation, fracture, muscle/ligamentous strain/sprain, spinal epidural hematoma, spondylolisthesis, spondylolysis

EVALUATION
- **High Yield History**
  — Red flags
    - Fevers
    - Nocturnal pain
    - Weight loss
    - Malignancy/TB
    - Age < 4yrs
    - Trauma
    - Back procedure
    - Coagulopathy
    - IV drug use
    - Immunocompromised
    - Steroid use
    - Neurologic symptoms (gait, bowel/bladder, weakness)
- **Exam**
  — Appearance: bruises, curvature (scoliosis)
  — Palpation: step-offs, bony/paraspinal tenderness
  — Neurologic: motor, sensation, deep tendon reflexes, gait
    - ALWAYS walk patient
  — Other: abdominal exam, CVAT, pelvic exam if indicated

- **Diagnostics** (not routine, based on suspicion)
  — Labs
    - Infection/inflammatory: CBC, ESR/CRP, +/– BCx
    - Neoplastic: CBC, CRP, LFTs, LDH, uric acid
    - Other: UA, UCx, urine pregnancy test, lipase
  — Imaging
    - Spine series XR
    - MRI if neurological impairment, concerning XR findings
  — Post void residual if concern for urinary retention

MANAGEMENT

Presentation	Exam	Diagnostics	Treatment Disposition
Discitis Disc inflammation, likely subacute infection Rare, 0-5yrs, subacute, irritability, gait abnormalities (refusal to crawl), +/– fever	Bony tenderness, pain or limitation w/flexion	Labs: WBC/ESR mildly ↑, BCx (for osteomyelitis) Imaging: XR often normal MRI (gold standard)	Admit for IV antibiotics, analgesia, immobilization
Spondylolysis Fracture of pars interarticularis, usually in lumbar spine Athletes, aching, worse w/sitting	Pain with hyperextension, limited flexion, hamstring tightness	Imaging: XR, MRI if high suspicion	Analgesia, rest, physical therapy
Spondylolisthesis Progression of spondylolysis with forward slippage of vertebral body (usually L5 on S1) Athletes, repetitive trauma, spondylolysis, persistent pain, +/– radiculopathy	Hyperextension pain, pain with straight leg raise, lumbar lordosis loss, Phalen-Dickson sign (knee-flexed, hip-flexed gait)	Imaging: As above	Analgesia, rest, physical therapy; Consult Neurosurgery if Grade > 1 on imaging or neurologic symptoms

DISPOSITION

- Benign cause: discharge with primary care follow-up
- Admit: requiring pain management, neurosurgery intervention, IV antibiotics

BEWARE

- ❗ Benign musculoskeletal back pain uncommon in < 4yrs
- ❗ Maintain HIGH index of suspicion for spinal epidural hematoma if trauma, coagulation disorders, anticoagulation therapy, vascular abnormalities
- ❗ Red flag symptoms or persistent pain > 2-4 weeks warrants work-up

2 ▶ Limp

BACKGROUND

- Abnormal gait from pain, weakness, injury, bone/joint pathology
  - Toddlers may present as refusal to bear weight or crawl
  - Infants may not be moving one leg
- DDx
  - Infection (see Orthopedic Infections)
  - Transient synovitis
  - Slipped Capital Femoral Epiphysis
  - Legg-Calve Perthes
  - Occult fracture
  - Trauma (fractures, strains/sprains, nonaccidental)
  - Malignancy
  - Sickle cell crisis or osteonecrosis
  - Congenital (clubfoot, hip dysplasia, limb length discrepancy)
  - Apophysitis (Osgood-Schlatter)
  - Arthritis (reactive, Lyme, juvenile idiopathic, HSP)
  - Growing pains
  - Muscular dystrophy
  - Acute rheumatic fever
  - Spinal conditions
  - Abdominal / genital pathology (appendicitis, psoas abscess, torsion, neuroblastoma)
- Legg-Calve-Perthes (LCP): idiopathic avascular necrosis of hip
  - Ages 2-12 yrs, peak 4-9 yrs, M > F, 10% bilateral
  - Insidious onset, mild thigh/knee pain, decreased hip abduction/internal rotation
  - Initial XR can be negative / subtle — maintain high index of suspicion
- Slipped Capital Femoral Epiphysis (SCFE): epiphysis slips off femoral neck at the physis
  - Appearance of ice cream falling off cone
  - Ages 11-16 yrs, M > F, obesity major risk factor, 20-40% bilateral
  - Hip/knee/groin pain without preceding trauma, chronic, worse with activity
- Transient synovitis: benign self-limited inflammation of hip joint
  - Unclear etiology, possibly post-viral
  - Typically age < 10 yrs, peak 3-6 yrs, M > F
  - Sudden onset unilateral hip/thigh/knee pain, leg abducted and externally rotated, able to range (unlike septic joint)
  - Well appearing, may have low-grade fever
  - Possible mild ↑ WBC, ESR, +/– effusion on US/XR
  - No synovial fluid bacteria if joint aspirated but may have mildly ↑ WBC
- Growing pains: unclear etiology
  - Benign recurrent bilateral lower extremity pain in young children
  - Often late in the day or at bedtime
  - Intermittently asymptomatic, normal exam, usually NO limp

EVALUATION

- **High Yield History**
  — Duration (chronic vs. acute), location (back v.s hip vs. leg vs. foot; muscle vs. bone), recent trauma or sports, fever
  — Malignancy: cyclical pain, worse at night, weight loss
  — Fracture, sprain/strain, apophysitis: constant pain, focal tenderness, worse with activity
  — Rheumatologic: morning stiffness
  — Transient synovitis: recent URI
  — Lyme: tick bite/outdoor activities, rash
- **Exam**
  — Vitals, growth curve, bruising/signs of trauma, back, abdominal, genital exam, rash
  — Extremity: gait, position of comfort (external rotation), point tenderness, redness, warmth, effusion, ROM, spasticity, gluteal fold symmetry (laying prone)
- **Diagnostics**: guided by history, exam, leading DDx
  — Labs
    - CBC, ESR/CRP, BCx
    - BMP, arthrocentesis, Lyme titers
  — Imaging
    - XR (AP and lateral)
      - AP pelvis and frog-leg lateral if considering hip pathology
      - Skeletal survey if concern for **NAT**
    - US for joint effusion but usually not diagnostic
    - MRI as indicated if initial XR nondiagnostic

MANAGEMENT

- Analgesia, rest, ice acutely, heat later, massage & physical therapy as indicated
- Transient synovitis: well-appearing, normal radiographs and labs if obtained, able to bear weight, give NSAIDs
- Fracture: splint or cast, follow-up with orthopedics
- Sprain/strain: rest, activity as tolerated, follow-up with PCP
- SCFE or LCP: orthopedics consultation, non-weight-bearing
- Septic arthritis, osteomyelitis — see Orthopedic Infections chapter
- Osgood-Schlatter, Sever's, and Pelvic Avulsions — see chapter

DISPOSITION

- Admit: SCFE if pre-operative, malignancy work-up needed, orthopedic infection, won't bear weight and unclear etiology
- Transient synovitis: discharge with follow-up next day for improvement

BEWARE

- ⚠ Image hips if knee/thigh pain to rule out referred pain from LCP, SCFE
- ⚠ Patients often report a red herring history of trauma with non-traumatic causes as they are considering possible causes
- ⚠ Red flags: febrile, adolescent with sudden limp, nocturnal pain, ataxia
- ⚠ Consider referred pain from abdominal, genital, back pathology
- ⚠ Consider NAT

3 ▶ Nursemaid's Elbow

BACKGROUND

- Radial head subluxation due to sudden longitudinal traction applied to the hand or wrist with the elbow extended and forearm pronated
  — Swinging or pulling/lifting child by the hand or wrist
- Radial head slips under annular ligament → traps ligament in radiohumeral joint
- Ages 1-4 yrs (annular ligament strengthens ~ age 5 yrs)
- Female, left arm predominance
- Presents with pain, not using affected arm

EVALUATION

- **High Yield History**
  — Arm traction (swinging, lifting, pulling)
  — Prior nursemaid's elbow (20% recurrence rate)
- **Exam**
  — Arm held adducted, pronated, elbow slightly flexed or fully extended
    - Unable to supinate forearm
  — Child keeps arm still and may protect arm with opposite hand
  — No or mild tenderness to palpation
  — No pain unless arm manipulated
  — No ecchymosis, erythema, edema, signs of trauma
- **Diagnostics**
  — XR not routinely needed
    - XR if swelling, history of a fall, point tenderness, not moving arm after reduction, inconsistent history
    - Spontaneous reduction may occur during positioning for XR

MANAGEMENT

- Reduction techniques
  - Hyperpronation
    - High success rate, may be less painful
    - Hyperpronate forearm with elbow flexed at 90 degrees
  - Supination with flexion
    - Supinate forearm then flex at elbow while applying pressure to radial head
- Often hear or feel a "click" when reduced
- Multiple attempts may be necessary
- Child will have full ROM 5-10 min after reduction
- If normal ROM not resumed, obtain XR and consider alternative diagnosis
- Operative reduction rarely needed if chronic subluxation that cannot be reduced

DISPOSITION

- Discharge
- Advise caretakers to avoid high-risk pulling / swinging / lifting maneuvers

4 ▶ Orthopedic Infections

OSTEOMYELITIS

- M > F, most common in infants, toddlers
- ↑ children vs. adults due to rich metaphyseal blood supply, thick periosteum
- Femur most common site
- Organisms: *Staphylococcus aureus* most common
  - *Haemophilus influenzae* now much less common due to vaccine
  - *Kingella kingae* in younger patients
    - Cause of culture negative infections
    - Needs blood culture medium to grow

SEPTIC ARTHRITIS

- Most common in children ~2 yrs
- Knee most common joint
- Organisms: *Staphylococcus aureus* most common pathogen in all ages
  - See treatment chart below for pathogens by age
- Can develop from osteomyelitis, especially in neonates (transphyseal vessels allow proximal spread into the joint)

EVALUATION

- **High Yield History**
  - Limp, ↓ use of affected extremity, fever without source
  - Osteomyelitis: history of trauma common
  - Septic arthritis: often preceded by osteomyelitis
    - Adolescent: sexual history, STIs
- **Exam**
  - Osteomyelitis: tenderness, warmth, +/– swelling overlying long-bone metaphysis, +/– fever
  - Septic hip: fever in 60-70%, ↓ ROM, severe pain with passive ROM
    - Septic hip held abducted and externally rotated
- **Diagnostics**
  - Labs
    - Osteomyelitis CBC (leukocytosis with left shift), ↑↑ ESR/CRP, obtain blood culture
      - Definitive diagnosis by aspiration/bone biopsy (orthopedics or interventional radiology)
    - Septic Arthritis: all of the above plus lactate
      - Lactate may be high in GPC or GNR infection
      - BCx + in 15-46%
      - Joint aspiration for definitive diagnosis: cell count and differential, gram stain, culture
        - WBC count > 50,000/mm^3
        - Fluid glucose level may be 50 mg/dL < serum glucose
  - Imaging
    - Osteomyelitis: XR with soft tissue edema early, metaphyseal hypodensity and lucencies late, may be normal in early disease
      - MRI key to evaluate for abscess
    - Septic arthritis: XR widened joint space, may even have subluxation
      - US can be helpful to evaluate for effusion
- **Kocher Criteria** (for hip joint, if 3/4 positive, > 90% have septic arthritis)
  - Serum WBC > 12,000cells/microL
  - ESR > 40 mm/hr
  - Inability to bear weight
  - Temperature > 101.3°F (38.5°C)

MANAGEMENT

- Osteomyelitis: IV antibiotics (vancomycin + 3rd generation cephalosporin as in table), consult orthopedics, infectious diseases specialist
  - If history of penetrating foot puncture, particularly through shoes, cover for *pseudomonas*
- Septic hip: arthrocentesis, consult orthopedics, infectious diseases specialist, IV antibiotics as below:

Age	Common organisms	Empiric Antibiotics
< 3mo	*Staphylococcus*, GBS	Vancomycin 15 mg/kg IV every 8 hrs **AND** 3rd generation cephalosporin: cefotaxime 50 mg/kg IV every 6-8 hrs or ceftriaxone (if > 28 days old) 50 mg/kg IV daily
6mo-5yr	*Staphylococcus*, *Kingella kingae*, *Streptococci*, *H. influenzae*	Vancomycin 15 mg/kg IV every 8 hrs **AND** First-gen cephalosporin: cefazolin 50 mg/kg every 8 hrs to cover *K. Kingae* (doesn't cover *H. influenzae*)
5-12yrs	*Staphylococcus aureus*, Strep spp	First-generation cephalosporin: cefazolin 50 mg/kg (max 2 g) IV every 8 hrs or if high community MRSA prevalence, vancomycin 15 mg/kg (max 1 g) IV every 8 hrs
12-18yrs	*S. aureus*, *N. gonorrhoeae**	Oxacillin 50 mg/kg (max 3 g) IV every 6 hrs **OR** Cefazolin 50 mg/kg (max 2 g) IV every 8 hrs **OR** 3rd gen cephalosporin for gonorrhea (ceftriaxone 50 mg/kg [max 1 g] IV daily); consider treating for chlamydia as well
Sickle cell disease all ages	*Salmonella*, gram negative organisms in addition to age-specific	Add ceftriaxone 50 mg/kg (max 1 g) IV every 12 hrs **OR** cefotaxime 50 mg/kg (max 1 g) IV every 8 hrs to age-specific coverage

**N. Gonorrhoeae*: migratory polyarthralgia, can have macular-papular rash, often has < 50,000 cells/mL on joint aspiration

DISPOSITION

- Osteomyelitis: Admit
- Septic Arthritis: Admit for surgical washout, synovial fluid cultures

BEWARE

- ⚠ No labs or imaging can rule out septic arthritis in a child
  — If truly suspicious, joint aspiration indicated
- ⚠ Because pus is chondrolytic, septic arthritis is a surgical emergency; articular damage begins within 8 hours of onset

5 ▶ Osgood-Schlatter, Sever, Pelvic Avulsions

BACKGROUND

- Overuse injuries in young athletes increasing due to overtraining, year-round sports, and improper conditioning
- Osgood-Schlatter: tibial tubercle apophysitis
  — Activities: running (sprinters), jumping (basketball, volleyball)
  — Often children/adolescents starting to play competitive sports (ages 10-15 yrs)
  — 20-30% bilateral, M > F
- Sever disease: calcaneal apophysitis
  — Running and jumping (basketball, soccer), flat-soled shoes
  — Pre-teens aged 9-12 yrs
  — 60% bilateral, M > F
- Pelvic avulsion: most commonly at hamstring insertion on ischial tuberosity but other sites possible
  — Typically older adolescents with forceful kicking sports or pushing off (soccer, sprinting, hurdles, ballet)
  — Often report a pop or snap before pain

EVALUATION

- **High Yield History**: previous history of same pain, sport(s) played (repetitive running/jumping), hours of sport practice and competition per week (overuse)
- **Exam**
  — Osgood-Schlatter
    - Tibial tubercle tenderness and bony prominence
    - Pain on resisted knee extension
  — Sever
    - Tenderness over calcaneus and Achilles' tendon insertion site
    - Typically no visible deformity; mild swelling possible

- Pelvic avulsion
    - Ischial tuberosity tenderness at site of hamstring insertion most common; other sites possible
- **Diagnostics:** Imaging
    - Osgood-Schlatter: imaging unnecessary; tibial tubercle irregularity and possible fragmentation if obtained
    - Sever: imaging unnecessary; usually normal if obtained
    - Pelvic avulsion: XR shows avulsed apophysis (compare to unaffected side)

MANAGEMENT

- Supportive: discontinue offending activity, rest affected extremities for 4-6 weeks, swimming is a good alternative activity / conditioning exercise
    - Analgesia: NSAIDs, ice after activity
    - Exercises: daily stretching and strength-training of affected tendons
- Osgood-Schlatter: knee sleeves/strapping to decrease tension on apophysis
- Sever: gel heel cup shoe inserts to decrease tension on Achilles tendon
- Pelvic avulsion: may need protected weight bearing with crutches and early ROM/stretching

DISPOSITION

- Discharge; follow-up with PCP or sports medicine physician for recovery and determination whether orthopedic referral is indicated (rare)
- Osgood-Schlatter and Sever self-limited but may take 1-2 years to resolve
    - Do not resolve until after growth has stopped

BEWARE

⚠ Should be indolent process that fits history of overuse, symmetric if bilateral
    - If anything odd, consider limb-threatening causes of pain such as osteomyelitis, septic arthritis, bone tumor

Section XVIII
Psychiatry

1 ▶ Autistic Child

AUTISM SPECTRUM DISORDER (ASD)

- Impaired sensory processing, communication, social interaction, +/− intellectual impairment
- 1/54 children with diagnosis
- Many prefer routine and predictability, restricted interests
  — ED is a difficult and dynamic environment
- Pediatric patients with ASD have 4x higher odds of unmet health care needs, up to 30× more likely to come to ED

EVALUATION

- **High Yield History**
  — Child's ability and method of communication (pointing, imitation, showing, verbal, nonverbal)
  — Likely triggers (sensitivity to light, sound, touch, other stimuli)
  — What calms or soothes child?
  — History of neurodevelopmental evaluation, formal assessments or diagnoses
  — Comorbid conditions (ADHD, GI disturbance, sleep or behavioral problems)
  — Medical and mental health history of family, siblings with ASD
- **Exam**
  — Observe family-patient and provider interaction, language ability
  — Patients often avoid eye contact, have repetitive/stereotypic behaviors
- **Diagnostics**
  — Dependent on presenting complaint but may be more difficult to obtain

MANAGEMENT

- Create low-stimulus environment: quiet, low light, reduce clutter and crowds
  — Single rooms and child life if available
- Allot extra time for challenging communication

- Have empathy for behavioral challenges; caregivers often know best strategies for calming child
- Weighted blankets, toys, electronic devices for distraction
- Minimize wait times
- Procedures - consider the following medications
  — Non-painful procedures
    - Midazolam 0.3 mg/kg (max 10 mg), IN or 0.5 mg/kg (max 20 mg) PO/SL
    - Dexmedetomidine 2-3 mcg/kg IN 30-60 min prior to procedure
  — Painful procedures: consider procedural sedation
- Maintain suspicion for common comorbid medical conditions: seizures, pica, GI complaints, migraines, asthma, allergies, sleep disturbances, metabolic disorders

DISPOSITION
- If new diagnosis of ASD suspected, ensure appropriate referrals to neurodevelopmental specialist

BEWARE
- ↑ sensitivity to medications: carefully monitor for side effects, especially after sedation; may have paradoxical reactions to benzodiazepines, diphenhydramine
- May be on psychotropic medications; beware possible interactions

2 ▶ Behavior

BACKGROUND
- Attention deficit hyperactivity disorder (ADHD): persistent pattern of inattention and/or hyperactivity that interferes with functioning
- Conduct disorder (CD): rule breaking, destroying property, hurting people and animals (< 18 yrs of age)
- Oppositional defiant disorder (ODD): defiant behavior against authority figures; features may overlap with CD
- Tic disorder: rapid, recurrent, non-rhythmic motor movements or vocalizations
  — Onset peak ages 4-6 yrs; peak severity ages 10-12 yrs
- Tourette disorder: motor and vocalization tics for > 1 yr
- Pediatric autoimmune neuropsychiatric disorder associated with streptococcal infections (PANDAS)
  — Acute onset of obsessive-compulsive disorder (OCD)/tics in childhood following Group A Strep infections
  — Presumed antibody mediated

- Night terrors
  - Occur early in night, child not easily aroused, does not remember once awake (different from nightmares)
  - Most often ages 3-7 yrs (as young as 18 mos), usually subside by 10 yrs

EVALUATION

- **High Yield History**: developmental and social history, medications, concerns for patient danger to self or others, collateral information
- **Exam**: VS, neurologic and mental status exams, signs of self-harm or abuse
- **Diagnostics**
  - Sudden new onset behavior: CBC, CMP, Utox, EKG, thyroid function tests
  - Sudden worsening in severity of behavior or tics: investigate for concurrent infections, other organic causes
  - EEG, neuroimaging if indicated by neurologic findings

MANAGEMENT

- Therapy mostly started as outpatient
- ADHD
  - Stimulants (amphetamine or methylphenidate derivatives); non-stimulant atomoxetine
    - Common side effects: appetite suppression, insomnia
    - Serious but uncommon side effects: mania, hypertension, cardiac dysrhythmias
  - Clonidine and guanfacine
    - Side effects: hypotension and sedation
- ODD/CD: Treatment focuses on family/school-based interventions
- Nightmares and night terrors: reassurance and caregiver education

DISPOSITION

- Discharge with caregiver reassurance and PCP follow-up
- Refer to qualified mental health professional if distressing or functionally impairing
- Admit if indicated for concurrent medical or psychiatric conditions

BEWARE

- Children with ADHD, ODD, CD high risk for depression, suicidality, risk-taking behaviors
- Tics in the context of declining motor or cognitive function warrant a full neurologic assessment and workup to evaluate for underlying pathology

3 ▶ Depression and Suicidal Ideation

BACKGROUND
- Second leading cause of death among 15-24 yrs old in U.S.
- Nearly 75% who complete suicide saw a doctor in last 4 months of life
- Red flags: social isolation, giving away belongings, conveying intent to peers or on social media, abuse

EVALUATION
- **High Yield History**
  — SIGECAPS: **S**leep, **I**nterest in activities, **G**uilt, **E**nergy level, **C**oncentration, **A**ppetite, **P**sychomotor changes, **S**uicidal ideation (SI)
  — Nonspecific somatic symptoms, declining school performance, risky behaviors
  — Risk factors: prior suicide attempts, stressors, chronic illnesses, psychiatric comorbidities, access to lethal means (firearms, drugs), sexual minority youths, contagion (SI/suicide in close contact), family history of mental illness
  — HEADDSSS assessment with patient alone (**H**ome, **E**ducation, **A**ctivities, **D**rugs, **D**iet, **S**exuality, **S**uicide, **S**afety)
  — Outpatient therapy, medications
- **Exam**:
  — Examine patients while they are wearing a hospital gown
    - Signs of injuries (cutting, ligature marks, bruises)
    - In abuse, bruises may be in covered areas such as shoulders, buttocks, thighs, abdomen, back
  — Consider ingestions, toxidromes
  — May have flat affect, psychomotor retardation
- **Diagnostics**:
  — Validated screening tools
    - Ask Suicide-Screening Questions (ASQ)
    - PHQ-9 Modified for Adolescents (PHQ-A)
  — Labs (routine labs unnecessary, rarely change management)
    - Urine: toxicology screen, pregnancy test if indicated
    - Blood: CBC, CMP, TSH if indicated
    - If concern for ingestion: ethanol, salicylate, acetaminophen, VBG, lactate, drug screen, other medication levels as indicated, EKG

MANAGEMENT

- Safety is top priority (self, staff, patient)
- Address concern for unpredictable, erratic, violent behavior first
- Involuntary hold if patient meets any criteria:
  — Risk for self-harm
  — Risk for harm to others
  — Unable to protect or care for self due to mental health (gravely disabled)
- If involuntary hold:
  — Remove belongings
  — Arrange close observation in ED
  — Consult Psychiatry for admission vs. safety plan and outpatient care

DISPOSITION

- Admit or observe: medically unstable
- Admit to Psychiatry: deemed unsafe for discharge but medically cleared
- If safe for discharge, secure Psychiatry follow-up and a clear safety plan

BEWARE

- Many conditions mimic psychiatric disorders: thyroid dysfunction, SLE, encephalitis, substance- or medication-induced mood disturbances, ADHD, etc.
- When talking to adolescents in distress, avoid trying to "fix it"

4 ▶ Eating Disorders

BACKGROUND

- ↑ in children and adolescents
- F > M, becoming more recognized among boys, minority groups, those with coexisting anxiety disorders
- Mortality (especially anorexia nervosa) 6-20% (among highest of any psychiatric disorder)
- Pathologies may include (but not limited to):
  — Anorexia nervosa
  — Bulimia
  — Avoidant/restrictive food disorder
  — Pica

EVALUATION
- **High Yield History**
  - Stunted growth, pubertal delay, irregular menses or amenorrhea, weight loss with unclear precipitant
  - Signs of compensatory behavior, binging/purging not always present
- **Exam**
  - Plot weight, height, BMI
  - Anorexia nervosa: sinus bradycardia, hypotension, orthostasis, hypothermia, facial wasting, oligomenorrhea, signs of hypothyroidism, lanugo
  - Bulimia: similar to anorexia, may include knuckle abrasions, dyspepsia, parotid gland enlargement, dental caries/ erosion
    - May not be underweight
- **Diagnostics**:
  - Labs: CBC, CMP, Ca, Mg, Phos, TSH/Free T4, UA
    - Hypokalemia, hypophosphatemia, hypochloremic metabolic alkalosis (vomiting), metabolic alkalosis or acidosis (laxative abuse)
    - May see leukopenia, anemia, thyroid dysfunction, renal insufficiency
  - EKG (prolonged QTc)
  - Consider echocardiogram if concern for significant mitral valve prolapse, pericardial effusion, cardiomyopathy

MANAGEMENT
- Electrolyte repletion if severe derangements
- Patients at risk of developing CHF with rapid IV fluid repletion
- Supportive care

DISPOSITION
- Admit: syncope, hematemesis, intractable vomiting, significant electrolyte abnormalities (Na, K, Cl, Mag, Phos), suicide risk
- Admit anorexia nervosa: bradycardia < 50 daytime / < 45 nighttime, hypotension (SBP < 90), hypothermia (< 35.6°C), orthostasis, arrhythmia, body fat < 10%, refusal to eat, failed outpatient treatment (< 75% ideal body weight despite treatment)
- Admit bulimia: K < 3.2 mEq/L, Cl < 88 mEq/L, esophageal tear, prolonged QTc, hypothermia, failed outpatient management
- Discharge: medically stable, appropriate outpatient resources, support available

BEWARE

- ⚠ Refeeding Syndrome: repletion of glucose causes insulin secretion and rapid intracellular shift of phosphorus, potassium, and magnesium
  - Hypophosphatemia in particular can lead to cardiopulmonary collapse
  - Be judicious with repletion in the ED: an IV bolus (20 mL/kg, max 1 L) can overload patients with severe cardiomyopathy
- ⚠ Screen for suicidal/homicidal ideation
  - 30-50% of those with an eating disorder also have major depressive disorder
  - 20% of eating disorder-related mortality from suicide

5 ▶ Managing the Agitated Child

BACKGROUND

- Up to 10% of children presenting with a primary psychiatric complaint require restraint
- Distinguish between organic vs. primary psychiatric causes of agitation

EVALUATION

- **High Yield History**
  - Collateral information from caretaker(s), medications, traumatic mechanisms, developmental history
  - Prior history of agitation and aggression
  - What provokes, what calms
- **Exam**
  - Early warnings: pacing, clenching, rocking, muttering, verbalizing distress
  - Signs of intoxication/withdrawal or toxidromes
- **Diagnostics**
  - Consider CK: agitation can → rhabdomyolysis
  - Other labs, UA, Utox, EKG, imaging if suspect organic cause

MANAGEMENT

- Maintain safety of patient and healthcare team
  - Give patient space (keep 2 arms' length)
  - Do not allow yourself to be trapped in room
- Nonpharmacologic measures should be attempted before pharmacologic
- Trauma informed care: assume trauma likely part of patient history
  - Minimize additional trauma

- Verbal de-escalation
  - Allows for the most individualized approach, minimizes risk of medication side effects, maintains trust in the physician/healthcare system
  - Decrease stimulation, environmental chaos
  - Provide basic needs (food, water, clothing, entertainment, silence)
  - Involve caretaker or favored staff member if appropriate
- Restraints
  - Physical: soft or hard, 2 or 4 point
    - Requires frequent reassessment for continued need
  - Chemical: see chart

Medication	Dose	Time to Peak Effect	Potential Adverse Effects
Diphenhydramine	PO/IM/IV: 1 mg/kg, max 25-50 mg	PO/IV/IM: 2 hrs	Can cause paradoxical agitation; Avoid in delirium
Lorazepam	PO/IM/IV: 0.05-0.1 mg/kg, max 0.5-2 mg	IV: 10 min PO/IM: 1-2 hr	Can cause paradoxical agitation; Avoid with olanzapine due to risk of respiratory suppression
Chlorpromazine	PO/IM/IV: 0.5-1 mg/kg, max 12.5-50 mg	PO: 30 min-1hr IM/IV: 15 min	QTc prolongation, hypotension
Haloperidol	PO/IM/IV: 0.05 mg/kg, max 2.5-5 mg	PO: 2 hr IM/IV: 20 min	QTc prolongation, extrapyramidal symptoms
Olanzapine	ODT: 0.1 mg/kg, max 2.5-10 mg IM: 1.25-5 mg < 10 yrs, 5-10 mg ≥ 10yrs	ODT: 30-60 min IM: 15-45 min	Can cause CNS and respiratory depression
Risperidone	PO: 0.005-0.01 mg/kg (0.25-1 mg/dose)	PO: 1 hr	Akathisia in higher doses

Adapted from Gerson, et. al

DISPOSITION

- Psychiatry consult

BEWARE

- Potential organic causes include meningoencephalitis, intoxication, medications
  - Medication reactions: serotonin syndrome, neuroleptic malignant syndrome, dystonic reactions, anticholinergics
- Chemical restraint medications may prolong QTc
  - Assess home medications' QTc prolongation potential

Section XIX
Pulmonary

1 ▶ Asthma

BACKGROUND
- ~ 1 in 11 children in U.S. have asthma
- Bronchospasm, airway inflammation → obstruction
- DDx: bronchiolitis, pertussis, FB aspiration, CHF, retropharyngeal abscess, anaphylaxis, pneumonia, cystic fibrosis, external compression (mediastinal mass, vascular ring/sling)

EVALUATION
- **High Yield History**
  - Triggers: household smoking, pets, allergens, weather, exercise, recent illness
  - Home controller/rescue medications, # prior ED visits, steroid courses, hospitalizations, intubations, ICU stays
  - Recent infection symptoms (fever, coughing)
  - Family Hx/PMH: atopy, eczema
- **Exam**
  - Vitals: respiratory rate, temperature, SpO2
    - Tachypnea can interfere with oral temp measurement
  - Pulmonary
    - Work of breathing: ability to speak in full sentences, accessory muscle use, nasal flaring, tracheal tugging, inter- and subcostal retractions, tripod positioning, belly-breathing, grunting
    - Expiratory wheezes, ↓ breath sounds in more severe obstruction
    - Stridor, rales, other focal findings may = another diagnosis
  - SpO2 often mildly ↓ due to VQ mismatch
    - Treatment → patient clinically improves, but ↓ SpO2 as open previously non-ventilated alveoli
  - Pulsus paradoxus: ↓ SBP by > 10 mmHg in inspiration compared to expiration = severe asthma

- **Diagnostics**
  - Routine ABG not indicated
    - SpO2, end-tidal CO2 for non-invasive monitoring
  - CXR
    - Choosing Wisely guidance: CXR in asthma patients "low-value"
    - Consider: first wheezing episode, fever > 39°C, persistent hypoxia, focal exam, poor treatment response

MANAGEMENT

Mild-moderate

- Albuterol: mainstay therapy; inhaled beta agonist bronchodilator
  - Nebulized 0.15-0.3 mg/kg (min 2.5 mg, max 10 mg) every 20 min
    - Often 2.5 mg for < 20 kg, 5 mg for > 20 kg
  - MDI 4-8 puffs every 20 min with spacer = efficacy to nebulized
  - Severe exacerbations: continuous nebulization 0.5 mg/kg/hr (max 20 mg/hr)
  - Side effects: tachycardia, tremors, headache, hypokalemia
- Ipratropium: anticholinergic, ↓ bronchoconstriction
  - Synergistic with albuterol
  - 0.25-0.5 mg nebulized or 4-8 puffs MDI with spacer every 20 min × 3
  - Often 0.25 mg for < 20 kg, 0.5 mg for > 20 kg
- Systemic corticosteroids: ↓ inflammation and relapse
  - Low threshold to give, proven ↓ hospitalizations
  - Prednisone 1 mg/kg/day (max 60 mg) for 5 days OR
  - Dexamethasone 0.3-0.6 mg/kg (max 16 mg) PO IV, IM; 2nd dose in 36-48 hrs **OR**
  - Methylprednisolone 1-2 mg/kg (max 125 mg) IV

Severe, add:

- Magnesium sulfate: smooth muscle dilator
  - Shown ↓ hospitalizations
  - 25-75 mg/kg IV over 20 min (max 2 g)
  - Watch for hypotension
- Epinephrine: alpha & beta agonist → bronchodilator, ↓ mucus
  - Consider nebulized racemic epinephrine 0.03 mL/kg (max 0.5 mL) of 2.25% solution in 5 mL NS if albuterol unavailable
  - IM 0.01 mg/kg (max 0.5 mg) of 1 mg/mL formulation
    - Opens bronchioles enough to permit inhaled medications to exert effect
  - Infusion 0.1-1 mcg/kg/min alternative to terbutaline

- Terbutaline: long-acting beta agonist
  — 10 mcg/kg SQ, IV (max 400 mcg), may repeat q20min
  — Continuous infusion 0.3-0.5 mcg/kg/min, titrate to max 3 mcg/kg/min

Other therapies
- Ketamine: bronchodilator at sedative doses
  — Preferred RSI sedative: 1-2 mg/kg IV
  — Subdissociative dose 0.1-0.3 mg/kg IV, particularly with BiPAP use
  — Beware: laryngospasm
- BiPAP, High-flow O2: PEEP prevents bronchiolar collapse
  — May improve nebulized medication delivery
- Theophylline: no longer recommended
- Heliox: helium + oxygen may improve laminar flow in refractory cases
  — Limited in hypoxic patients: ↓ efficacy with FiO2 > 30%

Impending respiratory failure
- Intubation: only if significantly worsening AMS, acidosis, hypercarbia, hypoxia
  — RSI medications / paralysis may → cardiopulmonary collapse given marked respiratory acidosis
    - Volume resuscitate first if possible
  — Ketamine 1-2 mg/kg IV
  — Succinylcholine 1.5 mg/kg IV or rocuronium 1 mg/kg IV paralytic
- Ventilator settings goals
  — SpO2 > 92%
  — Permissive mild hypercarbia, pH > 7.2
  — Consider slower rate, prolonged expiratory phase, low PEEP
- Post-intubation complications
  — DOPES: displacement, obstruction (mucus plugging), pneumothorax (↑ risk barotrauma in ventilated asthmatic), equipment failure, stacked breaths
    - Stacked breaths (auto-PEEP): incomplete exhalation → hyperinflation, can ↓ preload → hypotension
      * Disconnect and physically compress chest to promote exhalation
      * ↓ ventilator rate to allow complete exhalation

DISPOSITION
- Admit: persistent ↑ work of breathing, hypoxia, significant wheezing
- Discharge stable, appropriate response to treatment, close outpatient follow-up
  — Prescribe/refill controller and rescue medications, instructions on MDI with spacer use

BEWARE

- ⚠ Absent wheezing may = severe obstruction, poor air movement rather than ruling out asthma
- ⚠ Breath stacking may be etiology of ventilator high pressure alarms

2 ▶ Bronchiolitis

BACKGROUND

- Lower respiratory tract infection
  - Common causes: RSV *most common*, human metapneumovirus (HMV), rhinovirus, adenovirus, coronavirus, parainfluenza
  - Pathophysiology: airway epithelial cell invasion → cell necrosis, epithelial sloughing, small airway inflammation, mucus plugging, air trapping, atelectasis
- Seasonal: November - April, ↑January
- Children ≤ 2 yrs
- Incubation period: 4-6 days
- Spread: direct inoculation of mucus membranes or inhalation of large droplets
- Risk factors for severe disease
  - Prematurity, age < 12 wks, underlying cardiopulmonary disease, immunodeficiency, smoke exposure

EVALUATION

- **High Yield History**
  - Prodrome nasal congestion, cough, +/– fever → wheezing
  - Prior wheezing illness, apnea, cyanosis, ↓ feeding, ↓urine output
  - Prematurity, current post-conceptual age (chronologic age (wks) + gestational age at birth)
  - Use of palivizumab RSV prophylaxis in high risk
- **Exam**
  - Tachypnea, nasal flaring, grunting, retractions, wheezing, crackles, hypoxemia
  - Hallmark: minute-to-minute change in exam secondary to repositioning of debris/mucus within airway
  - Assess hydration
  - Infants < 2 mo may present with apnea only
  - SpO2 (continuous if concern for apnea)
- **Diagnostics**
  - *Clinical diagnosis*: routine labs/imaging not recommended

- PCR testing only if results would affect management
- UA +/− Ucx: febrile infants ≥ 39°C
- CXR: diagnostic uncertainty, severe, concern for complication (eg, pneumothorax, bacterial pneumonia)

MANAGEMENT

- Supportive care (suction, rehydration, antipyretics) mainstay
  - Nasal suctioning: deep suctioning may worsen airway irritation
- Supplemental oxygen only when SpO2 < 91% per AAP guidelines, others prefer higher cutoff depending on work of breathing
  - Humidified high-flow nasal cannula
- Treatments with unproven benefit
  - Nebulized hypertonic saline: may benefit hospitalized patients
  - Bronchodilators: consider if prior recurrent wheezing or strong family history of atopy/asthma
  - Racemic epinephrine: possible benefit for severe cases
  - Corticosteroids, chest physiotherapy
  - Antibiotics not indicated unless bacterial superinfection

DISPOSITION

- Admit
  - Oxygen saturation < 91% on RA
    - Some use higher cutoffs depending on follow-up, concomitant symptoms
    - Artificially ↑ SpO2 reported to clinicians increased hospitalizations without improving outcomes
  - Severe ↑ work of breathing
    - If tachypneic yet comfortable, tolerating PO, may discharge
  - Concern for apnea
    - Some support for ↑ risk in post-conceptual age < 48 wks
      - Controversial if no other reason for admission
    - Apneic episode(s) at home or in ED
  - Cannot maintain hydration/tolerate PO
- Discharge
  - Follow-up 48-72 hrs, supportive care (nasal bulb suction, hydration)
  - Expected cough/congestion duration 2-3 wks
  - Return precautions: cyanosis, grunting, severe nasal flaring or retractions, apnea, ↓urine output, lethargy, worsening course

3 ▶ Cough

BACKGROUND
- 8% of PED chief complaints
- Extensive differential from benign to deadly
- Acute: < 3 wks; chronic: > 4-8 wks; subacute between

EVALUATION
- **High Yield History**
  - Neonate
    - Congenital anomalies, GERD, CHF, pertussis, RSV
  - Associated symptoms: fever, sore throat, nasal discharge, sinus pain
    - URI, sinusitis, pneumonia, COVID-19
    - Serial URIs can mimic chronic cough
  - Onset
    - Choking episode → FB aspiration
    - Exercise or cold exposure → reactive airway disease (RAD)
    - Nocturnal → allergies, sinusitis, RAD
  - Character
    - Barking, seal-like → laryngotracheitis (croup)
    - Paroxysmal whooping, post-tussive emesis → pertussis
      - Infants may not whoop
    - Brassy with wheeze → tracheitis
    - High-pitched "tight" → asthma, bronchiolitis
    - Harsh barking/throat-clearing, resolves when asleep → "habit" cough
  - Duration
  - Ill or tuberculosis (TB) contacts
  - Personal or family Hx: allergies, asthma, GERD
  - Medications, anti-tussives
  - Tobacco, other irritant exposure
- **Exam**
  - Vitals, SpO2
  - Upper respiratory
    - Rhinorrhea, sinus tenderness, swollen turbinates
  - Lower respiratory
    - Wheezes, ronchi, crackles/rales

- — Signs of allergy
  - ▪ Boggy nasal mucosa, nasal crease, allergic shiner, cobblestoning
- — Otitis media can cause cough
- — Evidence of chronic hypoxia
  - ▪ Clubbing, CHF (edema, S3 gallop, hepatomegaly)
- **Diagnostics**
  - — Labs based on presentation
    - ▪ Respiratory PCR/culture including pertussis, COVID-19
    - ▪ TB testing
  - — CXR: focal lower respiratory findings, hypoxia, suspected TB, concern for FB

MANAGEMENT

- Supportive care: hydration with warm fluids, honey if > 1 yr old
- Anti-tussives not recommended in < 6 yrs
  - — Consider: cough preventing sleep, causing rib fractures, hypoxia
  - — Dextromethorphan 5-10 mg PO six times daily
- Viral URI: reassurance, supportive care
- Cough-variant/exercise-induced asthma
  - — Albuterol MDI trial
- Sinusitis
  - — Clinical diagnosis: purulent nasal discharge, facial congestion/fullness, fever, > 10 days unremitting symptoms
  - — Choosing Wisely guidance: avoid ABx in the ED for uncomplicated sinusitis
    - ▪ Mild/moderate: amoxicillin/clavulanate 22.5 mg/kg (max 875 mg) PO two times daily for 14 days
    - ▪ ABx failure/resistance: amoxicillin/clavulanate (use 600 mg/5 mL concentration) 45 mg/kg (max 2 g) PO two times daily for 14 days
- GERD
  - — H2-blocker
  - — Positioning: elevate head of bed or left lateral decubitus
    - ▪ Not for infants
    - ▪ Avoid postprandial supine position
- Pertussis
  - — Age ≤ 5 mos: azithromycin 10 mg/kg PO once daily for 5 days
  - — Age ≥ 6 mos: azithromycin 10 mg/kg (max 500 mg) PO once, then 5 mg/kg (max 250 mg) PO once daily for 4 days

- Suspected FB aspiration
  - Consult specialist to consider laryngoscopy/bronchoscopy
- Pneumonia: see chapter

DISPOSITION

- Discharge with close follow-up unless suspected FB aspiration, respiratory distress, hypoxia, young infant with suspected pertussis

BEWARE

- ! Recurrent pneumonia or FTT may = cystic fibrosis or immunodeficiency
- ! Pertussis → give close contacts post-exposure prophylaxis

4 ▶ Cystic Fibrosis (CF)

BACKGROUND

- Epidemiology
  - Autosomal recessive genetic disease
  - 1 in 25 Caucasians carrier → incidence 1 in 2500 births
  - Median life expectancy mid 20s – early 30s
  - All 50 states require newborn screening
    - ↑ blood test IRT (immunoreactive trypsinogen)
    - Positives confirmed with sweat chloride test
- Etiology
  - Genetic mutation on chromosome 7 affecting CFTR protein (cystic fibrosis transmembrane conductance regulator, many variants)
  - CFTR-related disorder = one copy of disease-causing mutation vs. two in full CF → intermediate sweat chloride levels, ↓ clinical manifestations
- Pathophysiology
  - Impaired chloride transport → altered water movement across epithelial cells → thickened GI/respiratory secretions, concentrated sweat
  - Affects respiratory tract, sweat glands, biliary epithelium, pancreatic exocrine function
  - Frequent pulmonary exacerbations caused by impaired mucociliary clearance, chronic bacterial colonization/infection
- If not diagnosed through newborn screening, commonly presents with meconium ileus, respiratory symptoms, or FTT
  - Later presentations adolescence & young adulthood: GI symptoms, new-onset DM, infertility

EVALUATION

- **High Yield History**
  - Pulmonary exacerbation
    - SOB, cough, chest pain / discomfort, sputum quality or quantity change, ↑ work of breathing
    - Appetite loss, fatigue, fevers
  - Distal intestinal obstruction
    - Infants: inability to pass stool after birth = meconium ileus
    - Children: vomiting, abdominal pain, constipation
  - Pancreatic insufficiency
    - Steatorrhea, pancreatitis, diabetes mellitus
    - Symptoms of fat-soluble vitamin deficiency
  - Prior complications
  - Current medications, recent antibiotics
  - Recent bacterial cultures & colonization history
- **Exam**
  - Vitals, SpO2, weight, growth curve
  - Dehydration (at risk for fluid and electrolyte loss)
  - Lung
    - Retractions, tachypnea, crackles, wheezing, ↑ tactile fremitus, hyperinflation, hypoxia, hypercapnia
  - Cardiac
    - CHF (crackles, hepatomegaly child, JVD & edema older) due to *cor pulmonale*
  - Abdomen
    - Abdominal distension, tenderness, tympany
    - Rectal prolapse, nephrocalcinosis, nephrolithiasis
  - Skin wrinkling of palms (aquagenic wrinkling) when immersed in water
- **Diagnostics**
  - Labs
    - Diagnosis confirmed by sweat chloride ≥ 60 mmol/L, gene sequencing
      - Sweat chloride 30-59 mmol/L intermediate
    - POC GLC, CBC, CMP, lipase, UA
    - +/- PCR respiratory panel, sputum culture, blood gas
  - Imaging
    - CXR: compare to prior, look for new infiltrates, pneumothorax
      - Chronic: bronchiectasis, especially perihilar/upper lobes

- CT thorax useful to assess disease progression over time
  - Rarely indicated in ED
- Abdominal imaging if suspect obstruction
  - Supine/upright KUB
  - CT abdomen: to localize stool inspissation
- Pulmonary function tests (PFTs): decreased FVC and/or FEV, compare to baseline

MANAGEMENT

- Consult CF specialist
- Pulmonary exacerbation — no standardized treatment protocol
  - Common organisms: *Haemophilus influenzae, Staph aureus, Pseudomonas aeruginosa, Aspergillus*
  - Antibiotics
    - Guided by recent sensitivities, CF specialist recommendations
    - Often double *Pseudomonas* coverage
    - Oral/inhaled or parenteral depending on severity of exacerbation
    - May require larger than typical doses
    - Common: aminoglycosides (IV or inhaled), ceftazidime, cefepime, piperacillin-tazobactam, ticarcillin-clavulanate, meropenem, aztreonam, fluoroquinolones
  - Oxygen supplementation
  - Bronchodilator: albuterol 0.15 mg/kg nebulized (max 10 mg) or 4-8 puffs MDI
  - Chest physiotherapy by RT helps airway clearance of pathogens
  - Mucolytics
    - 7% hypertonic saline, 4 mL nebulized
    - Dornase alfa 2.5 mg nebulized (requires specialized nebulizer)
    - N-acetylcysteine no longer recommended
  - May benefit from short course steroids for asthma-like exacerbation
    - Consult CF specialist
  - Noninvasive ventilation or mechanical ventilation for severe respiratory distress/failure
- Distal obstruction
  - Treatment depends on degree of obstruction
  - NGT, IV hydration
  - Simple enema vs. hyperosmolar contrast enema w/ guidance from radiology
  - GI/surgical consultation

- Dehydration, electrolyte losses
  — IV fluids, electrolyte repletion
    - Cautious fluids to avoid pulmonary edema
- Diabetes
  — Older adolescents, young adults with decline in pancreas function
  — Manage as for any diabetic

DISPOSITION
- Depends on symptoms, caretaker resources, nutritional status, recent health status
- Consult CF specialist early!

BEWARE
- Maintain high index of suspicion as not all patients diagnosed by newborn screen
  — Early diagnosis & treatment → better patient outcomes
- Critical to know patient's recent bacterial cultures/colonization status
- Early supportive care for respiratory distress with bronchodilators, chest physiotherapy followed by NIPPV to prevent intubation

5 ▶ Pneumonia

BACKGROUND
- Clinical categories
  — Community-acquired (CAP): not acquired in a healthcare facility
  — Hospital-acquired
  — Aspiration (consider in neuromuscular or seizure disorder)
- Majority of CAP in preschool-aged children is viral
- Common age-related causes
  — Neonate
    - Early (1st week): group B streptococci, non-typeable *H. influenzae, E. coli, Listeria monocytogenes*
    - Late: *E. coli, Staphylococcal spp, Chlamydia trachomatis, P. aeruginosa*
  — 1-3 mo: viruses, *Chlamydia trachomatis, B. Pertussis*
  — 3 mo-5 yrs: viruses, *S. aureus, S. pneumoniae*
  — ≥ 5 yrs: Mycoplasma, *S. pneumoniae, Chlamydia pneumoniae*
- Special groups
  — Cystic fibrosis: *P. aeruginosa, S. Aureus*
  — Immunocompromised: fungal (eg, *Pneumocystis jirovecii)*, CMV

- Aspiration: anaerobic oral flora
- Hospital-acquired: *S. Aureus*, Gram-negative bacilli

EVALUATION

- **High Yield History**
  - Cough (productive), fever, SOB, chest pain
  - Symptom duration, sick contacts: viral (influenza, COVID-19) & tuberculosis, immunizations (*S. pneumoniae* immunization protective)

Viral pneumonia more likely	Bacterial pneumonia more likely
• Gradual onset • Low grade fever • Bilateral perihilar CXR findings • Tachycardia, tachypnea out of proportion to fever • Wheezing • Rhinitis • GI symptoms	• Abrupt onset (except atypical → subacute) • High fever • Unilateral lobar CXR findings • Pleural effusion • No or prodromal URI symptoms • No wheezing • Abdominal pain • Toxic appearing

  - Atypical bacterial pneumonia
    - *C. Trachomatis*: afebrile, tachypneic, staccato cough, conjunctivitis, wheezing, hoarseness
    - Mycoplasma: sore throat, low grade fever, headache, cough, rash, myalgias, GI/neurological symptoms
- **Exam**
  - Vitals, SpO2
  - Lungs: focally ↓ breath sounds, focal crackles (rales) or rhonchi
    - ↑ work of breathing: retractions, tracheal tugging, grunting, nasal flaring
- **Diagnostics**
  - Labs
    - PCR respiratory panel (influenza, COVID-19)
    - +/− CBC, blood culture
      - Blood culture poor yield
      - Indications: age < 3 mo, antibiotic failure, progressive disease, suspected moderate-severe bacterial
    - Blood gas rarely needed
  - Imaging
    - CXR (2-view PA and lateral)
      - DO NOT obtain in well-appearing suspected viral pneumonitis
        - Can lead to ↑ ABx use from over-calling findings

- Viral: bilateral interstitial infiltrates, peribronchial cuffing, hyperinflation, atelectasis, no pleural effusion
- Bacterial
  - Unilateral focal consolidation, air bronchograms
  - Pleural effusion (empyema) or pneumatocele
  - Round pneumonia: seen exclusively in children due to poor development of interalveolar communications (pores of Kohn), which prevent lateral spread of infection
    - Usually *S. pneumoniae*
- Atypical bacterial pneumonia: bilateral interstitial infiltrates
— Consider CT chest w/IV contrast: complicated pneumonia
- Pneumatocele: common with staphylococcal, later in disease course
  - Differentiate from abscess
    - Pneumatocele thin smooth walls, clinically improving
    - Abscess thick irregular walls, air-fluid level, toxic appearing
- Parapneumonic effusion: common with streptococcal
- Necrotizing: consolidation with cavitation +/− air
- Lung US — ↓ ionizing radiation exposure
  - Viral: focal B lines & small subpleural consolidations < 1.5-2 cm
  - Bacterial: hepatization +/− dynamic air bronchograms, larger consolidations
  - US vs. CXR: ↑ sensitivity (96% vs. 87%), but ↓ specificity (95% vs. 98%)

MANAGEMENT

- Supplemental oxygen to keep SpO2 ≥ 95%
- Non-invasive ventilation (high-flow O2, BiPAP, CPAP) or intubation and mechanical ventilation PRN for hypoxia, hypercarbia, work of breathing, mental status
- Empiric antimicrobial therapy
  — < 3 mo (inpatient)
    - Post-conceptual age = gestational age at birth + chronological age (weeks)
    - Post-conceptual age > 44 wks: ceftriaxone 50 mg/kg IV daily
    - Corrected gestational age < 44 weeks: cefotaxime 50 mg/kg IV every 6-8 hrs
      - Ceftriaxone displaces bilirubin = kernicterus risk
      - If cefotaxime unavailable, ceftazidime 50 mg/kg IV every 8 hrs or cefepime 50 mg/kg IV every 8 hrs
    - Consider pertussis coverage if history of apnea or post-tussive emesis, ill contact with chronic cough, lymphocytosis on CBC

- Azithromycin 10 mg/kg/day PO for 5 days
  - \> 3 mo (inpatient)
    - Uncomplicated: ceftriaxone 50 mg/kg (max 1 g) IV daily +/– Azithromycin as above
    - Complicated: Ceftriaxone 50 mg/kg (max 2 g) IV every 12 hrs + MRSA coverage
      - Vancomycin 15 mg/kg (max 1 g) IV every 6 hrs OR
      - Clindamycin 10 mg/kg (max 450 mg) IV every 6 hrs
- Concern for hospital-acquired: cover *Pseudomonas*, *S. aureus*, *Enterobacteraciae*, anaerobes
  - Aminoglycoside + *Pseudomonas* coverage (piperacillin-tazobactam, meropenem, ceftazidime, or cefepime) +/– MRSA coverage (vancomycin)
- \> 3 mo (outpatient)
  - DO NOT prescribe ABx unless bacterial etiology suspected
  - Amoxicillin 45 mg/kg (max 1 g) PO two times daily for 10 days
  - ≥ 5 yrs: azithromycin 10 mg/kg (max 500 mg) day 1, then 5 mg/kg (max 250 mg) days 2-5 PO to cover atypical organisms
    - Atypical infection unlikely < 5 yrs
- Parapneumonic effusion
  - Small (< ¼ thorax opacified) may not require drainage
  - Ceftriaxone & metronidazole or beta-lactamase inhibitor, +/– MRSA coverage (vancomycin, clindamycin)
  - Consult pediatric pulmonologist or surgeon for management: pleural catheter with flushing, chest tube, fibrinolytics, VATs

DISPOSITION

- Admit
  - Age ≤ 3mo
  - Severe symptoms: respiratory distress, hypoxia, apnea, AMS
  - Suspected staphylococcal
  - Complicated (eg, effusion, pneumatocele)
- Discharge
  - Consider first dose antibiotic in ED
  - Follow-up 48-72 hr
  - Educate caretaker: supportive care (bulb suction, humidifier), return precautions, expected course

BEWARE

- Suspect FB aspiration in patients with recurrent lobar pneumonia
- Differentiating viral from bacterial CAP is difficult and they can coexist

6 ▶ Spontaneous Pneumothorax (PTX) & Pneumomediastinum

SPONTANEOUS PNEUMOTHORAX

BACKGROUND

- Air in pleural space without inciting traumatic/ iatrogenic event
- Primary Spontaneous PTX: usually apical bleb rupture
  - Typically tall, thin, healthy males
  - Risk factors: preterm infants, very loud music, smoking/cannabis, playing brass/woodwind instruments, inhalation drug use, snorting cocaine
  - Tension PTX: rare (1-3%)
- Secondary Spontaneous PTX: underlying disease, usually lung
  - Infection such as *Pneumocystis jirovecii*, pulmonary disease (asthma, cystic fibrosis), connective tissue disorders, malignancy, congenital, catamenial

EVALUATION

- **High Yield History**: chest pain, cough, dyspnea
- **Exam**: tachypnea, tachycardia, ↓ breath sounds, ↓ SpO2
  - Tension pneumothorax
    - Hypotension, tachycardia, mediastinal shift, JVD
- **Diagnostics**
  - CXR
    - Upright: absence of lung markings extending to chest wall
    - Sizing: visceral pleura of collapsed lung at lung apex to cupola (cervical pleura): ≤ 3 cm = small, > 3 cm = large
    - Supine: deep sulcus sign
  - POCUS
    - Absence of lung sliding
    - Lung point sign: near 100% specific

MANAGEMENT / DISPOSITION

- Avoid intubation/PPV → decompress PTX first
- 100% FiO2 to increase PTX absorption
- Tension PTX: finger thoracostomy or needle aspiration
  - Do not delay treatment for imaging

- Primary spontaneous PTX
  - Small size, clinically stable: 4-6 hrs observation, may discharge home with 12-48 hr follow-up if no progression on repeat imaging
    - Recurrence rate 50%
  - Large size or unstable: small bore catheter or chest tube, admit
    - Consider large bore chest tube if need PPV
- Secondary spontaneous PTX
  - Small size & clinically stable: admit, +/– chest tube
  - Large size or unstable: admit, large bore chest tube
  - Consult surgeon or pulmonologist if recurrent

SPONTANEOUS PNEUMOMEDIASTINUM

BACKGROUND
- Air in the mediastinal space with no traumatic/ iatrogenic event
  - Alveolar rupture → air tracks along bronchovascular sheaths to mediastinum → may follow fascial planes into neck
- Rare, self-resolves
- Risk factors: inhalation drug use (i.e. bongs, vaping), valsalva, coughing, vomiting

EVALUATION
- **High Yield History**: sore throat, dysphagia, chest pain, neck pain, dyspnea
- **Exam**: subcutaneous emphysema, neck/face swelling, wheezing, tachypnea, Hamman crunch = sound auscultated over cardiac apex (uncommon, ~12%)
- **Diagnostics**
  - CXR (2-view)
    - Linear lucency outlining mediastinal contour
    - Thymic wing sign
    - Continuous diaphragm sign
  - CXR & cervical soft tissue XR: subcutaneous emphysema

MANAGEMENT
- Analgesia
- Avoid valsalva
- Anti-tussives, antiemetics as needed
- Consider 100% oxygen to promote nitrogen washout

DISPOSITION

- Admit for observation to determine no deterioration, rule out esophageal perforation

BEWARE

- ⚠ Consider Boerhaave syndrome with vomiting → chest pain, subcutaneous emphysema
- ⚠ Can have both PTX and pneumomediastinum

7 ▶ E-Cigarette or Vaping Associated Lung Injury (EVALI/VALI)

BACKGROUND

- Acute inhalation lung injury attributed to e-cigarette use and/or dabbing (inhaling concentrated liquid)
- Still much unknown about cause, diagnosis, treatment, disease course
  — Vitamin E acetate, diluent used in tetrahydrocannabinol (THC) fluid/resin strongly implicated
  — Most patients endorse THC use, up to 14% nicotine only
- Epidemiology
  — 15% of patients < 18 yrs, median age 24 yrs
  — Higher risk among males, non-Hispanic white
- Long-term sequelae unknown
  — Some resolved cases → chronic pulmonary disease

EVALUATION

- **High Yield History**
  — Symptoms nonspecific
    - May present with GI symptoms only, respiratory symptoms later
    - GI: nausea/vomiting, diarrhea, abdominal pain
    - Respiratory: dyspnea, cough, pleuritic chest pain, hemoptysis
    - Constitutional: fever, malaise, myalgias
  — E-cigarette use and/or dabbing within last 90 days
  — Common comorbidities: ADHD, anxiety, depression, asthma, substance use
- **Exam**
  — Fever, tachycardia, tachypnea, hypoxia, hypotension, ↑ work of breathing, rales

- **Diagnostics**
  - Clinical diagnosis of exclusion
    - History of recent vape use (< 90 days)
    - Pulmonary infiltrates
    - No other cause identified
  - Labs (to exclude other disorders)
    - Leukocytosis (neutrophilic predominance), elevated ESR/CRP, blood cultures, respiratory PCR panel, COVID-19, Utox
    - Consider blood gas +/– procalcitonin to assess severity
  - CXR: diffuse bilateral, interstitial infiltrates
    - No pathognomonic infiltrate pattern
  - Consider CT Chest
    - Centrilobular ground glass opacities/nodules +/– subpleural sparing +/– pleural effusions
    - +/– CTPA (rule out pulmonary embolism)

MANAGEMENT

- Oxygen, non-invasive ventilation vs. intubation / mechanical ventilation PRN
- Empiric antibiotics for pneumonia +/– antivirals for influenza PRN
- Discontinue e-cigarette products
- Corticosteroids
  - Methylprednisolone 1 mg/kg (max 125 mg) IV daily as inpatient
  - Oral taper for outpatient

DISPOSITION

- Most patients admitted to PICU, especially if respiratory distress, hypoxia
- Criteria for outpatient management
  - Normal vital signs (SpO2 ≥ 95%)
  - No significant comorbidities
  - Good social support
  - Follow-up within 24-48 hrs
  - Pulmonary follow-up within 2-4 wks

BEWARE

- Relapse with resumption of vaping or during steroid taper
- Patients may present with mild symptoms but rapidly decompensate in 24-48 hrs

Section XX
Renal and Urinary System

1 ▶ Fluid and Electrolyte Disturbances

Electrolyte abnormality	Definition	Differential diagnosis
Hyponatremia	< 130 mEq/L	Vomiting/diarrhea, peritonitis, pancreatitis, burns, diuretics, osmotic diuresis, nephropathy, SIADH, water intoxication (overdiluted formula), CHF, renal failure, RSV infection
Hypernatremia	> 150 mEq/L	Concentrated infant formula, insensible water loss, head trauma, brain tumors, diabetes insipidus (DI)
Hypokalemia	< 3.5 mEq/L	Hyperaldosteronism, Bartter syndrome, hypomagnesemia, renal tubular acidosis (RTA), vomiting, diarrhea, administration of insulin/B-agonists, hypokalemic periodic paralysis
Hyperkalemia	> 5.5 mEq/L	Blood transfusion, K+ salt of PCN, oral intake, acute or chronic renal failure, adrenal insufficiency, burns, rhabdomyolysis, coagulopathy, tumor lysis syndrome, GI bleed, metabolic acidosis, pseudohyperkalemia (hemolysis)
Hypocalcemia	< 9 mg/dL	Hypoparathyroidism, vitamin D deficiency, hypomagnesemia, pancreatitis, sepsis, massive transfusion of citrated blood, phosphate enema toxicity
Hypercalcemia	> 10.5 mg/dL	Hyperparathyroidism, hyperthyroidism, vitamin D intoxication, thiazide diuretics, milk-alkali syndrome, sarcoidosis, bone malignancy, tumor lysis syndrome, inherited disorders

EVALUATION

- **High Yield History**
  - Feeding, how mixing infant formula
  - Hypo/hypernatremia
    - Asymptomatic until severe
    - Tremulousness, ataxia, doughy skin, hyperreflexia, confusion, seizure
  - Hypokalemia: weakness, cramps, hyporeflexia
  - Hyperkalemia: fatigue, paresthesias, palpitations
  - Hypocalcemia: weakness, paresthesias, irritability, Chvostek sign, Trousseau sign, tetany
  - Hypercalcemia: constipation, anorexia, abdominal pain
- Exam
  - Signs of dehydration
    - Delayed capillary refill, sunken fontanelle
    - Tachycardia, tachypnea, thready pulses
    - Irritability, lethargy, AMS
- Diagnostics
  - Labs
    - POC electrolytes, POC GLC
    - BMP, Ca^{2+}, PO_4^{3-}, Mg^{2+}, albumin
      - Frequent repeat electrolytes as correcting
      - Corrected Na^+ for hyperglycemia: Measured Na^+ + 0.024 × (serum GLC mg/dL − 100)
      - Corrected Ca^{2+} for hypoalbuminemia: Measured total Ca^{2+} + 0.8 (4 − serum albumin)
      - Ionized calcium = physiologically active form
    - Consider urine-specific gravity, urine Na^+, serum/urine osmolarity, Vitamin D, PTH
  - EKG
    - Hypokalemia: T-wave flattening, ST depression, U-waves, PAC/PVC
    - Hyperkalemia: peaked T-waves, PR prolongation, progressive QRS widening, "sine wave" may degenerate to asystole or VF
    - Hypocalcemia: QT prolongation, bradycardia
    - Hypercalcemia: QT shortening, bradycardia, heart block, sinus arrest

MANAGEMENT

- Dehydration
  - Oral rehydration
    - Mild (≤ 5%) 30-50 mL/kg
    - Moderate (≤ 10%): 60-80 mL/kg
    - Give 25% of fluid/hr × 4hrs
  - Severe: (> 10%) or AMS, persistent vomiting, acute abdomen/ileus, respiratory distress, shock:
    - 20 mL/kg of NS IV, repeat as needed
    - Difficult IV access: IO, consider NGT
  - Consider hypodermoclysis for mild to moderate + failed PO or difficult IV
  - Ondansetron 0.15 mg/kg PO, IV if vomiting (max 4 mg/dose)
- Hyponatremia
  - Acute (developed over < 48 hrs): gradually correct at ≤ 0.5 mEq/L/hr
    - Slow correction to reduce risk of osmotic demyelination syndrome
    - Na+ needed (mEq) = (0.6 × wt in kg)(desired Na+ - current Na+)
    - NS infusion (mL/hr) = (Na+ needed × 1000) / (154 × time(hrs))
      - Add to maintenance fluid rate
      - Rule of thumb: NS at 1.5x maintenance to raise 0.5 mEq/L/hr
  - Seizure, coma: correct rapidly with 3% hypertonic saline 3-5 mL/kg aliquots until neurologic status improves
  - SIADH: fluid restriction
- Hypernatremia
  - Gradually correct < 0.5 mEq/L/hr to decrease cerebral edema risk
  - Water deficit = (0.6 × wt(kg)) × (1 - [desired Na+/current Na+])
    - Give over 48 hrs, added to maintenance fluids
    - Rule of thumb: ½ NS at 1.25x maintenance
  - Suspected DI: ensure free access to water, consider DDAVP 0.02-0.08 mcg/kg (max 1 mcg) IV or SQ
- Hypokalemia
  - Consider treatment < 3.5 mEq/L or symptomatic
  - KCl 1-2 mEq/kg/dose PO preferred
  - If PO is contraindicated, increase [K+] in maintenance IV fluids to 40 mEq/L
  - If life-threatening hypokalemia or critically low, IV KCl 0.3 -1 mEq/kg (max 20-40 mEq) at rate 0.3-0.5 mEq/kg/hr (max rate 1 mEq/kg/hr)
    - Max PIV concentration: 80 mEq/L; max central line: 200 mEq/L

- Correct hypomagnesemia with MgSO4 25-50 mg/kg IV over 2-4 hrs (diluted to max concentration 200 mg/mL)
- Hyperkalemia
  - Asymptomatic or level < 7 mEq/L: stop K+ intake & K+- sparing medications, trend level closely
    - Renal dysfunction: sodium polystyrene sulfonate 1-2 g/kg PO/PR
  - Symptomatic or level ≥ 7 mEq/L

Hyperkalemia Emergent Therapy		
Therapeutic	Dose	Comments
Calcium gluconate 10% OR	50-100 mg/kg = 0.5-1 mL/kg IV/IO over 5 min	Give if significant EKG changes
Calcium chloride 10%	10-25 mg/kg = 0.1-0.25 mL/kg IV slow push	If cardiac arrest (faster onset); central line only
Insulin + glucose	IV insulin 0.1U/kg (max 10U) + dextrose 0.4 g/kg (4 mL/kg D10) over 15-30 min	Shifts potassium intracellularly
Sodium bicarbonate	1 mEq/kg IV over 15 min	
Albuterol	2.5-5 mg nebulized	

  - Consider loop diuretic to enhance K+ excretion, furosemide 1 mg/kg IV (max 40 mg)
  - Definitive treatment: hemodialysis
- Hypocalcemia
  - Consider treatment if level < 7.5 mg/dL or symptomatic
  - IV Ca2+ given over 2-5 min
    - Calcium gluconate 10%, 50-100 mg/kg = 0.5-1 mL/kg IV over 10-20 min
    - Calcium chloride 10%, 10-25 mg/kg = 0.1-0.25 mL/kg IV over 10-20 min
      - Requires central line, higher risk tissue necrosis with extravasation
  - Correct any hypomagnesemia with MgSO4 25-50 mg/kg IV over 2-4 hrs (diluted to max concentration 200 mg/mL)
- Hypercalcemia
  - Asymptomatic, mild (level < 12-14 mg/dL): treat underlying cause, avoid high Ca2+ diet, thiazide diuretics
  - Consider treatment if level > 12-14 mg/dL or symptomatic
    - Volume expansion with NS 20 mL/kg IV
    - Furosemide promotes Ca2+ excretion 1 mg/kg (max 40 mg) IV
    - Consider calcitonin to suppress bone resorption, hydrocortisone for vitamin D-related hypercalcemia, other drugs to decrease bone resorption (mithramycin, indomethacin, bisphosphonates) at discretion of Endocrinology consultant
  - ARF or dysrhythmias: hemodialysis
- Consult Nephrology, Endocrinology

DISPOSITION

- Admit for prolonged electrolyte repletion or comorbidity requiring further management
  - PICU for AMS, requiring frequent monitoring
- If discharged, close PCP follow-up

BEWARE

- ⚠ Sodium repletion: "low to high your pons will die (central pontine myelinolysis), high to low your brain will blow (cerebral edema)"
- ⚠ Pseudohyperkalemia: hemolysis from blood draw, prolonged tourniquet use, small-gauge needle use
- ⚠ Hypomagnesemia often associated with hypokalemia, hypocalcemia

2 ▶ Hematuria

BACKGROUND

- Abnormal # urine RBCs
  - Macroscopic (lower urinary tract) or microscopic (upper tract) (> 5 RBCs/HPF)
- Epidemiology
  - ED incidence 0.13%, > 56% identifiable cause
  - Incidental finding 0.41-4%
    - Most common: hypercalciuria (11-30%)
    - Concomitant proteinuria (0.06-0.7%) → higher risk of renal disease
- DDx
  - Glomerular causes
    - Primary
      - Glomerulonephritis (GN): post-strep, membranous proliferative, focal segmental, membranous, rapidly progressive
      - IgA nephropathy
      - Alport syndrome (kidney disease, hearing loss, eye abnormalities)
      - Thin glomerular basement membrane/familial - benign
        - URI → gross hematuria episodes
      - Acute interstitial nephritis (ibuprofen, diuretics, antibiotics)
    - Systemic: serum sickness, HUS, SLE, HSP, polyarteritis nodosa, Hep B/C, Goodpasture, granulomatosis with polyangiitis (Wegener's), TTP, infections

- Nonglomerular
  - UTI/pyelonephritis
  - Hemorrhagic cystitis
    - Infectious: bacterial, viral, parasitic
    - Drug-induced: cyclophosphamide
  - Hypercalciuria: idiopathic (most common), hyperparathyroid, immobilization, vitamin D intoxication
  - Nephrolithiasis
  - Vascular abnormalities: hemangiomas, renal vein/artery thrombosis, hereditary telangiectasia, AV malformations
  - Anatomic abnormalities: ureteropelvic junction obstruction, posterior urethral valves, urethral prolapse, urethral diverticula, polycystic kidney disease, multicystic dysplastic kidney
  - Trauma
  - Wilms tumor/other renal tumors
- Extrarenal
  - Sickle cell disease
  - Bleeding disorder: coagulopathies, hemophilia, Von Willebrand, thrombocytopenia
  - Nutcracker syndrome (left renal vein entrapment, commonly between aorta and SMA → impaired blood outflow)
  - Strenuous exercise
- Factitious
  - Drugs (rifampin, phenazopyridine, nitrofurantoin, metronidazole)
  - Foods (beets, blackberries, rhubarb, food coloring, mushrooms)
  - Catheterization does not result in hematuria > 3 RBC/HPF in adults
    - Pediatric data limited

EVALUATION

- **High Yield History**
  - Prior episodes, trauma, exercise, UTI symptoms, fever, flank pain, edema, oliguria, urine color, recent infection (throat, skin, GI), frequent bleeding (nosebleeds, hemarthrosis), abdominal pain, joint pain, rashes, pallor, medications, diet, foreign travel (*Schistosoma haematobium*)
  - Timing
    - At start of urine stream → distal source (urethra)
    - Throughout stream → bladder, ureter, or kidneys
    - At end of stream → bladder source

- Color
  - Glomerular: brown (tea/cola colored)
  - Lower urinary tract/vascular bleeding: pink/red, clots
- PMH: sickle, bleeding disorder, previous umbilical catheters, birth asphyxia (corticomedullary necrosis)

- **Exam**
  - Hypertension: GN, Wilms tumor, polycystic kidneys, vasculitis, anatomic obstruction
  - Fever: infection
  - HEENT: oropharyngeal erythema (post-strep GN), hearing loss (Alport)
  - Abdominal exam: masses, CVAT, trauma, lower abdominal tenderness, ascites
  - GU: trauma, varicocele (nutcracker syndrome), penile discharge, irritation
  - Extremities: joint swelling
  - Skin: rash (HSP), pallor, petechiae (HUS), ecchymoses (coagulopathy)
  - Edema of face, scrotum, sacrum, extremities

- **Diagnostics**
  - Urine dipstick/UA
    - + blood but negative RBCs → myoglobin
    - CPK: rule out rhabdomyolysis
  - Trauma: cutoff for further work-up controversial, generally > 50 RBC/HPF obtain CT
  - Casts and dysmorphic RBCs associated with glomerular etiology
  - Proteinuria > 2+ associated with glomerular disease
  - UCx if fever, dysuria, leukocyte or nitrite +
  - Spot urine Calcium/Cr ratio for hypercalciuria
    - Ratio > 0.2 in children > 6 years or 24 hr urine calcium > 4 mg/kg/day considered positive
  - CBC, BMP with BUN, Cr
    - Consider complement (C3, C4, total), ASO titers, throat culture if proteinuria / history of possible strep infection
    - Consider Hgb electrophoresis
  - Imaging
    - None: asymptomatic with normal Cr, BP, no proteinuria/casts
    - US to rule out malignancy, cystic disease if gross hematuria; may detect urolithiasis, tumors, renal parenchymal disease, hydronephrosis, Nutcracker syndrome, bladder inflammation/polyps, posterior urethral valves
    - CT abdomen/pelvis with contrast for trauma, urolithiasis not diagnosed on US
    - Retrograde urethrogram if concern for urethral trauma

MANAGEMENT
- Treat underlying etiology
- Hypertension: antihypertensives if > 95th% for gender/age/height with glomerular disease to prevent end organ damage — consult pediatric nephrologist
- Consultation
  - Nephrology: glomerular disease, hypercalciuria/urolithiasis (metabolic workup), hemoglobinopathies, systemic causes (SLE, TTP, Goodpasture), unexplained persistent hematuria
  - Urology
    - Kidney stone > 5 mm, failure to pass, hydronephrosis, infection
    - Gross hematuria with no glomerular involvement
    - Vascular/anatomic abnormalities, tumor, Nutcracker syndrome, hematuria from recurrent UTIs

DISPOSITION
- Admit: intra-abdominal injury, uncontrollable hypertension, oliguria, renal failure, need for IV hydration/analgesics, uncontrollable bleeding
  - Consider for edema, proteinuria, RBC casts, systemic illness
- Asymptomatic isolated microscopic hematuria: follow up outpatient for repeat UA ×2 within 2 wks

BEWARE
- High index of suspicion for significant renal disease in patients with sickle cell, rheumatologic disorders, HSP, hepatitis, Goodpasture, granulomatosis with polyangiitis
  - Monitor BP, renal function

3 ▶ Hemolytic Uremic Syndrome

BACKGROUND

- Epidemiology: ↑children < 3-5 yrs, can affect any age
- Etiologies
  — Shiga-toxin producing *E. Coli O157:H7* (STEC) responsible for ~90%
    - Sources: contaminated raw fruits/vegetables, undercooked beef, deli meats, unpasteurized milk/juice, community pools
  — Other: *Shigella, Campylobacter, Pneumococcus*, HIV
  — Rarer non-infectious causes: hereditary complement-mediated HUS, medications, SLE, antiphospholipid syndrome, pregnancy
- Pathophysiology
  — AGE bacteria infect colonic endothelium → endothelial sloughing
    - Resultant exposed basement membrane pro-thrombotic
  — Partial/complete vessel occlusion → RBC shearing and hemolytic anemia, organ ischemia (most common kidneys +/− brain, liver, heart, pancreas)
- Presents 5-14 days after diarrhea onset with triad of microangiopathic hemolytic anemia (MAHA), thrombocytopenia, acute kidney injury (AKI)
  — Often within 1-2 days of diarrhea resolving

EVALUATION

- **High Yield History**
  — Recent AGE – bloody diarrhea, pallor/fatigue, decreased urine output, abdominal pain
    - ABx for diarrhea (↑ risk of HUS if STEC infection)
  — Exposures (food, community pool, daycare, sick contacts)
- **Exam**
  — Anemia/thrombocytopenia: tachycardia, pallor, bruising, petechiae
  — Renal dysfunction: hypertension, edema, high-output heart failure suggestive
  — Abdominal tenderness
- **Diagnostics**
  — Labs: CBC + peripheral smear, Coombs, bilirubin, haptoglobin, LDH, reticulocytes
    - MAHA (Coombs negative, Hgb < 10 mg/dL, low haptoglobin, ↑ LDH, indirect bilirubin, and reticulocytes, schistocytes/burr/helmet cells on smear)
    - Thrombocytopenia
      ◆ Renal function tests, K+: AKI
      ◆ Coags: normal
      ◆ Extrarenal manifestations: ↑ troponin, transaminases, lipase

- UA: +/– proteinuria, hematuria
- Stool studies
    - Shiga toxin: PCR most reliable
    - *E coli O157:H7*: can isolate STEC from stool, via serology
    - Stool culture

MANAGEMENT

- Consult Nephrology
- Avoid ABx, antimotility, nephrotoxic medications
- Renal failure
    - Early fluid resuscitation correlated with improved outcomes
    - Correct metabolic abnormalities
    - Hypertension: fluid restrict, give anti-hypertensives
    - Dialysis frequently required
- Transfuse PRBCs if Hgb < 7, platelets if actively bleeding
    - Avoid rapid transfusion as intravascular expansion disrupts fluid balance

DISPOSITION

- Admit PICU
- Once discharged, monitor for late renal effects (hypertension, proteinuria, end-stage renal disease)

BEWARE

- 10-30% never have bloody diarrhea
- 30% will not have positive STEC/serotest in stool
- Complications: hypertension, seizures, hyponatremia/hypocalcemia, intussusception, bowel perforation, toxic megacolon

4 ▶ Hypertension

Category	1 to 12 yrs	13 yrs or older	Management
Stage 1 hypertension	BP 95%* to 95%* + 12	130/80 to 139/89	Outpatient work-up unless symptomatic
Stage 2 hypertension	BP ≥ 95%* + 12	BP ≥ 140/90	Expedited outpatient work-up; if symptomatic = emergency
Hypertensive emergency	BP > 95%* + 30	BP > 180/120	As below for emergency

*95% = 95th percentile for age, sex, height

- Urgency: WITHOUT end-organ damage (headache, nausea, vomiting)
- Emergency: WITH end-organ damage
  - Encephalopathy most common
  - Papilledema, retinal hemorrhage / exudate, heart failure, renal insufficiency
  - Also BP ≥ 95th percentile + 30 even if asymptomatic
- Primary/essential hypertension: underlying pathology NOT identified
  - Diagnosis of exclusion
  - Risk factors: high BMI, sedentary lifestyle, high-salt/high-caloric diets
- Secondary hypertension: underlying pathology
- White-coat hypertension: repeat after rest period
  - Persistently elevated → further evaluation

EVALUATION

- **High Yield History**
  - Renal: frequent UTIs, dysuria, unexplained fevers
  - Endocrine: weight loss, sweating, palpitations
  - OSA, obesity, pregnancy, medication/drug use, history of kidney issues or umbilical artery catheterization
  - End-organ damage: dizziness, confusion/AMS, nausea/vomiting, vision changes, chest pain, shortness of breath, hematuria
- **Exam**
  - Check cuff size
    - Too narrow = falsely high
    - Too wide = falsely low
  - Eye: retinal hemorrhages, disc edema
  - CHF: peripheral edema, crackles, hepatomegaly

- Renal disease: renal artery bruit, renal mass, edema
- Hyperthyroidism or catecholamine excess: diaphoresis, tachycardia, goiter, proptosis, tremor
- Aortic coarctation: absent/decreased femoral pulses
- **Diagnostics**
  - Labs: CBC, BMP, urinalysis, urine drug screen, urine pregnancy
  - Imaging
    - CXR: cardiomegaly, heart failure
    - Renal US w/Doppler: renal artery stenosis, tumor
    - CT head if severe headache, neurologic findings, papilledema
  - EKG for hypertrophy

MANAGEMENT
- Consult with pediatric nephrologist or cardiologist
- Hypertensive emergency
  - Reduce blood pressure by no more than 25% in first 8 hrs
    - Normalize over 3-4 days to maintain adequate cerebral perfusion
  - Medications (start at lower dose, titrate slow)
    - Labetalol 0.2-1 mg/kg IV bolus (max 40 mg/dose) followed by 0.25-3 mg/kg/hr infusion (caution in asthma)
    - Hydralazine 0.1-0.2 mg/kg IV (max 20 mg/dose)
    - Nicardipine 30 mcg/kg (max 2 mg) IV bolus, followed by 0.5-1 mcg/kg/min (max 4-5 mcg/kg/min)
    - Esmolol 100-500 mcg/kg IV bolus over 1 min, followed by 100-500 mcg/kg/min
  - Address end-organ damage
- Hypertensive urgency
  - Oral medications (given in consultation with specialist)
    - Isradipine 0.05-0.1 mg/kg/dose (max 5 mg)
    - Clonidine 2-5 mcg/kg (0.8 mg max)
  - Treat underlying conditions

DISPOSITION
- Admit hypertensive emergency to PICU
- Asymptomatic mild hypertension, hypertensive urgency → discharge with follow-up

BEWARE
- Oral nifedipine in children unpredictable effect, risk of hypotension, rebound hypertension

5 ▶ Nephrotic and Nephritic Syndromes

BACKGROUND

- Nephritic syndrome—immune complex deposition → inflammation of the nephrons → hematuria, proteinuria, oliguria, edema, hypertension
  — Annual incidence very low; M > F; ages 3-7 yrs (unlikely < 2 yrs)
  — Poststreptococcal glomerulonephritis (PSGN) most common acute glomerulonephritis
    - Recent strep pharyngitis or cellulitis
    - Timely treatment does not clearly decrease incidence
- Nephrotic syndrome—increased permeability across the glomerular filtration barrier resulting in massive proteinuria (> 50 mg/kg/day) → hypoalbuminemia (< 3 g/dL), edema, and hyperlipidemia
  — Annual incidence in < 16 yrs is 2/100,000
  — Idiopathic most common
    - Unclear pathogenesis
      ◆ Podocyte effacement and injury due to genetic, infectious, or drug-induced causes
    - Light microscopy minimal changes, focal segmental glomerulosclerosis, or mesangial proliferation
  — High rate of recurrent episodes

EVALUATION

- **High Yield History**: edema, urine changes (color, hematuria, foamy), recent strep infection, SLE, Hodgkin lymphoma, HSP, HIV, obesity, family history of kidney disease
  — PSGN: tea/cola-colored urine
- **Exam**
  — ↑ blood pressure (see Hypertension chapter)
  — Edema
    - Gravity dependent (periorbital early in the day, lower extremity later, sacral if reclining)
    - May resolve as day progresses
  — Ascites: consider paracentesis to r/o spontaneous bacterial peritonitis
  — Pleural effusion
  — Signs of specific underlying disease (rash of SLE, HSP)
- **Diagnostics**
  — UA w/microscopy
    - Nephritis: hematuria, RBC casts, proteinuria

- Nephrotic syndrome: proteinuria +/– hematuria
    - Urine Protein Excretion = Spot total urine protein / urine creatinine
        - \> 3 mg protein per mg creatinine (300 mg protein per mmoL creatinine) indicates nephrotic range proteinuria
- Labs: CBC, BMP, LFTs, albumin, PT/INR, PTT, lipid panel
    - Nephrotic syndrome: low albumin, hyperlipidemia
    - Consider:
        - ASO titer, rapid strep antigen test
        - Complement levels (C3, C4, CH50) low in PSGN
        - HIV, Hepatitis B/C, EBV
        - ANA, anti-dsDNA

MANAGEMENT

- Consult Nephrology (renal biopsy)
- PSGN: supportive care, ABx
    - Amoxicillin 50 mg/kg PO daily × 10 days (max 1 g/dose)
- Nephrotic syndrome
    - Fluid restriction (caution: ↓ effective circulating blood volume)
    - Na+-restricted diet (2-3 mEq of Na+/kg/day with 2000 mg/day max)
    - Diuretics
        - Furosemide 0.5-1 mg/kg (max 40 mg/dose, can give up to 2 doses)
        - Use with caution, closely monitor BUN and creatinine
    - Albumin
        - 0.5-1 g/kg IV over 4 hrs
        - Use salt-poor 25% albumin
    - Steroids only in consult with Nephrology
    - Mobilization important to avoid thromboembolic complications

DISPOSITION

- Nephrotic syndrome: admit if signs of hypovolemia, uncontrolled fluid loss anticipated (due to AGE, for example), significant hypertension, oliguria or renal insufficiency, bacterial peritonitis, to give albumin + furosemide therapy
- PSGN: admit if hypertension (may develop hypertensive emergency), renal insufficiency

BEWARE

- ❗ Children with nephrotic syndrome are usually immunocompromised (urinary loss of immunoglobulins) which predisposes to severe bacterial infection (particularly encapsulated bacteria)
  — Consider 23-valent and heptavalent conjugated pneumococcal vaccination
- ❗ Nephrotic syndrome also → hypercoaguable state due to losses of antithrombin, protein S, and plasminogen, leading to ↑ thromboembolism risk

6 ▶ UTI and Pyelonephritis

BACKGROUND

- Urinary tract infection (UTI)
  — Retrograde ascent of GI bacteria via perineum, instrumentation; hematogenous spread
  — Lower UTI: cystitis, urethritis
  — Upper UTI: pyelonephritis
- Prevalence in febrile children: < 2 yrs 7%; < 5 yrs 3.4%
- Most common serious bacterial illness (SBI) of infants < 3 mo
  — Risk of bacteremia 1.5-9.8%
- Risk factors: fever > 39°C, symptoms > 24-48 hrs, female, uncircumcised male, vesicoureteral reflux, bladder dysfunction, constipation, malnutrition, renal transplant, prior UTI
- DDx
  — Neonates: pneumonia, bacteremia, meningitis
  — Young child: irritation (bubble bath, tight clothing, harsh detergent), chemical urethritis, vaginitis, balanitis, child sexual abuse
  — Adolescent: STI, irritation (douching)

EVALUATION

- **High Yield History**
  — Classic UTI symptoms less frequent in kids
    - Infants: fever, fussiness, lethargy, feeding intolerance, FTT
      ◆ Neonates: may present with jaundice only
    - Older children: dysuria, frequency, urgency, suprapubic discomfort, hematuria, flank/back pain
  — Abdominal/flank pain, vomiting, systemic signs → pyelonephritis
    - Presume upper UTI in young febrile children with UTI

- Wiping (front to back in girls), hygiene, masturbation, constipation
- Prior UTI (including resistant organisms), known urinary obstruction, recent instrumentation, recent ABx, sexual activity/abuse, pregnancy

- **Exam**
  - Vital signs, appearance (toxicity → urosepsis)
  - Capillary refill, color, perfusion
  - Suprapubic tenderness, CVAT
  - Careful abdominal exam as UTI symptoms may occur with appendicitis due to ureter irritation by inflamed appendix
  - GU exam: discharge, foreign bodies, vaginitis, balanitis, tight phimosis, epididymitis, orchitis, labial fusion

- **Diagnostics**
  - Younger, stable children with fever without source: decision to test based on balancing pretest probability with risk/discomfort of invasive testing
    - UTIcalc and AAP algorithm provide guidance on when to test
  - Labs
    - Urine dipstick, microscopic urinalysis, culture
      - Urine dipstick: if nitrites and leukocyte esterase concordant, UTI effectively ruled in or out (84% PPV and 95% NPV)
        - Nitrites (> 90% specificity for UTI) suggest infection with Gram negatives (most commonly *E. Coli*)
      - UA: pyuria = ↑ WBC (> 5-10/HPF) and uropathogen bacteriuria
        - If both negative, UTI excluded
        - Lower specific gravity = lower cutoff (3 WBC/HPF at specific gravity < 1.010) to optimize sensitivity
      - Urine culture: number of CFUs/mL debatable but generally > 50,000 catheterized specimen, > 100,000 clean catch
        - Gold standard
      - Collection methods vary based on age
        - Suprapubic aspiration least contamination but rarely performed
        - Urethral catheterization in diapered children
        - Urine bag when catheterization not possible: labial adhesions, phimosis, caretaker refusal
          - Risk of contaminated sample
        - Clean catch if toilet-trained
    - Broader sepsis work-up in toxic appearing/suspected pyelonephritis: CBC, BMP, blood cultures, CRP, procalcitonin

- Adolescent/sexually active
  - Urine NAT for gonorrhea, chlamydia
  - Wet mount for trichomonas, bacterial vaginosis, candida
  - Pregnancy test
- Imaging
  - Only if alternate diagnosis suspected (nephrolithiasis, appendicitis)
  - Refer all < 2 yrs with first febrile UTI, recurrent UTI for outpatient renal US

MANAGEMENT

- ABx per local susceptibilities/resistance patterns; include *E. coli* coverage
  - Empiric therapy until culture results available
    - Use prior culture susceptibilities to guide choice
    - Consider different class if recently on antibiotics
  - IV antibiotics for infants < 2 mo (↑risk of bacteremia), toxic, pyelonephritis + pregnant, sepsis, failed outpatient antibiotics, immunocompromised, risk for resistant organisms, inability to tolerate PO
    - Ceftriaxone 50 mg/kg IV once daily (max 2 g/dose) for > 28 days old
    - Cefotaxime or ampicillin + gentamicin for neonates
  - Oral ABx for young febrile infants without urinary tract abnormalities, recurrent infection
    - Widespread resistance to ampicillin and amoxicillin, ↑ resistance to TMP/SMX, 1st gen cephalosporins: use regional antibiograms
    - If afebrile, immunocompetent, non-toxic
      - Cephalexin 50 mg/kg PO two times daily, longer course if recurrent UTI or < 2 yrs
      - Nitrofurantoin used in female adolescents 100 mg PO two times daily
        - Ineffective against bacteremia, pyelonephritis, complex
      - Treatment duration: < 2 yrs 7-10 days, child 5-7 days, adolescent/adult 3-5 days
    - If febrile or pyelonephritis, 2nd/3rd generation cephalosporins first line agents (but do not cover enterococcus) for 10-14 days
      - Cefuroxime 15 mg/kg two times daily
      - Cefdinir 14 mg/kg PO once daily
  - Children > 6 yrs: consider phenazopyridine for analgesia 4 mg/kg every 8 hrs for 2-3 days (max 200 mg/dose), do not continue > 3 days → risk of methemoglobinemia

DISPOSITION

- Admit: infants < 2 mo, pregnant with pyelonephritis, immunocompromised, intractable vomiting/dehydration, renal insufficiency, toxic appearing
  - Consider for: known urinary tract abnormality, urinary tract obstruction, ureteral stents/other foreign body
- If discharged, follow up with pediatrician in 24-48 hrs

BEWARE

- Pyuria without UTI ("sterile pyuria") can occur in adolescents with STIs, appendicitis, Kawasaki, MIS-C
- Ensure tolerating PO prior to discharge
- Uncircumcised males < 2 yrs and all males < 6 mo = UTI nearly as prevalent as in females

Section XXI
Rheumatology & Vasculitides

1 ▶ Acute Rheumatic Fever

BACKGROUND
- Children age 5-15 yrs
- Very rare in U.S. and other developed countries
- Autoimmune reaction against endocardial tissue and cardiotoxicity from Streptolysin O
  — Follows only streptococcal pharyngitis, not skin or other infections

EVALUATION
- **High Yield History**
  — Fever, arthralgias, pharyngitis (1/3 have no history of sore throat)
  — Usually 2-3, up to 6wks after streptococcal pharyngitis
- **Exam**
  — Polyarthritis/arthralgia, commonly knees, ankles, wrists
  — Cardiac: mitral/aortic regurgitation, pericardial friction rub
  — Subcutaneous nodules, symmetric, firm, painless, most common at elbow
  — Sydenham chorea: rapid, irregular, involuntary movements
  — Erythema marginatum: transient pink rash with ring-like lesions on trunk and extremities
- **Diagnostics**
  — Jones criteria: 2 major or 1 major + 2 minor plus evidence of preceding strep pharyngitis

Major Criteria	Minor Criteria
• Joints: migratory polyarthritis of large joints • Cardiac: carditis (clinical or on echo) • Nodules, subcutaneous • Erythema marginatum • Sydenham chorea	• Fever ≥ 38.5°C or ≥ 38° if high risk • Arthralgias • ESR ≥ 30 mm/hr low risk, ≥ 60 mm/hr mod-high risk, CRP ≥ 3.0 mg/dL • EKG - prolonged PR, non-specific

- Labs
    - CBC, ESR, CRP
    - Antistreptolysin O titers ↑ or rising
    - Throat culture
- EKG
- Imaging
    - CXR for cardiomegaly
    - Echocardiogram: pericardial effusion, atrial myxoma, CHF

MANAGEMENT

- Antibiotic therapy
    - Initial: antibiotics to eradicate strep pharyngitis
        - IM benzathine penicillin 600,000U ≤ 27kg, 1.2 millionU > 27 kg OR
        - Amoxicillin 50 mg/kg (max 1 g) PO once daily for 10 days
    - Prophylaxis against recurrence/long-term rheumatic heart disease
        - IM benzathine penicillin as above every 21-28 days preferred
        - Penicillin VK PO 250 mg two times daily ≤ 27 kg, 500 mg two times daily > 27 kg
        - Sulfadiazine PO 500 mg daily ≤ 27 kg, 1 g daily > 27 kg
        - Azithromycin 5 mg/kg (max 250 mg) PO daily
        - Duration of prophylaxis
            - If no carditis: 5 years or until 21 yrs old
            - If carditis w/o residual heart disease for 10 years or until 21 yrs old
            - If carditis with residual heart disease (valvular carditis): 10 years or until 40 yrs old
- Bed rest/activity limitation acutely
- Carditis
    - Standard heart failure management with cardiologist input
    - Prednisone 1-2 mg/kg/day often given, although not supported by evidence
- Arthritis: NSAIDs
- Chorea: carbamazepine or valproate (consult Neurology)

DISPOSITION

- Admit, consult Cardiology

2 ▶ Henoch-Schonlein Purpura

BACKGROUND

- Immune-mediated vasculitis: IgA deposits in small vessels
- Often preceding URI (Group A strep common) or GI infection
- 90% < 10 yrs, peak incidence 4-6 yrs, M=F, uncommon in summer
- Complications
  - Anemia from hemorrhage into skin, GI tract, urine
  - Kidney disease → hypertension, nephrotic syndrome, renal insufficiency
  - GI hemorrhage, bowel ischemia/necrosis, bowel perforation, intussusception
  - Rare: ICH, pulmonary hemorrhage, uveitis, keratitis, pancreatitis

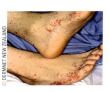

EVALUATION

- **High Yield History**
  - Recent URI
  - Rash typically first symptom, eventually seen in all patients
  - Within 1-2 wks of rash onset: abdominal pain (50%), arthralgias (75%)
  - Hematuria, BRBPR, melena
- **Exam**
  - Vitals: hypertension (renal involvement)
  - Skin: painless palpable purpura on extensor surfaces of lower extremities
    - May have dependent or periorbital edema
  - Abdomen/GU: tenderness (variable), heme positive stool, scrotal tenderness
  - Joints: transient migratory arthritis (hips, knees, ankles most common)
    - Typically no warmth, erythema, effusion
  - Neuro: assess for changes in behavior or mental status, r/o ICH
- **Diagnostics**
  - Labs: CBC, CMP, lipase, PT/INR, PTT, ESR, UA
    - Mild leukocytosis, eosinophilia, normal platelet counts and coagulation studies, ↑ ESR, microscopic/gross hematuria, proteinuria
  - Imaging
    - US: intussusception, bowel wall thickness, hematomas, peritoneal fluid
    - CT Head non-contrast if AMS

MANAGEMENT

- Supportive, acetaminophen for joint pain (NSAIDs if no renal involvement or GI bleed)
- Severe symptoms: prednisone 1-2 mg/kg (max 60-80 mg) PO daily with input from specialist
- May require antihypertensive therapy
- Management of renal disease in consultation with nephrologist

DISPOSITION

- Admit: unable to orally hydrate, severe joint or abdominal pain, significant GI bleeding, hypertension or renal insufficiency
- Discharge: PCP follow-up within week for urine and blood pressure monitoring

BEWARE

- ❗ HSP does not cause thrombocytopenia/coagulation abnormalities
  - Consider ITP or leukemia if these are present or if patient has bleeding gums, bruising, petechiae, pallor, fatigue
- ❗ Rash may initially mimic urticaria

3 ▶ Juvenile Idiopathic Arthritis

BACKGROUND

- Persistent arthritis in ≥ 1 joint lasting ≥ 6wks in children ≤ 16 yrs
- Unknown cause, genetic susceptibility
- Classifications: pauciarticular, polyarticular, systemic

EVALUATION

- **High Yield History**
  - Polyarticular: low-grade fever, malaise, morning stiffness (TMJ, hip, fingers), "gelling" (stiffness after prolonged sitting), myalgias
  - Family history

- **Exam**

	Pauciarticular	Polyarticular	sJIA
Epidemiology	F > M Type I – females Type II – males	F > M	F = M
Joint exam	≤ 4 joints affected Type I – large joints Type II – axial	≥ 5 joints affected within 6mo of onset Symmetric, large and small joints	Arthralgias → Arthritis, Synovitis
Other	I – iridocyclitis (photophobia, redness, tearing, miosis, blurred vision) II – acute anterior uveitis (often ANA+)		Fever ≥ 102.2°F for ≥ 2wks, salmon-colored maculopapular transient rash, serositis (pleural, pericardial effusion), lymphadenopathy, hepatosplenomegaly, torticollis (cervical involvement)

- **Diagnostics**
  - Clinical diagnosis of exclusion
  - Labs: CBC (↑WBC, anemia), CMP, ↑ferritin/ESR/CRP
    - May have +ANA, +RF, +HLA-B27
  - Imaging
    - US: cortical erosions, synovial thickening, effusions
    - XR: soft tissue swelling, periarticular erosions, narrowed joint spaces
    - CXR: pleural effusion
    - Echocardiogram: pericarditis, effusion
  - Arthrocentesis may be done to rule out septic arthritis

MANAGEMENT

- NSAIDs
  - Ibuprofen 10 mg/kg (max 400 mg analgesic, 800 mg anti-inflammatory) PO every 6 hrs
  - Naproxen 5-7.5 mg/kg/dose (max 500 mg) PO every 12 hrs
  - Aspirin no longer drug of choice due to adverse effects
- Nonpharmacologic pain management: heat packs, immobilization

- Rheumatologist consult may recommend:
    - Moderate-severe disease: steroids, methotrexate, IL-1/IL-6 inhibitor (anakinra)
    - Disease-modifying antirheumatic drugs (DMARDs): hydroxychloroquine, sulfasalazine, leflunomide, cyclosporine, IL-1/IL-6 inhibitors, TNF-alpha inhibitors

DISPOSITION

- Admit: initial diagnosis, systemic symptoms
- Consult Rheumatology, Ophthalmology

BEWARE

(!) ANA + children < 7 yrs → high risk uveitis

(!) Macrophage Activation Syndrome severe complication of sJIA: DIC, hemophagocytosis, hepatic inflammation, seizures/coma
   - Treated with high dose methylprednisolone 30 mg/kg (max 1 g) IV

4 ▶ Kawasaki Disease

BACKGROUND

- Self-limited systemic vasculitis of unknown etiology
- 80% children < 5 yrs, peak age 18-24 mo
    - Race: Japanese > other Asian > Black > White
    - Uncommon in summer months
- DDx: viral exanthem, scarlet fever, EBV infection, COVID-19 MIS-C, rheumatologic disease, adenovirus

EVALUATION

- **High Yield History**
    - Abrupt, high fever (≥ 102°F × ≥ 5 days)
        - Confirm daily, measured
    - Uncharacteristically inconsolable/irritable
    - Ask about recent symptoms (conjunctivitis) even if not currently present

- **Exam**

Diagnostic Findings	
C	Conjunctivitis (bulbar, non-exudative)
R	Rash (variable), desquamation ~2 wks after fever onset
A	Adenopathy (cervical, 1.5 cm, single unilateral)
S	Strawberry tongue; cracked red lips
H	Hand/foot swelling, erythema of palms/soles
Burn	5+ days of fever

- **Diagnostics**
  — Labs
    - CBC: leukocytosis, elevated platelets
    - CMP: transaminitis, hypoalbuminemia, hyponatremia
    - Elevated ESR/CRP
    - UA: sterile pyuria
    - Blood, urine, throat cultures: rule out other diagnoses
  — Imaging
    - Echocardiogram to assess for coronary aneurysms
    - Biliary ultrasound if suspect gallbladder hydrops
- Diagnostic criteria
  — Classic: fever ≥ 5 days + 4 of 5 diagnostic findings
    - Can make diagnosis on day 4 of fever if 4 diagnostic findings
  — Incomplete: fever ≥ 5 days + 2-3 diagnostic findings or infant ≤ 6 mo with unexplained fever ≥ 7 days → screen with labs
    - CRP ≥ 3.0 mg/dL or ESR ≥ 40 mm/hr AND
    - 3 or more of: anemia for age, platelets ≥ 450,000 after 7th day of fever, albumin ≤ 3 g/dL, elevated ALT, WBC ≥ 15,000/mm3, urine WBC ≥ 10/HPF
    - OR echocardiogram with coronary aneurysm
      ◆ Perform echocardiogram if meets ESR/CRP criteria and desquamation develops

MANAGEMENT

- Infectious diseases, cardiology specialists consult
- IVIG 2 g/kg over 10-12 hrs; most effective in first 7-10 days of illness
- Aspirin: high dose 80-100 mg/kg/day or moderate dose 30-50 mg/kg/day PO divided q6hrs until afebrile, then low dose 3-5 mg/kg/day
  — Contraindications: varicella, influenza

- Complications
  - Gallbladder hydrops: cholecystectomy if perforated, supportive otherwise
  - Uveitis: ophthalmic corticosteroids
  - Arthritis: supportive
  - KD shock syndrome: fluid boluses, inotropic agents
  - Coronary aneurysms: low dose aspirin for thrombosis prophylaxis
  - Recurrent disease: retreatment with IVIG vs. immunologics

DISPOSITION
- Admit
- Echocardiogram at 2 wks and 6-8 wks post-discharge
  - Discontinue aspirin if normal echocardiogram at 6-8 wks
  - If coronary artery abnormalities, continue aspirin indefinitely

BEWARE
- Consider incomplete KD if prolonged fever and 2-3 cardinal findings
- Findings may have resolved prior to ED presentation
- Children outside age 6mo-5yrs often present atypically
- Patients with prior KD at risk for myocardial ischemia due to aneurysms, aneurysmal rupture

5 ▶ Systemic Lupus Erythematosus

BACKGROUND
- Chronic autoimmune disease with multisystem inflammation, broad range of clinical features, ongoing disease-related damage
- Serious complications: infection, cardiovascular disease, renal disease
- F > M, ↑ in non-Caucasians

EVALUATION
- **High Yield History**
  - Nonspecific constitutional symptoms typical: fever, headaches, weight loss, fatigue, anorexia, arthralgias
    - May present as prolonged fever of unknown origin
  - Neurological symptoms range from headaches to seizures, stroke, psychosis
  - May have Raynaud phenomenon

- Diagnosis requires at least 4 of 11 American College of Rheumatology Criteria

Diagnostic Criteria
Malar rash
Photosensitivity
Discoid rash
Oral ulcers
Serositis: pleuritis, pericarditis
Arthritis
Nephritis / proteinuria
Neurological disorder: seizure, psychosis
Hematological disorder (see labs)
Antinuclear antibodies (ANA) +
Immunologic disorder (see labs)

- **Exam**
  — Hypertension common initial finding due to renal glomerular involvement
  — Oral/nasal ulcers, nonscarring alopecia
  — Classic malar rash (butterfly distribution across the face sparing nasolabial folds) or rarely discoid rash (scaly, crusty patch on forehead or scalp)
  — Pericarditis: pleuritic, positional chest pain (better with leaning forward), pericardial friction rub, tachycardia
  — Arthralgias, arthritis
  — Lymphadenopathy, hepatosplenomegaly
- **Diagnostics**
  — Labs
    - CBC (hemolytic anemia, thrombocytopenia, leukopenia, lymphopenia), CMP (kidney and liver function)
    - ↑ESR, normal CRP (↑CRP if patient also has serositis or active infection)
    - Immune: ANA, anti-dsDNA, anti-Smith, antiphospholipid antibodies, lupus anticoagulant, low complement (C3, C4)
    - Blood cultures, UA, urine culture if febrile without source
  — Imaging
    - CXR: evaluate for pulmonary infection, pleural or pericardial effusion
  — EKG: evaluate for thromboembolism, pericarditis in patient with chest pain, shortness of breath

MANAGEMENT
- Hydroxychloroquine 5 mg/kg (max 400 mg) PO daily
- Symptomatic treatment with analgesic NSAIDs
- Moderate-severe disease: long-term corticosteroids, other drugs with Rheumatology input
- Patients on chronic corticosteroids who present with infection require stress-dose steroids
  — Hydrocortisone 25 mg IV infants, 50 mg IV children, 100 mg IV teens

DISPOSITION
- Admit: acute flare, fever and neutropenia, severe complication
- Discharge otherwise with Rheumatology input and close follow-up

BEWARE
- ❗ Treat fever seriously in this immunocompromised patient population!
- ❗ Complications of chronic steroid use: infection, avascular necrosis
- ❗ Macrophage Activation Syndrome severe complication: high fever, DIC, hemophagocytosis, hepatic inflammation, seizures/coma
  — Treated with high dose methylprednisolone 30 mg/kg (max 1 g) IV

Section XXII
Toxicology

1 ▶ Caustic Substances

BACKGROUND
- Most are accidental and are among pediatric & elderly populations
  — ~ 4% intentional for self-harm
- Common substances - household supplies:
  — Acids: Toilet/drain cleaners, acetic acid, hydrofluoric acid
  — Alkalis: Ammonia, lye, detergents, bleach, oven cleaner, hair relaxers
- Routes of exposure
  — Ingestions, skin, ocular
- Pathophysiology
  — Acids
    - Coagulation necrosis of tissue proteins
    - Strong odor and pain
    - Can be absorbed systemically
  — Alkalis
    - Liquefaction necrosis and deeper injury by dissolving fats in cell membranes
    - Colorless & odorless, no immediate pain

EVALUATION
- **High Yield History**
  — Product, timing, amount, duration, last meal, suicidal intent
    - Is the container available?
  — Symptoms
    - Common: pain, dysphagia, photophobia (ocular exposure)
    - Concerning: difficulty breathing, peritonitis, hemodynamic instability
- **Exam**
  — Oropharyngeal: drooling, burns, edema

- Ocular: photophobia, red eye, conjunctival swelling/blanching
- Lungs: stridor, hoarseness, retractions
- Abdomen: peritoneal signs
- Skin: erythema, burns

- **Diagnostics**
  - Labs
    - pH of ingestant/ocular discharge, CBC, BMP, Ca2+ level for hydrofluoric acid exposure
  - Imaging
    - CXR
    - Perforation: KUB upright or CT scan w/water-soluble contrast urgently or delayed esophagram 24 hrs post ingestion
  - EKG
    - Hydrofluoric acid exposure: hypocalcemia (prolonged QT)
  - Procedures
    - Nasopharyngoscopy for airway visualization
    - No concern for perforation: flexible endoscopy within 12-24 hrs

MANAGEMENT

- Oropharyngeal
  - ABCs, IV, NPO, ENT/GI consult, esophagoscopy/endoscopy
    - Early intubation: respiratory distress, stridor, voice changes
  - Activated charcoal, gastric lavage contraindicated
  - Avoid vomiting
    - Ondansetron 0.15 mg/kg (max 4 mg) IV PRN
- Skin
  - Copious irrigation
  - Monitor pH
  - Consult burn specialist
- Ocular
  - Copious irrigation
    - Morgan lens/IV tubing, any IV solution
    - Endpoint: when pH is neutralized
  - Ophthalmology consult
- Psychiatry consultation for suicidal ideation
- Poison control consultation for assistance in management

DISPOSITION

- Asymptomatic patients
  — Observe minimum 6 hrs; length depends on the exposure
    - Must tolerate PO fluids prior to discharge
  — May need GI follow-up for prognostic esophagoscopy
- Symptomatic patients
  — Admit to ICU: concern for airway compromise, high grade esophageal/gastric exposure
  — Surgical intervention: hollow viscus perforation, full-thickness burns
  — Significant burns: transfer to Burn Center

BEWARE

- Patients that look well may have severe injuries
- Small ingestions can be as serious as larger ingestions
- Ocular exposure to acid/alkali = true ophthalmic emergency

2 ▶ Common Pediatric Ingestions

BACKGROUND

- Majority < 5 yrs
  — Exploratory behavior; hand-to-mouth activity
- Adolescents commonly intentional
  — Suicidality, recreational, overdose
- Consider neglect or abuse

EVALUATION

- **High Yield History**
  — Potential toxins accessible to patient
    - Medications: prescription/OTC, family & visitors
    - Household substances
    - Herbals/supplements
    - Recreational drug use
  — Timing, amount/total in container before ingestion
  — Symptoms

- **Exam**
  - Vitals, AMS
  - Pupils: miosis/mydriasis
  - Skin: dry, moist/diaphoretic, color
  - HEENT: moist vs. dry mucous membranes, secretions
  - Lungs: wheezes, crackles (bronchospasm/bronchorrhea)
  - Abdomen: bowel sounds, bladder size (urinary retention)
  - Neurologic: reflexes, fasciculations, paralysis
- **Diagnostics**
  - POC GLC
  - Labs: CBC, CMP, blood gas, urine pregnancy, PT/INR, PTT, +/− serum osm, lactate
    - Toxicology screens
      - Utox
      - Acetaminophen, salicylate, ETOH
      - Drug-specific levels PRN (lithium, digoxin, iron)
  - Imaging
    - CXR +/− neck XR, KUB
      - Radiopaque FB (coins, button batteries)
        - Esophageal coins present *en face* on AP view
        - Tracheal coins present sideways on AP view, *en face* on lateral view
        - Button batteries: "step off" or "double halo" signs
      - May visualize iron pills, enteric coated tablets, heavy metals
  - EKG
    - Specific QRS, QTc findings may suggest toxidrome/ingestion

MANAGEMENT

- ABCs, remove any visualized FB
- Activated charcoal
  - 1 g/kg (max 50-100 g) PO
  - Indications: ingested drug absorbed by charcoal (most are)
    - Best if given early
  - Contraindications: aspiration risk, AMS, intestinal obstruction, non-absorbable substances (heavy metals, toxic alcohols, caustics, lithium)
- Whole bowel irrigation
  - Polyethylene glycol 20-40 mL/kg/hr in < 6 yrs (max 0.5 L/hr); adolescents 1 L/hr; PO or NGT until rectal effluent is clear

- Indications: possibly useful for heavy metals (iron), extended release preparations, foreign objects (drug packets)
- Contraindications: preceding diarrhea, ileus/obstruction, perforation
• Specific antidotes

DISPOSITION

- Depends on ingestion and presentation
- Consider psychiatry consult for intentional ingestion
- Consult Poison Control Center

SPECIFIC SUBSTANCES

Acetaminophen (APAP)
- Pathophysiology: CYP450 enzymes (mainly in liver, kidney) oxidize APAP to toxic metabolite: N-acetyl-p-benzoquinoneimine (NAPQI)
  - Glutathione detoxifies; once exhausted, NAPQI causes cellular toxicity
- Toxic dose acutely or over 24 hrs (depends on age/weight)
  - Infants/toddlers may tolerate up to 200 mg/kg without toxicity
  - Older: > 150 mg/kg or > 10 g
- Symptoms:
  - Stage 1 (first day): usually asymptomatic, or nausea, vomiting, abdominal pain
  - Stage 2 (days 2-3): usually no-mild symptoms, hepatotoxicity: ↑ AST/ALT, bili
  - Stage 3 (days 3-4): acute liver necrosis, nausea, vomiting, abdominal pain, jaundice, encephalopathy; ↑ AST/ALT, synthetic liver dysfunction, coagulopathy (↑ PT/INR)
  - Stage 4 (day 5+): deterioration and death OR recovery
- Exam: tachycardia, dehydration, jaundice, abdominal/RUQ tenderness
- Diagnostics
  - Labs: standard as above, lactate/blood gas if ill appearing
  - Measure APAP level at least 4 hrs after ingestion
    - Use Rumack-Matthew nomogram to evaluate toxicity risk
      - Not useful for chronic/repeated ingestions
- Management
  - Activated charcoal may be beneficial
  - NAC: N-acetylcysteine: glutathione substitute
    - Most effective within 8 hrs of ingestion
    - Indications
      - APAP level > 150 mcg/mL at 4 hrs after ingestion
      - ↑ AST/ALT with any detectable APAP level

- ◆ APAP ≥ 150 mg/kg ingested and no available level within 8 hrs
- ◆ Timing of ingestion unknown (> 24 hrs) and ↑ AST/ALT and/or any detectable APAP level
- ▪ Dosing
  - ◆ Consult Poison Control Center or Medical Toxicologist
  - ◆ PO
    - ∗ Load 140 mg/kg, max 15 g
    - ∗ Maintenance 70 mg/kg (max 7.5 g) every 4 hrs
  - ◆ IV
    - ∗ Load 150 mg/kg (max 15 g) over 60 min
    - ∗ Second dose 50 mg/kg (max 5 g) over 4 hrs
    - ∗ Third dose 100 mg/kg (max 10 g) over 16 hrs
- **Disposition**
  - Discharge asymptomatic patients not meeting indications for NAC
  - Admit if treated with NAC
  - Consider transfer to transplant center if encephalopathy, fulminant hepatic failure, profound lactic acidosis, renal failure

Alcohols

- Sources
  - Ethanol
    - ▪ Most common intoxicant worldwide
    - ▪ Alcoholic beverages, household products (mouthwash, perfumes)
  - Methanol
    - ▪ Colorless liquid with "alcohol" odor
    - ▪ Solvents, antifreeze, wood alcohol, paint stripper, windshield washer fluid
  - Ethylene glycol
    - ▪ Sweet taste
    - ▪ Sources similar to methanol
  - Isopropyl alcohol
    - ▪ Commonly used as disinfectant
    - ▪ Rubbing alcohol, hand sanitizers
- Symptoms/Exam
  - Progressive CNS depression from intoxication to coma
  - Respiratory or hemodynamic compromise, tachypnea from acidosis
  - Nephrotoxicity/calcium oxalate crystals with ethylene glycol
  - Late vision symptoms (blurry vision/blindness) with methanol
  - Hemorrhagic gastritis with isopropyl alcohol

- Diagnostics
  - Standard labs/EKG as above + POC GLC
  - Blood alcohol level; toxic alcohol levels (ethylene glycol, methanol) not immediately available
  - Anion gap
    - ↑ in ethanol (if ketoacidosis), ethylene glycol, methanol
    - Normal with isopropyl alcohol
  - Serum osmolality, calculated osmolality, osmolar gap
    - ALL toxic alcohols increase osmolar gap
- Management
  - Ethanol, Isopropyl alcohol
    - Supportive care: ABCs, rehydration/IVF
  - Methanol
    - Fomepizole: 15 mg/kg IV over 30 min, then 10 mg/kg q12hrs
    - Ethanol: given if fomepizole unavailable, goal blood alcohol 100 mg/dL
    - Folic acid 1-2 mg/kg IV q4hrs
    - Correction of acidosis with bicarbonate (goal pH 7.45-7.5)
  - Ethylene glycol - treat as above for methanol with addition of:
    - Thiamine 25-50 mg IV
    - Pyridoxine 50 mg IV
    - Magnesium 50 mg/kg IV
  - Consider hemodialysis for methanol/ethylene glycol: persistent acidosis, level ≥ 50 mg/dL, renal failure
- Disposition
  - Admit patients with detectable toxic alcohol ingestions
  - ICU: significant acidosis, evidence of end-organ damage, airway concerns

Iron

- Sources: prenatal/multivitamins
  - % elemental iron determines toxicity
- Pathophysiology: direct injury to gastric mucosa → volume loss, intestinal ischemia, necrosis in extreme cases, impaired cellular metabolism, ↑ capillary permeability
- Toxic dose: mild < 20 mg/kg elemental iron, severe > 60 mg/kg
- Symptoms/Exam
  - Stage 1 (first 6 hrs): nausea, vomiting, abdominal pain, diarrhea
  - Stage 2 (6-24 hrs): latent/quiescent phase, ↓ GI symptoms
  - Stage 3 (6-72 hrs): shock, lactic acidosis, dehydration, hypovolemia

- Stage 4 (1-5 days): hepatic necrosis & failure
- Stage 5 (weeks): GI scarring, strictures, stenosis, obstruction
- Diagnostics
  - Standard labs as above
  - Serial serum iron levels
    - 4-6 hrs post-ingestion, 8 hrs for extended release
    - 300-500 mcg/dL: GI symptoms
    - > 500 mcg/dL: systemic toxicity
  - KUB: radiopaque pills (low sensitivity)
- Management
  - Consider whole bowel irrigation for large overdoses
  - Deferoxamine iron chelator
    - Indications: shock, acidosis, toxic-appearing, level > 500 mcg/dL
    - Consult Poison Control Center or Medical Toxicologist for dosing
    - Hydrate patient first; may cause hypotension
- Disposition
  - Discharge: asymptomatic for 6 hrs
  - PCU/ICU: most admitted to monitor hemodynamics, coagulopathy, mental status

Salicylates

- Sources: aspirin, oil of wintergreen, pepto-bismol, many OTC preparations
- Pathophysiology: uncouples oxidative phosphorylation → ↑ metabolic rate, hyperthermia, impaired gluconeogenesis
- Toxic dose 150 mg/kg, severe 300 mg/kg
- Symptoms/Exam
  - Vomiting, tinnitus/hearing loss, tachypnea, hyperventilation, hyperthermia, diaphoresis, hypotension, AMS, seizure, coma, shock
- Diagnostics
  - Standard labs/EKG as above
  - Salicylate (ASA) level
    - Toxicity at > 30-50 mg/dL
    - Peak usually 6 hrs after absorption
  - Repeat BMP, ASA levels every 2 hrs until ASA levels peak
  - Blood gas: mixed acid-base disturbance

- Respiratory alkalosis earliest sign
      - Anion gap metabolic acidosis
- Management
  — IVF with dextrose (hypoglycemia risk)
  — Activated charcoal if no aspiration risk
  — Plasma alkalinization: IV sodium bicarbonate
      - Indications: anion gap acidosis and suspect serious toxicity
      - Bolus 1-2 mEq/kg
      - Drip 150 mEq (3 amps) in 1L D5W at 2-3 mL/kg/hr
      - Goal serum pH 7.45-7.50
  — Hypokalemia, hypomagnesemia require aggressive repletion
  — Try to avoid intubation (difficult to match minute ventilation)
      - Risk of worsening acidosis
      - Consider bicarbonate bolus peri-intubation
  — Indications for hemodialysis
      - Persistent or worsening acidosis, renal failure, pulmonary edema, AMS, significantly elevated ASA level
- Disposition
  — Discharge: asymptomatic for at least 6hrs, normal labs, ASA < 30 mg/dL at peak, AND no ingestion of enteric-coated/extended-release tablets
  — Admit all others to appropriate level of care (SDU, ICU)

BEWARE

⚠ Maintain extremely high index of suspicion for all pediatric ingestions

⚠ Ask about all substances accessible to patient, visitors' medications, OTC/household/herbal products

⚠ Repeat labs until levels peak; a single negative level does not rule out toxicity

3 ▶ Gases

BACKGROUND

GASES	Carbon monoxide (CO) Odorless, colorless, tasteless	Cyanide (CN) Colorless, some may detect "bitter almond" smell
Sources	Incomplete combustion of carbon-containing material, household fires	• CN salts used in industry and plastics • Apricot, peach kernels
Risk	Colder months (faulty heaters, outside gas-generators, stoves used indoors)	Exposure often during fires and industrial accidents
Mechanism	Impairs oxygen delivery to cells by binding to hemoglobin	Rapidly uncouples mitochondrial electron transport chain
High Yield History	• Persistent or recurrent headaches or flu-like symptoms, esp. if occurring at a single location and improving when elsewhere • Families/groups with same symptoms • Patient found down with unexplained cardiovascular collapse	Exposures: fire, industrial, dietary, experimental medical treatments
Common symptoms	• Mild/moderate: dull headache, dizziness, nausea, blurred vision • Severe: coma, dysrhythmias, cardiovascular collapse • May misdiagnose as infant colic	Rapid onset headache, ataxia, confusion, coma, seizures, dysrhythmia, cardiovascular collapse
Exam	Nonspecific, ataxia, "cherry red skin" usually found post-mortem	Tachycardia with hypotension, AMS

EVALUATION

- **Diagnostics**
  — CO: COHb blood level obtained from blood gas with co-oximetry
    - 0 - 5% COHb normal in non-smoker
    - Lactate, troponin, EKG, cardiac monitoring
  — CN: CN levels typically a "send-out" lab
    - Lactate > 8mmol/L suggests CN toxicity in fire victim
    - Anion gap acidosis
    - EKG: dysrhythmias, ST abnormalities

MANAGEMENT

- CO
  - 100% oxygen (non-rebreather mask or intubation)
    - Consider for all symptomatic
    - Endpoint: COHb < 5% and symptoms resolved
  - IVF for hypotension, inotropes for cardiac depression
  - Hyperbaric indications
    - Syncope, coma, seizure, AMS/neurologic deficit, CO exposure over 24 hrs, COHb > 25%
    - Consult Poison Control Center or Medical Toxicologist
- CN
  - Antidotes
    - Hydroxocobalamin preferred: 70 mg/kg (max 5 g) IV
    - Cyanide Antidote Kit
    - Sodium nitrite: dosing varies by weight, Hgb; see instructions
      - Do not give if suspected concurrent CO toxicity
    - Sodium thiosulfate 25% solution 1.65 mL/kg (max 50 mL) IV
  - High flow O2 regardless of SpO2

DISPOSITION

- CO
  - Admit: severe toxicity, persistent symptoms
  - Discharge: mild initial symptoms, resolved with treatment, normal COHb level
  - Follow-up in 1-2 wks
- CN: Admit

BEWARE

- Concurrent CO and CN toxicity can occur in fire victims
- Do not wait for CN level result to treat suspected CN toxicity
- Sodium Nitrite in the cyanide antidote kit works by inducing methemoglobinemia
  - Contraindicated in fire victims also exposed to CO
  - Nitrites can cause significant hypotension

4 ▶ Methemoglobinemia

BACKGROUND

- Causes
  - Topical anesthetics
    - Benzocaine: teething products, benzocaine spray
    - EMLA
  - Antibiotics/antimalarials: rifampin, dapsone, hydroxychloroquine, chloroquine, quinolones, sulfonamides (sulfamethoxazole)
  - Metoclopramide
  - Nitrites, nitrates (well water)
  - Phenazopyridine
  - Oxidant stress
    - Diarrhea-induced methemoglobinemia, typically in < 4 mo olds
    - Hereditary/genetic: usually presents at birth
- Pathophysiology
  - Oxidizing substance converts hemoglobin iron from ferrous (Fe^{2+}) → ferric (Fe^{3+}) state which forms methemoglobin (MetHb)
  - MetHb is unable to bind oxygen → left shift of oxyhemoglobin dissociation curve → hypoxia, cyanosis

EVALUATION

- **High Yield History**
  - Medications, including OTC topical sprays/gels
  - Recent illness including diarrhea
  - Dietary (well water)
  - Prior / family history
  - Symptoms: headache, tachypnea, SOB, cyanosis, lethargy, seizure
- **Exam**
  - SpO_2 often reads 82-86% regardless of PaO_2
  - Cyanosis, hypoxia NOT responsive to oxygen, tachypnea, AMS
    - Patients may appear cyanotic with 1.5 g/dL of MetHb
      - 5 g/dL needed for cyanosis in deoxyhemoglobin
  - Chocolate colored blood

- **Diagnostics**
  - Labs
    - CBC, blood gas with co-oximetry for MetHb level
    - Severely anemic = sicker at lower MetHb levels
    - Standard toxicology labs, lactate, troponin if ill appearing

MetHb level (%)	Signs & Symptoms
0-3	Asymptomatic
3-20	Usually asymptomatic or: cyanosis, skin discoloration, chocolate-brown blood
20-50	Mild/Moderate: fatigue, SOB, headache, syncope, tachycardia
50-70	Severe: respiratory failure, lactic acidosis, myocardial damage, seizure, shock coma
> 70	Fatal

MANAGEMENT

- ABCs, IVF
- Remove offending agent
- Methylene blue
  - Symptomatic and/or MetHb level > 30%
  - 1-2 mg/kg IV over 5 min
  - May be repeated in 1 hr if repeat MetHb level remains > 30%
  - Contraindicated in patients with G6PD deficiency
    - Can precipitate hemolysis
- Consider exchange transfusion or hyperbaric oxygen for G6PD deficient or unresponsive to methylene blue
- Consider Vitamin C IV or PO in conjunction with methylene blue
  - Works too slowly for treatment of acute, acquired methemoglobinemia
- Consult Poison Control Center or Medical Toxicologist

DISPOSITION

- Depends on symptom severity and response to treatment

BEWARE

- ⚠ Consider in cyanotic/hypoxic patient not responsive to oxygen therapy
- ⚠ Asymptomatic patient with methemoglobinemia may appear cyanotic
- ⚠ Anemic patients may have significantly elevated MetHb or be symptomatic but not appear cyanotic

5 ▶ One Pill Can Kill

BACKGROUND

- Drugs highly toxic in small amounts
  - Alpha 2-adrenergic agonists: clonidine, oxymetazoline, glaucoma eye drops
  - Beta blockers
  - Calcium channel blockers (CCBs)
  - Iron (see Common Pediatric Ingestions chapter)
  - Oil of wintergreen (see Common Pediatric Ingestions chapter: salicylates)
  - Opioids (see Recreational Drugs chapter)
  - Sodium channel blockers
    - Chloroquine
    - Class I antiarrhythmics
    - Tricyclic antidepressants
  - Sulfonylureas

EVALUATION

- **High Yield History**
  - Timing, quantity (estimated amount missing from bottle)
  - Accessible medications (family, visitors)
- **Exam**
  - Vitals
  - Mental status, pupils, muscle tone, reflexes
- **Diagnostics**
  - POC GLC
  - CBC, CMP, UA, Urine pregnancy, Utox, APAP, ASA, ETOH
  - EKG

MANAGEMENT (GENERAL)

- Decontamination (see Common Pediatric Ingestions)
  - Activated charcoal unless contraindicated, can mix with milk/soda
    Consider whole bowel irrigation, especially if extended release formulation
- Airway: may need prompt intubation if risk for aspiration
- Hypoglycemia
  - Dextrose 0.5 g/kg IV = 5 mL/kg D10W

- Hypotension
  - IVF 20 mL/kg NS
  - Vasopressors: norepinephrine, epinephrine, titrate to effect
- Bradycardia
  - Consider atropine, transcutaneous/transvenous pacing
- Seizures
  - Benzodiazepines, phenobarbital, levetiracetam (see Seizures chapter)
  - Phenytoin not recommended for toxicologic-induced seizures
- Drug-specific antidotes for known ingestion
- Consult Poison Control Center or Medical Toxicologist

MANAGEMENT (SPECIFIC SUBSTANCES)

Beta-blockers

- Metoprolol, labetalol, propranolol
  - Propranolol may also act as a Na+ channel blocker
- Beta-blockade → ↓ HR, ↓ gluconeogenesis, CNS depression
- Symptoms: AMS, bradycardia, hypotension, hypoglycemia
- EKG: AV block
- Management
  - If not improving with supportive care, consider:
    - Glucagon: 0.05 mg/kg (max 5-10 mg) IV over 1-2 min then 0.05 mg/kg/hr (max 5 mg/hr)
    - High dose insulin 1 U/kg bolus IV, then 0.5 U/kg/hr
      - Add glucose to maintain euglycemia
      - Serially measure/correct lytes, glucose
    - Calcium gluconate IV
      - 30-60 mg/kg (0.3 mL/kg of 10% solution) over 10 min OR
    - Calcium chloride IV (best via central line)
      - 10-20 mg/kg (0.1-0.2 mL/kg of 10% solution) IV over 10 min

Calcium Channel Blockers (CCB)

- Verapamil, diltiazem, amlodipine, nicardipine, nifedipine
- Ca2+ channel blockade → vasodilation, ↓ HR, and at high doses ↓ insulin secretion
- Symptoms: AMS, hypotension, bradycardia, hyperglycemia
- EKG: AV block

- Management
  - Calcium gluconate or calcium chloride at higher doses outlined above
  - High dose insulin + glucose as above
  - Glucagon as above

Alpha$_2$-adrenergic agonists

Medication	Formulation	Common indications
Clonidine	Oral, patch	Hypertension, opioid withdrawal
Guanfacine	Oral	Hypertension, ADHD
Brimonidine Apraclonidine	Eye drops	Glaucoma
Tetrahydrozoline Naphazoline Oxymetazoline	Eye drops Nasal spray	Decongestant

- Presynaptic alpha2-receptor agonist → ↓ synaptic catecholamine release
- Symptoms
  - AMS, sedation, lethargy, coma
  - Hypotension (may initially have transient hypertension), bradycardia
  - Respiratory depression, miosis, hypothermia
- Management
  - Naloxone 0.4-2 mg IV/IM/SQ/IO q2min PRN, up to 10 mg
    - Neonates: 0.1 mg/kg
    - If effective, redose in 30min-1hr or start a drip

Chloroquine and hydroxychloroquine

- Uses: malaria, autoimmune disease, COVID-19
- Na+ channel blocker
- Toxicity at 10 mg/kg
- Symptoms
  - AMS, seizures, coma
  - Cardiopulmonary arrest
  - Hypokalemia due to intracellular shift
- EKG: ↑ PR, ↑ QRS, ↑ QTc, Torsades, ventricular arrhythmias

- Management
  - Diazepam 2 mg/kg IV over 30 min if seizing, ↑ QRS/QTc, hypotension, arrhythmia
  - Sodium bicarbonate 1-2 mEq/kg IV to alkalinize blood to pH 7.45-7.55 to ↓ drug binding to myocardium & counteract Na+ channel blockade
    - Additional doses PRN widened QRS
    - Monitor for & treat hypokalemia
  - Replete Mg2+, may need overdrive pacing or cardioversion if Torsades
  - Monitor K+, replete cautiously (max 15 mEq/hr) for K+ < 3 mEq/L

Oral hypoglycemics

- Sulfonylureas: glipizide, glyburide, glimepiride
  - Stimulate pancreas to release insulin
- Hypoglycemia may be delayed up to 24 hrs post-ingestion
- Symptoms: dizziness, fussiness, lethargy, seizure, focal neurologic deficit
- Management
  - POC GLC hourly
  - Oral glucose or food
  - IV dextrose if GLC < 60 mg/dL
  - Octreotide 1-2 mcg/kg (max 50 mcg) IV/SQ every 6-12 hrs to ↓ insulin release
  - Consider glucagon 0.5 mg for < 20 kg, 1 mg for ≥ 20 kg IV/IM/SQ as temporizing measure
    - Short-acting, may repeat in 15 min if no response
    - Will not work if hepatic glycogen stores depleted

Tricyclics antidepressants

- Imipramine, desipramine, amitriptyline, nortriptyline
- Serotonin & norepinephrine reuptake inhibitor
  - Also Na+channel blocker, anticholinergic, α-antagonist
- Toxicity at > 10-20 mg/kg
- Symptoms
  - AMS, hallucinations, seizure, coma
  - Tachycardia, hypotension
  - Fever (early), hypothermia (late)
  - Anticholinergic toxidrome
- EKG: ↑ QTc, wide QRS, PVCs, V-tach, AV block, R > 3 mm in aVR

- Management
    - If not improving, consider:
        - Sodium bicarbonate 1-2 mEq/kg IV as above for chloroquine
            - Additional doses PRN widened QRS
            - Monitor for & treat hypokalemia
    - Anti-epileptic if seizing, avoid phenytoin
    - AVOID: physostigmine, quinidine, procainamide

DISPOSITION
- Admit
- Observation period prior to discharge if
    - Known ingestion well below toxic dose
    - Chloroquine ingestion, asymptomatic after 6hrs monitoring

BEWARE
- Dilution (having patient drink lots of water) is NOT recommended, can ↑ rate of pill dissolving and/or passage into GI tract
- Always consider suicide attempt/self-harm, child abuse (especially if unusual age for typical exploratory/accidental ingestions, eg, < 1 yr or 6-12 yrs) neglect/home safety (especially if prior ingestion history)

6 ▶ Recreational Drugs

BACKGROUND
- ~ 1/3 teens report using an illicit drug and 2/5 have consumed alcohol
    - Most common: alcohol, marijuana, amphetamines, inhalants
- Disclosure laws of what must be disclosed to parents vary by state

EVALUATION
- **High Yield History**
    - Discuss in private with the patient; clearly state what will be confidential
    - Ask parent/guardian what prescription or recreational drugs are available that their child may have taken, and when
    - Siblings, peer friends may provide additional history
- **Exam**: toxidromes vary by substances
    - Vitals (core temperature — sympathomimetics, anticholinergics), mental status, pupil size, nystagmus, diaphoresis vs. absence of axillary sweat, lung and bowel sounds, venipuncture wounds (track marks) if IV drug use suspicion, reflexes, ataxia

- **Diagnostics**: keep broad differential; do not limit workup solely to drug use
  - Labs
    - POC GLC
    - CMP: electrolytes, renal function, anion gap acidosis
    - CK: rhabdomyolysis from sympathomimetics or prolonged down time with opiate overdose
    - Blood gas: respiratory failure in AMS
    - Utox
      - Screen young children with AMS/agitation/bizarre behavior for unintentional recreational drug exposure
      - False positives due to cross-reactivity with other substances
  - EKG: widened QRS or prolonged QTc
  - CXR: aspiration in AMS

MANAGEMENT (GENERAL)

- ABCs, supportive care, observation as drug wears off
- Agitation
  - Quiet environment
  - Benzodiazepines first line for violent or severely agitated
    - See Managing the Agitated Child chapter
- Hydration: dehydration, rhabdomyolysis
- Counseling: offer substance abuse rehabilitation resources

MANAGEMENT (SPECIFIC SUBSTANCES)

Anticholinergics

- Diphenhydramine, hyoscine/scopolamine, dimenhydrinate, Jimson weed (plant containing atropine and hyoscine)
- Symptoms / toxidrome
  - Mydriasis, flushed skin, "marble mouth" garbled speech, AMS, dry mucous membranes, absence of axillary sweat, tachycardia, urinary retention
  - DDx diaphoresis in sympathomimetic, dry in anticholinergic
- Management
  - Consider physostigmine as diagnostic test in consultation with the Poison Center or Medical Toxicologist if normal EKG, no hypotension

Benzodiazepines
- Xanax, Valium, Ativan, Librium, "(Bars of) Xannies/Zannies"
- Symptoms
  — AMS, drowsiness, slurred speech
  — If alcohol, opiate co-ingested: respiratory depression
- Management
  — Flumazenil reverses intoxication but can precipitate seizure in chronic users
    - May use for iatrogenic benzodiazepine toxicity (procedural sedation)
      - 0.01 mg/kg (max 0.2 mg) IV
    - Not routinely recommended for AMS patient with unknown cause

Marijuana / THC edibles
- Many forms and routes
  — Marijuana leaves smoked, THC oil/resin smoked, THC cartridges in vaporizers
  — Eaten in baked goods, candies/chocolates, butters, cookies, mints, beverages
- Available OTC in some states
- Symptoms vary by user and product
  — Acute toxicity: tachycardia, ↓ coordination, sedation, agitation/paranoia/panic
  — Young children can become obtunded with tachycardia and can rarely experience apnea, hypotonia, bradycardia
- Management
  — Reduce environmental stimulation
  — Benzodiazepines for uncontrollable agitation

Opiates
- Prescription pills more common than IV drug use in pediatrics
  — Look for fentanyl patch
- Symptoms/toxidrome
  — Miosis, respiratory depression or apnea, somnolence, ↓ GI motility, bradycardia, hypotension
- Management
  — Airway management PRN
  — Naloxone for respiratory depression or apnea
    - 0.1 mg/kg IV/IM/SQ/IN (max 2 mg), may repeat PRN every 2-3 min
      - May require redosing with long-acting opiates
    - Full reversal can → agitation, goal = sufficient ventilation

Psychedelics
- Ketamine, PCP, LSD, Ecstasy/MDMA (also has sympathomimetic qualities)
- Symptoms
  — AMS (agitation/sedation), hallucinations, tachycardia, hypertension, nystagmus (ketamine, PCP)
- Management
  — Benzodiazepines for agitation
  — Cooling for hyperthermia

Sympathomimetics
- Cocaine, amphetamines
- Routes: IN, injection, smoking, oral
- Symptoms/toxidrome
  — Cardiac: dysrhythmias, ↑ myocardial oxygen demand, cocaine can → coronary vasospasm, act as a Na+ channel blocker
  — Agitation, delirium, tachycardia, hypertension, diaphoresis, mydriasis, seizures, hyperthermia
- Management
  — Hyperthermia
    - Ice-water immersion
    - Mist and fan (requires *large* fan)
    - Ice packs to groin, axilla
    - Monitor core temperature to avoid hypothermia
  — Agitation: benzodiazepines

Synthetic cannabinoid and synthetic cathinones
- Cannabinoids
  — Psychoactive substance sprayed onto inert organic matter and smoked ("fake weed")
  — Brand names and contents vary, most well-known: Spice, K2
- Cathinones
  — "Bath salts" orally ingested, insufflated, smoked or injected
- Symptoms vary by psychoactive substance used in production
  — May present similarly to sympathomimetic, anxiety, hallucinations
- Management: supportive, no reversal agent

DISPOSITION

- Discharge if symptoms resolve and no significant organ injury
- Observation/admission if prolonged AMS, agitation, psychosis

BEWARE

- ❗ Don't miss hyperthermia in patient with normal oral temperature
- ❗ Don't miss unintentional intoxication in children with unexplained AMS/agitation/bizarre behavior
- ❗ The drug patient thinks they took may differ from what they actually took

Section XXIII
Trauma

1 ▶ Abdominal Trauma

BACKGROUND

- Epidemiology
  - ~25% of pediatric patients with major trauma
  - Leading cause of unrecognized fatal injury
- Anatomy and physiology
  - Relatively large abdominal organs → ↑ blunt abdominal trauma
  - Thick visceral capsules → may limit hemoperitoneum and US sensitivity
  - Less abdominal fat, elastic ligamentous attachments → ↑ vulnerability to acceleration-deceleration / hollow viscus injury
  - ↑ surface area:volume ratio → ↓ internal volume over which force is dissipated
- Common mechanisms of injury
  - MVA
    - Waddell's triad (pedestrian vs. auto)
      - Ipsilateral (side of impact) femoral shaft fracture
      - Ipsilateral intrathoracic or intra-abdominal injury
      - Contralateral head injury
    - Seat belt injury
      - Erythema, ecchymosis, or abrasion across lower abdomen secondary to lap belt restraint
      - Chance fracture: flexion-distraction type injury of lumbar spine → vertebral body anterior wedge fracture +/− transverse posterior element fracture +/− distraction of facet joints/spinous processes
      - Solid organ injury, bowel perforation, mesenteric injury, and/or bladder injury
  - Handlebar injury
    - Circular epigastric bruising secondary to handlebar impact
    - Associated with solid organ injury (including pancreas), intestinal injury (duodenal hematoma), abdominal wall hernia

- Sports: isolated solid organ or intestinal tract injury
- NAT: abdominal injury second to head injury as cause of death in NAT

EVALUATION

- **High Yield History**
  - Mechanism of Injury
    - MVA
      - Airbags, seatbelt/car seat, speed, damage to vehicle, multi-system trauma, rollover, fatalities among other occupants
    - NAT
      - Mechanism, developmental milestones compatible
- **Exam**
  - Abdominal wall abrasions, bruising
  - Abdominal / flank tenderness
  - Peritoneal irritation: involuntary guarding, rebound, distention, rigidity
  - Lower chest wall injury
  - Pelvis tenderness, instability, crepitus
  - Rectal exam: mass, lacerations, blood, sphincter tone, high-riding prostate
  - Unexplained hypotension
- **Diagnostics**
  - Labs
    - CBC, BMP, LFT, lipase, TxS/C
    - Urine — gross hematuria indicator of potential serious injury
      - Controversial: microscopic hematuria ≥ 50 RBC/HPF may harbinger pediatric intra-abdominal injury
  - Clinical decision rule
    - PECARN → classified as low risk & may forgo CT if all are met:
      - No vomiting after injury
      - No GCS < 14
      - No evidence of abdominal or thoracic wall trauma
      - No abdominal pain or tenderness
      - Normal breath sounds
  - Imaging
    - CXR, pelvic XR
    - FAST in children → low sensitivity but high specificity
      - Positive FAST examination → need abdominal CT
      - Negative FAST, however, does not exclude intra-abdominal injury

- CT abdomen/pelvis with IV contrast - indications
  - Multi-system trauma
  - AMS or intoxication
  - Concerning exam findings
  - ↓ hemoglobin
  - AST > 200 IU/L or ALT > 125 IU/L (lower cutoffs sometimes used, especially for NAT)
  - Gross hematuria, consider in microscopic hematuria > 50 RBC/HPF

MANAGEMENT
- ABCs
- NPO, consider OGT/NGT
- Unstable patient
  - IV warm NS or LR 20 mL/kg (max 1L) then reassess
  - Transfuse PRBCs 10 mL/kg aliquots for fluid-refractory
    - If need > 40 mL/kg, consider massive transfusion protocol, surgical exploration
- Consult Surgery
- Spleen/liver injury
  - Fluid resuscitation, admit for monitoring with serial abdominal exams/labs
  - Non-operative management > 95%, consider interventional radiology/embolization
- Pancreatic injury
  - Least commonly injured solid organ, usually focal upper abdominal trauma, e.g. from handlebars
  - Amylase, lipase more specific indicators > 2 hrs after trauma
- Duodenal hematoma
  - Acute symptoms often mild/nonspecific → maintain high index of suspicion
  - CT insensitive → observation/serial examination crucial
- Intestinal injury
  - XR: free air; initial CT may be normal or subtle findings only
  - Observation/serial examination important for diagnosis
    - Admit for significant seatbelt sign
- Renal/bladder injury
  - Microscopic hematuria < 50 RBC/HPF is common after blunt trauma, may not require further investigation if isolated finding
    - Follow UA as outpatient to ensure hematuria clears

DISPOSITION

- PICU vs. SDU based on stability, need for serial exams
- Discharge if no suspected injury with close follow-up, strict return precautions

BEWARE

! Complete exposure during survey (including diaper)
! Hypotension is a LATE SIGN

2 ▶ Burns

BACKGROUND

- Common mechanisms
  — Scald → burn with splash pattern
  — Flame
  — Hot object → sharply demarcated burn in shape of object
  — NAT
    - Burns involving genitals, buttocks, perineum
    - Contact burns on dorsum of hand (cigarette burns)
    - "Stocking" or "glove" distribution - extremity held in hot water
    - Burns inconsistent with history, developmental capacity

EVALUATION

- **High Yield History**
  — Circumstances: flash/explosion, structure fire, enclosed space, steam injury
  — Time/duration of exposure, material burned/chemicals involved, throat symptoms, voice changes, visual impairment
  — Associated injuries
- **Exam**
  — Burn depth
    - Superficial: epidermis → pink, painful
    - Superficial partial thickness: upper dermis → pink, blisters, painful
    - Deep partial thickness: lower dermis → yellow, waxy, ↓ sensate
    - Deep full thickness: subcutaneous → pale / charred, waxy / leathery, no bleeding, insensate
  — BSA calculation
    - Superficial (non partial thickness) burns not included

- Rule of Nines for older pediatric patients
- Lund-Browder chart better for children < 10 yrs
- Palm with fingers in < 10 yr = 1% BSA, palm without fingers in ≥ 10 yr
— Signs of potential airway compromise/need for prophylactic intubation
  - Soot in nares, carbonaceous sputum (not absolute indication for intubation)
  - Severe burns of face/mouth, singed nasal/eyebrow hairs
  - Circumferential burns of the neck
  - Stridor/wheezing
  - Progressive respiratory difficulty
  - Inability to protect airway (profuse secretions, AMS)
  - Significantly elevated CO-Hb levels
— Complicated: circumferential, crossing major joints, compartment syndrome
- **Diagnostics**
  — Labs
    - CBC, CMP, Mg, PO4, CPK, UA, lactate
    - Blood gas, CO-Hb level if house fire or enclosed space
  — Imaging PRN for associated trauma, secondary or inhalation injury

MANAGEMENT

- ABCs
  — Early airway management PRN
  — NPO; NGT for major burns > 20% BSA
- Fluid resuscitation for major burns
  — Parkland Formula ATLS Revision
    - (2-4 mL × weight (kg) × % BSA burned) of LR first 24hrs
      - Half infused over first 8 hrs
      - Second half over next 16 hrs
      - Add hourly maintenance fluids to rate

Adults, children > 14 yrs	Children < 14 yrs	Electrical Injury (all ages)
2 mL/kg × % BSA burned	3 mL/kg × % BSA burned Add dextrose if ≤ 30 kg	4 mL/kg × % BSA burned

  — Adjust fluid resuscitation to maintain urinary output 1 mL/kg/hr for children < 30 kg, 0.5 mL/kg/hr for older children
    - Place urinary catheter

- Pain management
  — Morphine 0.1 mg/kg (max 4-10 mg) IV or fentanyl 1 mcg/kg (max 50 mcg) IV: frequent reassessment and redosing PRN important
  — Consider procedural sedation for line placement, debridement, dressing changes
- Monitor and maintain normothermia, normoglycemia
- Remove constricting items (clothes, jewelry)
- Burn care
  — If being transferred to a burn center
    - Large wounds: cover with dry, sterile drapes
    - Smaller wounds: cover with moist, sterile, saline-soaked dressing
  — ED wound management
    - Appropriate pre-treatment analgesia
    - Clean with sterile saline
    - Debride ruptured blisters
      - Debridement of intact blisters controversial
        - Consider for over mobile joints
    - Topicals
      - Face: Bacitracin
      - Periorbital: Erythromycin ophthalmic ointment
      - Body: 1% silver sulfadiazine cream or bacitracin
        - Do not use silver sulfadiazine in < 2mo
      - External ear: 11.1% mafenide acetate
    - Consider synthetic and biological membranes
    - Consult regional burn center for preferred management
  — Surgery consultation if fasciotomy/escharotomy possibly needed
- Consider CO, cyanide toxicity
  — Assess CO with blood gas with co-oximetry, treat with 100% O2
  — Suspect cyanide: ↑ lactate level, unexplained acidosis
    - Treat with hydroxocobalamin
- Tetanus immunization

DISPOSITION

- Burn center transfer criteria
  — Partial thickness burns > 10% TBSA
  — Third degree burns (any %, any age)
  — Burns of face, hands, feet, genitalia, perineum, circumferential, over major joints

- Electrical / chemical burns, associated trauma / inhalation injury
- Patients with complicated medical or social conditions
- Patients not meeting transfer criteria may require admission (pain control, suspected NAT)
- Discharge/follow-up for minor burns
  - Burn care instructions and return recommendations
  - Follow up 24-48 hrs for wound re-evaluation
  - Education
    - Water heater temperature ≤ 120°F if young kids
    - Safe kitchen practices

BEWARE

- Maintain high index of suspicion for NAT
- Always consider airway inhalation injury; have low threshold for intubation
- Consider abdominal compartment syndrome, need for neck / chest wall escharotomy for ventilatory insufficiency
- Prophylactic antibiotics NOT indicated in early post-burn period

3 ▶ Electrical Injury

BACKGROUND

- Pathophysiology
  - Electrical energy (tissue damage) → thermal energy (burns) → mechanical energy (blunt trauma)
  - Damage to high resistance tissues (bone, tendon, fat, dry skin) > damage to low resistance tissues (muscle, nerves, vasculature, moist skin)
- Children = 20% of electrical injuries
  - Low voltage, household appliances
  - Oral commissure burns from chewing on electric cord
- Alternating (AC) vs. Direct current (DC)
  - AC envelops body, travels within tissues, more damaging
  - DC flows through body out to ground, less tissue damage

EVALUATION

- **High Yield History**
  - Source
    - Household (sockets, appliances, cords): AC, low voltage
    - Power lines: AC, high voltage
    - Lightning: DC (10-120 million V)
  - Amount of energy (voltage, amperage, resistance, duration of contact)
    - High (> 1000V) vs. low (< 1000V) voltage
    - Tissue contacted, moisture
  - Secondary injury from blast / trauma
- **Exam**
  - Burns
    - Oral commissure burns in children
    - Check hands, feet
    - Lichtenberg figures, skin fern-like patterns on skin can appear from lightning (NOT true burn)
  - Blunt trauma
    - Primary & secondary survey for associated injuries
    - Ears (hearing, perforated TM, hemorrhage)
  - Cardiac dysrhythmias
    - Atrial fibrillation (most common in ED); Vfib, Asystole (most fatal)
  - Neurologic injury
    - AMS, CVA, seizures, coma, respiratory arrest (high voltage)
  - Orthopedic
    - Fractures, dislocations (contractions from AC)
    - Compartment syndrome
    - Rhabdomyolysis
  - Vascular injury
    - Aneurysm, pseudoaneurysm (delayed presentation)
- **Diagnostics**
  - Labs: CBC, CMP, lactate, troponin, CPK, UA
  - Imaging
    - XR/CT PRN suspected associated injuries
    - CTA PRN suspected vascular injuries
  - EKG, cardiac monitoring on every patient

MANAGEMENT
- ABCs
- Primary and secondary trauma survey: immobilize spine if thrown
- Burn care (see burn chapter)
- Cardiac monitoring
  — Low voltage injury, normal EKG → low risk of delayed dysrhythmia = No need for prolonged monitoring
- Rhabdomyolysis: hydration +/– urinary alkalinization
- Consult Surgery: fasciotomy for compartment syndrome

DISPOSITION
- Discharge: asymptomatic, low voltage injury, normal EKG
- Admit to Burn Center: high voltage injury, symptomatic low voltage injury

BEWARE
- Labial artery hemorrhage possible 2-3 wks after oral commissure burns with eschar formation
- Despite subtle findings, deeper injury may be present
  — Pain out of proportion
  — Unexplained lactic acidosis
  — Rhabdomyolysis

4 ▶ Extremity Trauma

BACKGROUND
- ~ 800,000 pediatric orthopedic injury ED visits annually
  — 10-25% fracture (fx) → 15-25% growth plate injuries
  — Upper > lower extremities
  — Falls, sports/recreation, bike, scooter, MVA, pedestrian struck, NAT
- Pediatric anatomy / physiology
  — Immature pliant bones (less dense, more porous, ↓ mineral and ↑ collagen, thicker periosteum) → specific fx patterns
    - Plastic deformation: longitudinal stress along shaft, bowing with intact periosteum
    - Greenstick: incomplete fx; one cortex fx, second cortex bowed
    - Buckle/torus: compressive force along shaft, most common distal radius; angulation of cortex at metaphysis/diaphysis junction

- Pediatric ligaments stronger than bones → avulsion fx > sprains
- Growth plates open in children: Salter-Harris classification
  - Physeal fracture classification
    - Type I: Physis only, tender with often normal XR
    - Type II: Physis & metaphysis, most common
    - Type III: Physis & epiphysis intraarticularly
    - Type IV: Physis, metaphysis, epiphysis
    - Type V: Crush injury to physis, worst prognosis
  - Progressive risk of growth arrest or deformity I → V

Salter-Harris Classification

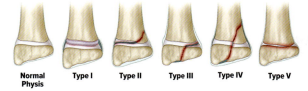

	Elbow Ossification Center	~ Age of Ossification
C	Capitellum	1
R	Radial Head	3
I	Internal (*medial*) Epicondyle	5
T	Trochlea	7
O	Olecranon	9
E	External (*lateral*) Epicondyle	11

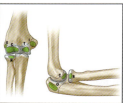

EVALUATION

- **High Yield History**
  - Timing, mechanism, direction / magnitude of force, prior injuries
  - Associated symptoms: numbness, paresthesias, weakness
- **Exam**
  - Skin integrity; remove any splints/bandages
  - Palpate entire limb: pain, tenderness, swelling, deformity
  - Examine joint above and below injury: effusion, passive/active ROM
  - Evaluate circulation: pulses, skin color, temperature, capillary refill
  - Thorough motor and sensory exam

Hand Exam		
Nerve	**Sensory**	**Motor**
Radial	First dorsal web space	"Thumbs up" sign
Ulnar	Volar aspect of little finger	Spread fingers against resistance
Median	Volar aspect of index finger	"Ok" sign

- Specific findings
    - Physeal point tenderness → growth plate injury
    - Snuff box tenderness → scaphoid fx
    - Base of 5th metatarsal tenderness → avulsion fx
- Compartment syndrome: pain out of proportion, pallor, paresthesias, pulselessness, paralysis
    - Classic signs / symptoms unreliable in young children
    - Consider with increasing analgesia requirements, anxiety, agitation
- **Diagnostics**
    - Minimum 2-view XR, joint above and below injured area
        - Large anterior (sail sign) / any posterior fat pad in elbow → occult fracture

COMMON INJURIES

- Ankle sprain
    - Ottawa Ankle Rule (applicable in children > 5 yrs, 98.5% sensitivity); XR if any of:
        - Tender over posterior edge or tip of lateral or medial malleolus or 6 cm proximal
        - Base of 5th metatarsal or navicular
        - Inability to ambulate immediately after injury and on evaluation
    - Treatment
        - Mild sprains → RICE, crutches PRN, analgesia, early ROM exercises as tolerated
        - Moderate sprains → splint/short leg cast, reevaluate in 2 wks
        - Orthopedic referral for symptoms > 8 wks
- Fractures
    - Clavicular fx: most common pediatric fx
        - Birth trauma, fall on shoulder, direct blow, fall on outstretched hand (FOOSH)
        - Non displaced/minimally displaced → simple sling × 1-2 wks for pain control
        - Very proximal or distal, displaced, dislocated, skin tenting → orthopedics
    - Supracondylar fx majority of pediatric elbow fx, lateral condylar fx
        - FOOSH, supracondylar with elbow hyperextension (fall off monkey bars)
        - Abnormal fat pads, anterior humeral line does not bisect mid-capitellum
        - No/mild displacement → long arm splint/cast, orthopedics follow-up; otherwise, consult Orthopedics

- Radius & ulna fx
  - Buckle or greenstick fx of distal radius most common
    - Splint or short arm cast, orthopedics follow up for greenstick
  - Complete, angulated, Salter-Harris physeal, displaced
    - Reduce and splint, orthopedics follow-up vs. consult
  - Monteggia fx-dislocation: most missed serious elbow fx
    - Ulnar fx with radial head dislocation
      - Suspect if line through mid-radius doesn't bisect capitellum
    - Consult Orthopedics
  - Galeazzi fx-dislocation
    - Distal radius fx with distal radioulnar joint dislocation
    - Consult Orthopedics
- Scaphoid fx: most common carpal fx
  - FOOSH or direct trauma
  - Wrist pain, tenderness at anatomic snuffbox & with thumb axial loading
  - Thumb spica splint/cast for 4-8wks, even with normal XR
  - Orthopedic follow-up; If proximal or displaced, orthopedic consult
- Femur fx
  - Suspect NAT if < 5 yrs, especially non-ambulatory
  - Externally rotated, refusal to bear weight, orthopedic consult
    - < 5 yrs: Pavlik harness, spica cast
    - > 5 yrs: long leg splint, traction
- Tibia & Fibula
  - Toddlers fx: non-displaced tibial shaft spiral or oblique fx
    - Rotation of the child's body around fixed foot
    - Not typically NAT
    - Splint or walking cast for 2-3wks
  - Tillaux fracture: Salter Harris Type III anterolateral distal tibia fx
    - Teens during period of partial physeal closure, consult Orthopedics
  - Triplanar fx: Salter-Harris Type IV anterolateral distal tibia fx
    - Teens during period of partial physeal closure, consult Orthopedics

- Dislocations
  - See Nursemaid's Elbow chapter
  - Elbow dislocation
    - Posterior most common; 10% involve neurologic injury
    - FOOSH, elbow held in flexion, shortened forearm
    - Closed reduction
    - Long arm posterior splint, orthopedic follow-up
  - Shoulder dislocation
    - Anterior > 90%
    - Abduction, extension, external rotational force
    - Evaluate for axillary nerve involvement
    - Multiple reduction techniques
    - Post reduction XR to confirm anatomic placement, assess for traumatic fx
    - Sling/shoulder brace after reduction, orthopedic follow-up
  - Patellar dislocation
    - Pivot knee on fixed lower leg, patella displaced laterally, knee held in flexion
    - May have associated lateral femoral condyle or medial patella margin fx
    - Reduction: gently extend knee while directing pressure medially on patella
    - Knee immobilizer, orthopedic follow-up

MANAGEMENT

- Pain management
  - Ice/elevation
  - NSAID and/or acetaminophen
  - Opiates PRN; intranasal fentanyl for young children without IV
  - Consider procedural sedation or hematoma block for reductions
- Splinting/casting
  - Most stable fractures can be splinted by ED with urgent orthopedic follow-up for reduction and casting
- Reduction
  - Significantly displaced/angulated fx → prompt orthopedic consult
  - Neurovascular compromise → emergent reduction by ED
- Open fx
  - Antibiotic prophylaxis, tetanus update, debridement and foreign material removal, immobilization, emergent orthopedic consult

- Consult Orthopedics

Discharge, Orthopedics in 1 week	Urgent Orthopedic consult	Emergent Orthopedic consult
• Stable fx, relocated shoulder or patellar dislocation with normal neurovascular status • No Orthopedics referral for nursemaid's elbow	• Salter-Harris III, IV, V fx • Tillaux, triplane fx • Displaced, angulated, complete fx without neurovascular compromise • Plastic deformation • Greenstick fx • Patellar sleeve fx • Tibial tuberosity avulsion, tibial spine fx • Elbow dislocation	• Open fx • Fx with neurovascular compromise • Compartment syndrome • Knee dislocation • Hip dislocation

BEWARE

❗ Consider NAT in every infant/young child with fx, especially humerus, femur

5 ▶ Head and Neck Trauma

BACKGROUND

- Falls, MVA, sports or recreational injuries, NAT
- Pediatric anatomy
  — Relatively larger head → lacerations/hematomas
  — Thinner cranium → skull fx
  — Open sutures → less ICP increase, delays injury recognition
  — Larger head volume → ↑ shear forces
- Common injury patterns
  — Isolated scalp hematoma, commonly forehead
  — Skull fx
    - Linear skull fx most common
    - Basilar skull fx: periorbital ecchymosis (raccoon eyes), postauricular ecchymosis (Battle sign)
  — ICH
    - Subdural, epidural, subarachnoid, intracerebral
  — Blunt trauma
    - Diffuse axonal injury, cerebral contusion

- Concussion
  - One or more: physical, cognitive, emotional, sleep changes

EVALUATION

- **High Yield History**
  - Mechanism
    - Fall (witnessed, height, surface struck)
    - MVA (speed, vehicle damage, airbags, seatbelts, multi-system trauma)
    - Sports/Recreational (protective gear)
    - Consider non-traumatic causative factors: syncope, seizure, intoxication
  - Symptoms
    - LOC and duration, amnesia, perseveration, disorientation/confusion, gait instability, post-traumatic seizure, vomiting, headache
    - Improvement or deterioration
  - PMH
    - Neurologic, developmental, psychiatric disorders, previous concussions, coagulation disorders, medications
- **Exam**
  - C-spine evaluation
  - GCS with frequent re-evaluation (see Quick Reference section)
  - Baseline pupil size, reactivity
  - Secondary survey
    - Facial/scalp hematomas, open/depressed/signs of basilar skull fx, hemotympanum, CSF otorrhea/rhinorrhea
    - Increased ICP/herniation syndromes
      - Bulging fontanelle
      - Anisocoria or dilated, unresponsive pupils
      - ↓ GCS
      - Cushing's triad: hypertension, bradycardia, irregular respirations
- **Diagnostics**
  - Labs: POC GLC, CBC, BMP, PT/INR, PTT, TxS, Utox, alcohol
  - Imaging
    - GCS 14-15
      - PECARN risk stratification: to identify those who do NOT need a head CT vs. other clinical decision-making tools (CATCH, CHALICE, NEXUS II)
        - Having PECARN risk factor does not automatically = CT
        - \> 2 yrs: normal mental status, no LOC, no severe mechanism, no vomiting, no severe HA, no signs of basilar skull fx

- < 2 yrs: normal mental status, normal behavior per caregiver, no LOC > 5 seconds, no severe mechanism, no or frontal-only scalp hematoma, no palpable skull fx
- Severe mechanism: fall > 3 ft in < 2 yrs, > 5 ft ≥ 2 yrs, ejection, rollover, fatality involved, auto vs. pedestrian, high-impact object
  - GCS ≤ 13, skull fx, AMS → neuroimaging
    - CT head non-contrast (and C-spine if not cleared)
    - CTA if penetrating injury

MANAGEMENT

- TBI goals: maintain normal BP, HR, SpO2, temperature, PaCO2, PaO2, glucose
- Major head trauma
  - Treatments / diagnostics after sensory, motor, mental status exam if possible
  - Airway: intubate for airway protection, expected course, generally GCS ≤ 8
    - Ventilator settings
      - PaCO2 35-40 mmHg
      - FiO2 < 60% as tolerated to prevent O2 toxicity
  - Elevated ICP
    - Elevate head of bed to 30°
    - Hyperosmolar agents
      - Mannitol 0.25-1 g/kg usual (max 2 g/kg) IV over 20-30 min
      - Hypertonic 3% saline 2.5-5 mL/kg IV over 10-15 min
  - Post-traumatic seizures
    - See Seizures chapter for treatment
    - Impact seizures right after head impact more common in children, usually self-limited
  - Neurosurgery consult: intracranial injury, depressed or basilar skull fx, need for emergent decompression/evacuation or invasive ICP monitoring
- Minor head trauma
  - Analgesia: acetaminophen and/or NSAIDs (avoid opioids)
  - Ondansetron 0.15 mg/kg (max 4 mg) IV/PO PRN nausea
  - Dizziness usually resolves with rest
    - Refer to physiotherapist or concussion clinic if severe

DISPOSITION

- Admit: significant injury, unremitting vomiting
- Discharge
  - Minor head trauma after normal CT or observation period

- Concussion: concussion symptoms often resolve in 7-10 days, may last months
    - Physical / cognitive rest until symptoms resolve
    - Graded return to learn, return to play programs prior to medical clearance
    - Family education: ATT Concussion Awareness Tool, CDC HEADS UP Concussion Resources https://www.cdc.gov/headsup, anticipatory guidance on sleep, fatigue, mood

PENETRATING NECK INJURIES

BACKGROUND
- High risk injuries
- Severity predicted by depth of injury: superficial to the platysma or violating

EVALUATION
- **High Yield History**: mechanism, other injuries, SOB
- **Exam**
    - Stridor, respiratory distress, shock, rapidly expanding hematoma → airway compromise
    - Wound: length, depth (platysma violation), location, foreign bodies
    - "Hard signs" of arterial injury: hypotension, pulsatile bleed, expanding hematoma, thrill/bruit, hematemesis/hemoptysis, neurologic deficit
    - "Soft signs:" venous oozing, non-expanding hematoma, subcutaneous air, hoarseness, dysphagia
    - Neurologic exam
- **Diagnostics**
    - Platysma violated: neck CT angiogram if stable and without hard signs
    - Consider observation without CT if stable, no hard or soft signs

MANAGEMENT
- OR if unstable or hard signs for stabilization and exploration/endoscopy
- Early consideration to secure airway PRN
- IV antibiotics: suspected esophageal injury or contaminated wound

DISPOSITION
- Discharge after observation: superficial injury without other significant injuries, stable, no vascular injury hard or soft signs
- Admit: emergent surgical, other concerns

BEWARE

- ⚠ Previously taught "Zones" of the neck dictating imaging and management may be unreliable as wounds may traverse multiple zones; safer to assess depth of injury, hard/soft signs
- ⚠ Prepare for difficult intubation, with cricothyrotomy/transtracheal jet ventilation backup

DENTAL TRAUMA

BACKGROUND

- Primary teeth erupt 6 mo-3 yrs
- Permanent teeth replace/erupt 6-16yrs

EVALUATION

- **High Yield History**
  - Time of injury, loose teeth, hot/cold intolerance, jaw malocclusion, associated head/neck injury
- **Exam** (see Quick Reference section)
  - Concussion: tender but no increased mobility/displacement; no bleeding
  - Subluxation: abnormal mobility but no displacement; possible bleeding
  - Luxation
    - Lateral: displaced palatal/lingual direction; often bleeding
    - Extrusive: displaced vertical direction; often bleeding
    - Intrusion: forced into the alveolus, usually locked without any mobility; appears shortened; often bleeding
  - Avulsion: complete displacement out of socket with severed periodontal ligament, often fractured alveolus

Dental Fractures (Ellis Classes)			
Ellis I	Superficial enamel	Chipped tooth, painless	Low risk, Outpatient dental follow-up
Ellis II	Enamel & dentin	Yellow at fx line, tender, sensitive to air / temperature	Infection risk. Cover (dental cement), consider antibiotics, dental follow-up 24-48hrs
Ellis III	Pulp	Pink/red at fx line, very painful	Dental emergency (dentist within 24-48hrs), antibiotics

- **Diagnostics**
  - XR (panorex if available): assess all teeth, alveolar bone
  - Maxillofacial CT: concern for facial fx
  - Consider CXR: aspirated teeth

MANAGEMENT

- ABx: open fx, avulsed permanent teeth (penicillin; clindamycin if allergic)
- Analgesia
- Suspected jaw fracture: jaw tenderness, alveolar disruption, posterior tooth fracture, malocclusion; oral surgery consult/referral
- Primary teeth
  - Concussion/Subluxation: No immediate treatment
  - Lateral/External luxation: if minor (< 3 mm), gentle repositioning; if > 3 mm or bite interference, referral to dentist
  - Intrusive luxation: No immediate treatment, refer to dentist to assess permanent tooth above
  - Avulsion: No immediate treatment; do not reimplant tooth
  - Fracture: as above per Ellis injury type
- Permanent teeth
  - Concussion/subluxation: No treatment indicated, soft diet
  - Lateral/external luxation: if minor reposition tooth, stabilize with a flexible splint for 4 weeks; if > 3 mm or bite interference, referral to dentist
  - Intrusive luxation: no immediate treatment, the tooth will typically re-erupt gradually on its own
  - Avulsion: reimplant clean tooth within 30 min if possible; if unable, store tooth in appropriate media with immediate dental referral
    - Balanced salt solution, milk, or patient saliva (do not use water)
  - Fracture: as above per Ellis injury type

BEWARE

- ⚠ Account for all missing teeth
- ⚠ Avoid touching root of avulsed tooth to preserve remaining tissue

6 ▶ Non-Accidental Trauma

BACKGROUND

- Epidemiology
  - 680,000 children/year, underestimation — many cases unrecognized/unreported
  - High risk
    - Younger children most vulnerable, highest morbidity/mortality
    - Poverty and lack of resources significant risk factors
    - Children with disabilities 2x risk
      - Behavioral problems (ADHD, conduct disorder) → physical abuse
      - Physical limitations or dependence → neglect
      - Deafness or blindness → sexual abuse
    - Caregiver characteristics: substance abuse, mental illness, intimate partner violence, younger age, lower education

EVALUATION

- **High Yield History**
  - Suspicious historical elements
    - Inconsistent with injury type
    - Incongruent with child developmental capabilities
    - Changing over time or amongst caregivers
    - Trauma history missing or doesn't explain injuries
  - Trafficking historical clues
    - Unusually high number of sexual partners
    - Accompanied by controlling individual (refuses to let them speak, interprets for them, refuses patient privacy)
    - Unwilling/hesitant to answer questions about injury or illness
- **Exam**
  - Remove ALL clothing and examine thoroughly
  - Bruises
    - ANY bruising in a non-ambulatory child or infant
    - Bruising on the TEN areas (Trunk, Ears, Neck) in children < 4 yrs
    - Patterned bruises (hand, object)
  - Subconjunctival hemorrhages
  - Oral injuries: frenulum tears
  - GU exam

- Sexual assault diagnosis relies on history + complete exam
  - Findings often normal or nonspecific
  - Perihymenal bruises
  - Hymenal abrasions, lacerations, complete transections
  - Vaginal lacerations
- Other injuries: head trauma, skull fx, rib fx, long bone fx, male GU trauma, burns
- Concerning injury patterns
  - Abusive head trauma ("shaken baby syndrome")
    - Subdural or epidural hematomas
    - Retinal hemorrhages (typically bilateral)
    - Spinal cord hemorrhage
  - Skull fractures
    - Eggshell pattern
    - Fractures in multiple planes crossing suture lines
    - Occipital fractures
  - Rib fractures: posterior, bilateral
  - Abdominal trauma
    - Liver lacerations (most common in NAT)
    - Pancreatic contusions, lacerations
    - Small bowel hematomas (nonaccidental > accidental trauma)
    - Isolated splenic, renal injuries (uncommon in NAT)
  - Extremity trauma: concerning fractures
    - Any in non-ambulatory child
    - Unexplained
    - Multiple in various states of healing
    - Classic metaphyseal "corner" or "bucket handle"
    - Highly predictive for abuse in infants
    - Proximal tibia, distal femur, proximal humerus
  - Burns
    - Thermal burns from scalds or contact (most common)
      - Immersion burns
        - Symmetrical, uniform depth
        - Sparing of flexor surfaces
        - Stocking/glove pattern
        - Absence of splash marks

- Contact burns
  - Branding type injury with distinct margins
  - Cigarette burns → 1 cm diameter
- Neglect accounts for the vast majority of child maltreatment cases worldwide
  - Encompasses physical, medical, educational, emotional, dental and other areas of child's well-being
  - Unkempt, failure to thrive, poor caregiver attachment
- Trafficking
  - Tattoos or branding
  - Inappropriate clothing for weather/location
  - Signs of physical abuse or unexplained injuries
  - Evidence of STI and/or repeated unwanted pregnancies
  - Retained foreign bodies
  - Evidence of drug abuse

- **Diagnostics**
  - Labs
    - Physical abuse
      - Trauma workup per protocol
      - Consider labs to rule out bleeding and bone disorders (coagulation studies, platelets, renal function, vWF antigen, Ristocetin cofactor, Factor VIII & IX levels, vit D and calcium levels)
      - Abdominal trauma: ALT/AST, lipase
    - Sexual abuse
      - STI screening (HIV, RPR, urine gonorrhea & chlamydia, hepatitis panel); urine pregnancy test
      - Evidence collection (see below)
    - Consider Utox
  - Skeletal survey
    - Head-to-toe radiographic assessment
    - Recommended in all children < 24 mo with injuries or high suspicion
    - Recommended selectively in children 2-5 yrs based on extent of injuries and developmental capabilities
    - Consider repeating in 2 wks to assess for initially missed fx

- CT head non-contrast
  - Consider in infants with high suspicion for abuse even in absence of neurological symptoms
  - Recommended if neurological symptoms or AMS
- CT abdomen/pelvis w/ contrast:
  - Recommenced if evidence of traumatic injury to the abdomen
  - Consider in asymptomatic children with abnormal LFTs (AST/ALT > 80) or pancreatic enzymes

MANAGEMENT

- Reporting: physicians are mandated reporters
- Consult child abuse specialists
- Sexual Assault Response Team/Center
  - Evidence collection for legal implications
  - Post-exposure prophylaxis for STI, pregnancy

DISPOSITION

- Dependent on patient condition/safety
- Do not discharge if question of patient safety, even if cleared by Child Protective Services

BEWARE

⚠ Mimics
  - Congenital dermal melanocytosis ("Mongolian spots")
    - Mistaken for bruises
    - Typically on sacrum/buttocks, bluish undertone, fade over time
  - Rickets: Vitamin D deficiency leading to fx (may be multiple fx)
  - Phytophotodermatitis: skin reaction caused by contact with chemical in certain foods + UV light exposure
    - Citrus fruits (limes), carrots, celery, parsley
    - Mimics burns
  - Inborn errors

⚠ Child abuse occurs in all socioeconomic groups; maintain a high index of suspicion

7 ▶ Spinal Trauma

BACKGROUND

- Spinal injuries children < adults
- Cervical most common in children
  — Anatomy: large head leading to different fulcrum
  — Infants: C2-3; 5-6 yrs: C3-4; 8-10 yrs: C5-7 (adult-like)
- Mechanisms: MVA, fall, sports, diving injuries, NAT, penetrating: bullets, knives, hanging or clotheslining type injury

EVALUATION

- **High Yield History**
  — Time and mechanism of injury, respiratory difficulty, predisposing conditions (Down syndrome — atlantoaxial instability)
  — Neck or back pain, paresthesias, numbness, weakness, incontinence, torticollis
- **Exam**
  — Neurologic: detailed motor, sensory and reflex exam by myotome and dermatome, anogenital reflexes
  — Spinal cord syndromes
    - Spinal shock
      - Transient traumatic paresis or paralysis
      - Flaccidity, areflexia, loss of anal sphincter control
      - Bulbocavernosus reflexes return first
    - Central cord
      - Hyperextension injuries, athletes
      - Motor weakness arms > legs
      - Shawl distribution pain & temperature sensation loss
    - Brown-Sequard
      - Hemisection of cord, penetrating trauma, rare
      - Contralateral loss of pain and temperature and ipsilateral motor weakness/plegia below lesion
    - Anterior cord
      - Crush injury or compression from a hematoma
      - Loss of motor and pain/temperature below lesion level

- **Diagnostics**
  - Clinical decision rules for need for imaging
    - PECARN: cervical spine imaging if any of:
      - AMS
      - Focal neurologic deficits
      - Complaint of neck pain
      - Torticollis
      - Substantial torso injury
      - Predisposing condition (Down syndrome)
      - High-risk MVA
      - Diving accident
    - NEXUS (validated in > 8 yrs) cervical spine clinically cleared if none of:
      - Neurologic deficits
      - Midline spinal tenderness
      - AMS
      - Intoxication
      - Distracting injury
  - Plain films
    - AP, lateral, odontoid view (3 views): 90% sensitive for unstable injuries
      - Upper C-spine pseudosubluxation common in young children
      - Soft-tissue swelling: soft tissue width > ½ adjacent vertebra width
      - Lateral most important view
      - Swimmer's view: adjunct to lateral to visualize C7-T1
    - Flexion-extension views for suspected ligamentous injury no longer thought useful
  - CT without contrast, more sensitive, preferred if high suspicion
    - High energy mechanism, AMS, neurologic deficits, distracting injury, head/facial injuries
    - Image entire spine (cervical, thoracic, lumbar) if any fx found as non-contiguous second fx common
  - MRI
    - Assess neurologic deficits without radiologic abnormalities
      - SCIWORA (spinal cord injury without radiographic abnormality)
    - Suspected soft-tissue or ligamentous injury, cord transection/edema, epidural hematoma

MANAGEMENT

- Priorities: ABCs, spinal stabilization, identify and prevent injury progression
- Spinal immobilization
  - Occiput recess/torso pad to achieve neutral neck position < 8 yrs
  - Pediatric sized cervical collar
- Types of fx/injuries
  - Stable fx
    - Odontoid type I
    - Spinous process
    - Unilateral facet dislocation
    - Isolated transverse process
    - Wedge with no retropulsion
    - Burst (may also be unstable)
    - Clay-Shoveler's
  - Unstable fx ("Jefferson Bit Off A Hangman's Thumb")
    - Jefferson
    - Bilateral facet dislocation
    - Odontoid type II and III (Dens)
    - Atlanto-occipital dissociation
    - Hangman's
    - Teardrop
    - Chance (see abdominal trauma chapter)
  - SCIWORA
    - < 8 yrs may present with initial or later symptoms of cervical cord injury without radiographic evidence
    - Acceleration-deceleration or rotation injury
    - Immobilization, MRI, neurosurgery consult
  - Atlantoaxial rotatory subluxation
    - Traumatic torticollis
    - Normal neurologic findings
    - Mild - immobilization, Severe — may require traction/surgical intervention
- Neurosurgery consultation as indicated

DISPOSITION

- Admit: unstable fx, suspected SCIWORA, Neurosurgery intervention
- Discharge: stable injury not requiring neurosurgical intervention

- Discharge with surgical follow-up: CT negative with persistent midline tenderness (home with soft c-collar, analgesia)

BEWARE

⚠ Consider early intubation with spinal injuries level C5 and higher

⚠ Hypotension: consider both hemorrhagic and neurogenic shock

8 ▶ Thoracic Trauma

BACKGROUND

- Thoracic injuries children < adults
- Multi-system trauma common, thoracic trauma presence ↑ mortality 20×
- Mechanisms of injury: blunt (> 80%), penetrating (< 20%)
- Anatomy
  - Compliant rib cage: rib fx uncommon
    - Lung, heart vascular injury more common
  - Mobile mediastinum: rapid tamponade development with pneumothorax (PTX)
- Injuries
  - Rib fx, flail chest, pulmonary contusion, PTX, hemothorax (HTX), myocardial contusion, pericardial and/or vascular injury

EVALUATION

- **High Yield History**
  - Mechanism, chest / back pain, cough, respiratory difficulty, SOB, abdominal pain, AMS
- **Exam**
  - Abnormal SpO2
  - Respiratory distress
  - Decreased / absent breath sounds
  - Distended neck veins → tension PTX, cardiac tamponade, traumatic asphyxia
  - Tracheal deviation → tension PTX
  - Focal tenderness / crepitus over bony prominences
  - Crepitus (subcutaneous air) → PTX, tracheo-bronchial tree injuries, esophageal perforation
  - Asymmetric (paradoxical) chest rise → flail chest, PTX, diaphragmatic injury
  - Penetrating wounds, ecchymoses, abrasions
    - Open chest wall wounds → sucking PTX
  - Muffled heart sounds, murmur, gallop → cardiac tamponade, contusion

- **Diagnostics**
  - Labs
    - CBC, CMP, PT/INR, PTT, TxS, lactate, troponin
  - Imaging
    - CXR
      - Less sensitive than US or CT, but most pediatric thoracic injuries can be identified by CXR + US
    - US / FAST
      - US nearly as sensitive as CT to identify PTX, HTX; more sensitive for pericardial effusion
      - Normal FAST does not rule out life-threatening injuries
      - Consider echocardiogram for suspected cardiac injury
    - CT chest w/contrast
      - Often overutilized in pediatric chest trauma
      - CT angiogram for suspicion of great vessel, tracheo-bronchial, esophageal injuries
  - EKG

MANAGEMENT

- ABCs, oxygen
- Analgesia
- Tension PTX
  - Needle decompression
    - 14 g (child) to 18 g (infant) angiocath, 2nd intercostal space (ICS), mid clavicular line
  - Tube thoracostomy
    - Maximum chest tube size = $4 \times$ uncuffed ETT size
    - 5th ICS at level of the nipple, anterior to mid-axillary line
    - Avoid breast tissue
  - Fluid resuscitation
- Simple PTX
  - Consider pigtail catheter for PTX without HTX
  - Tube thoracostomy for large or combined PTX/HTX
- Open PTX
  - Initial placement of occlusive dressing with tape on three sides
  - Definitive therapy: tube thoracostomy

- HTX
  - Fluid resuscitation
  - Tube thoracostomy
  - Potential indications for thoracotomy, massive transfusion protocol
    - Initial output of > 20 mL/kg (1.5 L in adolescents)
    - Continued output > 1-2 mL/kg/hr (200 mL/hr in adolescents)
- Flail chest or pulmonary contusion
  - Stable
    - Incentive spirometry, pulmonary toilet, analgesia
    - BiPAP, CPAP, or high flow O2
  - Respiratory failure
    - Intubation with PEEP
- Cardiac contusion: observe on monitor, treat dysrhythmia or cardiogenic shock
- Cardiac tamponade
  - Fluid resuscitation, surgery consult
  - ED pericardiocentesis if in extremis
  - Emergently to OR
- Aortic injury: aggressive BP control, emergently to OR
- Great vessel injury
  - Fluid resuscitation, transfusion PRN
  - Surgical intervention
- Tracheobronchial tree injury
  - Tube thoracostomy for large PTX
  - Surgical consultation
- Traumatic arrest from penetrating chest trauma: consider ED thoracotomy

DISPOSITION

- Admit
  - Significant injury; transfer to pediatric trauma center PRN
  - Significant mechanism of injury with normal work-up: consider admission for cardiac monitoring, observation, serial exams
- Discharge with close follow-up: minor mechanism of injury, normal exam and work-up

BEWARE

- Traumatic asphyxia, commotio cordis, tension pneumothorax more common in children
- Silent hypoxemia and/or tachypnea may be only sign of significant thoracic injury

Index

A

Abdominal pathology 193
Abdominal trauma 325
Abnormal uterine bleeding 156
Abscess 70
Acute gastroenteritis 127
Acute rheumatic fever 293
Acute scrotum 161
Adrenal insufficiency 110
Agitated child 255
Airway equipment 3
Airway management 31
Anaphylaxis 86
Anemia 165
Angioedema 86
Antibiotic allergic reactions 74
Apophysitis 247
Appendicitis 129
Arrythmias 53
Arthritis (juvenile idiopathic) 296
Arthritis (septic) 244
ARVC/ARVD 55
Asthma 257
Ataxia 221
Athlete's foot 77
Autism spectrum disorder 249

B

Back pain 239
Bacterial tracheitis 95
Balanitis 162
Behavior 250
Biliary atresia 131
Biliary pathology 130
Bites (mammals) 115
Bites (spiders) 120
Bleeding disorders 167
Bowel obstruction 132
Bradyarrhythmias 53
Branchial cleft cysts 104
Bronchiolitis 260
BRUE 198
Brugada 54
Burns 328

C

Candidiasis (oral) 99
Caustic exposures 303
Cellulitis 70
Central venous catheter 37
Chicken pox 82
Choledochal cysts 131
Common pediatric dosages 4-11
Congenital dermal melanosis 216
Congenital heart disease 56
Congenital neck masses 104
Constipation 134
Cough 262
COVID-19 190
CPVT 55
Cradle cap 74, 217
Croup 94
Crying infant 199
Cutis marmorata 216
Cystic fibrosis 264

D

Deep neck infections 101
Dental anatomy 16
Dental trauma 342
Depression 252

Dermatitis 72
Dermatologic conditions 69
Developmental milestones 14
Diabetic ketoacidosis. 107
Diaper dermatitis 73
Diaphragmatic hernia. 194
Discitis. 239
DOPES. 12
Down syndrome 147
DRESS 75
Drug rashes 74
Dysmenorrhea 156
Dysrhythmias 21

E

Eagle Barrett syndrome 197
Eating disorders 253
Eczema Herpeticum 83
EKG interpretation 51
Elbow ossification. 334
Electrical injuries 331
Electrolyte disturbances. 275
Encephalitis 184
Enteral feeding tube complications. . 136
Envenomation (marine) 116
Envenomation (snakes) 118
Epididymitis 162
Epiglottitis. .96
Epistaxis 92
Equipment sizing 2
Erysipelas 70
Erythema infectiosum 82
Erythema multiforme 75
Erythema toxicum 216
eVALI 273
Exam tips (pediatrics) 18

F

Febrile neonate/infant 201
Female-specific GU concerns 155
Fever of unknown origin 179
Fifth Disease 82
Fluid disturbances 275
Folliculitis 70
Foreign body removal 39
Fungal infections 76
Furncles/Carbuncles 70

G

Gases 312
German measles 81
GI bleeding 138
Gianotti-Crosti syndrome 83
Glasgow Coma Scale (pediatric) 2
Glucose metabolism 105

H

H's and T's 22
Hair apposition 43
Hand-foot-mouth disease 81
Harlequin color change 216
Head trauma 338
Headache 223
Hemangiomas 84
Hematuria 279
Hemolytic uremic syndrome 283
Hemophilia 167, 169
Henoch-Schonlein Purpura 295
Hernias 195
HOCM 54
Hypercalcemia 275
Hypercyanotic episode 62
Hyperkalemia 275
Hyperleukocytosis 173

Index **355**

Hypernatremia	275
Hypertension	285
Hyperthermia	121
Hyperthyrodism	113
Hypocalcemia	275
Hypoglycemia	105
Hypokalemia	275
Hyponatremia	275
Hypothermia	123
Hypothyroidism	112

I

Idiopathic thrombocytopenic purpura	170
Immunization schedule	13
Imperforate hymen	157
Impetigo (bullous and non-bullous)	69
Inborn errors of metabolism	150
Infective endocarditis	63
Infestations	78
Inflammatory Bowel Disease	142
Influenza-like illness	183
Ingestions	305
Intraosseous access	36
Intussusception	143
ITP	170

J

Jaundiced neonate	204
Juvenile idiopathic arthritis	296

K

Kawasaki disease	298

L

Labial adhesion	159
Laceration repair	41
Laryngomalacia	97
Laryngotracheal pathology/ complications	94
Lice	78
Limp	241
Long QT Syndrome	54
Lumbar puncture	44
Lupus	300
Lyme disease	79
Lymphadenitis	102
Lymphangiomas	104
Lymphangitis	70

M

Male-specific GU concerns	160
Maltreatment	344
Marfan syndrome	148
Mastoiditis	91
Measles	81
Meningitis	184
Meningococcemia	188
Methemoglobinemia	314
Milia/miliaria	217
MIS-C	190
Molluscum contagiosum	83
Mononucleosis	181
Muscular dystrophy	148
Myocarditis	66

N

Neck trauma	341
Necrotizing enterocolitis	196
Neonatal acne	217
Neonatal herpes	217
Neonatal resuscitation	25
Neonatal skin findings	216
Nephritic syndromes	287
Nephrotic syndromes	287
Neutropenic colitis	172

Neutropenic fever 171
Non-accidental trauma 344
Normal EKGs, pediatric 53
Normal feeding/elimination/growth . .211
Nursemaid's elbow 243

O

Oncologic emergencies 171
One Pill Can Kill 316
Orbital cellulitis 231
Orthopedic infections 244
Osgood-Schlatter 247
Osteomyelitis 244
Otitis externa 89
Otitis media 90
Ovarian torsion 157

P

PALS 21
Papular acrodermatitis 83
Paralysis 221
Paraphimosis 163
Pericarditis .65
Peritonsillar abscess 101
Pharyngitis 100
Phimosis 164
Phytophotodermatitis 74
Pierre-Robin Sequence 148
Platelet disorder 167
Pneumomediastinum 271
Pneumonia 267
Pneumothorax (spontaneous) 271
Prader-Willi syndrome 149
Premature baby (post-NICU) 213
Preseptal cellulitis 231
Priapism 164
Procedural sedation/analgesia 47
Prune belly syndrome 197

Pulseless arrest 22
Pyelonephritis 289
Pyloric stenosis 145
Pyogenic granuloma 85

R

Recreational drugs 320
Red eye 234
Resuscitation 21
Resuscitation medications 5
Retropharyngeal abscess 101
Return to school guidelines 17
Ringworm 76
Rocky Mountain Spotted Fever 80
Roseola infantum 82
Rubella 81
Rubeola 81

S

Salter-Harris fractures 334
Scabies 78
Scarlet fever 71
Seborrheic dermatitis 74, 217
Sedative agents 49
Seizures 225
Septic arthritis 244
Severs 247
Shock 27
Sickle Cell Disease 175
Sinusitis 93
Skin infection - bacterial 69
SLE 300
Spinal cord compression 175
Spinal trauma 348
Staphylococcal scalded skin
 syndrome 71
Stevens-Johnson Syndrome 76
Stroke 227

Submersion injuries 125
Suicidal ideation 252
Superior vena cava syndrome 174
Systemic lupus erythematosus 300

T

Tachyarrhythmias 53
Teeth chart 16
Testicular torsion 161
THE MISFITS 207
Thoracic trauma 351
Thrush 99
Thyroglossal duct cysts 104
Thyroid disorders 112
Tinea capitis 77
Tinea corporis 76
Tinea pedis 77
Tinea versicolor 77
Toxic epidermal necrolysis (TEN) 76
Tracheitis 95
Tracheomalacia 97
Tracheostomy complications 98
Transient neonatal pustular
   melanosis 218
Trauma, abdominal 325
Trauma, extremities 333
Trauma, head/neck 338
Trauma, spinal 348
Trauma, thoracic 351
Treacher Collins syndrome 149
Tumor Lysis syndrome 173
Turner syndrome 147

U

Umbilical cord issues 218
Umbilical vein catheter 38
Urethral prolapse 158
Urticaria 86
UTI 289

V

Vaccination schedule 13
Vaginitis 158
Vaping-associated lung injury 273
Varicella zoster 82
Vascular access 36
Vascular lesions 84
Ventilator settings 11
Viral exanthems 80
Vital signs 1
Vitamin K deficiency 167
von Willebrand disease 167
VP shunt 229

W

Weight by age 1
Williams syndrome 148
Wolff-Parkinson-White 54
Wound management 44

Z

Zipper injury 164